Quick Reference to Child and Adolescent Forensics

Mary E. Muscari, PhD, CPNP, APRN-BC, CFNS, is an associate professor at the Decker School of Nursing, State University of New York (SUNY) at Binghamton (Bing-hamton University). Muscari has been a pediatric nurse practitioner (PNP) since 1980, when she earned her MSN/PNP from Columbia University. She earned a post-master's certificate in psychiatric nursing and a PhD, both from Adelphi University; a post-master's certificate in forensic nursing (2003) from Duquesne University; and has additional forensic education as a sexual assault nurse examiner, a legal nurse consultant, and a medicolegal death investigator. She attended the Sudden Unexpected Infant Death Investigation (SUIDI) Academy (2007) through the Centers for Disease Control and Prevention. Muscari has worked clinically as a PNP in a variety of environments, and has served on the Pennsylvania Sex Offender Assessment Board (2005–present) and as a private consultant on child health/mental health, parenting, and forensic issues.

Kathleen M. Brown, PhD, APRN-BC, FAAN, is a practice assistant professor at the University of Pennsylvania School of Nursing as well as a practicing women's health nurse practitioner (NP) for 23 years and a sexual assault nurse examiner for the Philadelphia County, Pennsylvania, Sexual Assault Response Team. Additionally, she is a postgraduate student of Dr. Robert Sadoff at the University of Pennsylvania School of Medicine in the Applications of Forensic Psychiatry curriculum. She has been a coinvestigator in four funded research studies: two for the National Institute of Justice and two for the National Institute of Nursing Research. Her dissertation research on leaving abusive relationships was funded by American Women's Health, Obstetric and Neonatal Nursing (AWHONN).

Quick Reference to Child and Adolescent Forensics

A Guide for Nurses and Other Health Care Professionals

MARY E. MUSCARI, PhD

KATHLEEN M. BROWN, PhD

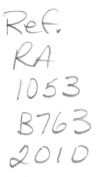

SPRINGER / PUBLISHING COMPANY
New York

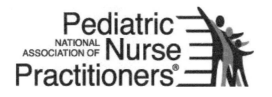

Springer Publishing Company, LLC
11 West 42nd Street
New York, NY 10036
www.springerpub.com

Acquisitions Editor: Margaret Zuccarini
Project Manager: Laura Stewart
Cover Design: Mimi Flow
Composition: Apex CoVantage, LLC
ISBN: 978-0-8261-2417-3
E-book ISBN: 978-0-8261-2418-0

10 11 12 13 / 5 4 3 2 1

The author and the publisher of this Work have made every effort to use sources believed to be reliable to provide information that is accurate and compatible with the
standards generally accepted at the time of publication. Because medical science is
continually advancing, our knowledge base continues to expand. Therefore,
as new information becomes available, changes in procedures become necessary.
We recommend that the reader always consult current research and specific
institutional policies before performing any clinical procedure. The author and publisher shall not be liable for any special, consequential, or exemplary damages resulting,
in whole or in part, from the readers' use of, or reliance on, the information contained
in this book. The publisher has no responsibility for the persistence or accuracy of
URLs for external or third-party Internet Web sites referred to in this publication and
does not guarantee that any content on such Web sites is, or will remain, accurate or
appropriate.

Library of Congress Cataloging-in-Publication Data

Muscari, Mary E.
   Quick reference to child and adolescent forensics : a guide for nurses and other
health care professionals / Mary E. Muscari, Kathleen M. Brown.
       p. ; cm.
   Includes bibliographical references and index.
   ISBN 978-0-8261-2417-3 (alk. paper)
1. Medical Jurisprudence. 2. Nurses. I. Brown, Kathleen M., 1950– II. Title.
   [DNLM: 1. Forensic Medicine—methods. 2. Adolescent. 3. Child Abuse.
4. Child. 5. Crime Victims. 6. Juvenile Delinquency. 7. Violence.
W 700 M985q 2010]
   RA1053.B763   2010
   614'.1—dc22   2010002839

Printed in the United States of America by the Hamilton Printing Company

To Mike Barrett and the crew at Minooka Subaru
where this book was birthed and nurtured—in their waiting area—
all while we were experiencing the best customer service in the country.

And to Margaret Zuccarini, the editor who has been with this project since it was just an
idea and whose expert guidance and support have made it a reality. Margaret enabled this
book to become a guide that can, we hope, minimize some of these horrible forensic
problems that happen to the most innocent of victims—our children, including those
children who also have traveled onto the pathway of offending.

Contents

Foreword

Forensics is a cutting-edge topic, especially for today's pediatric health care providers. Far too often, children become victims or perpetrators of violence. Some children fall victim to bullies, sexual predators, and even their own parents, while other children become bullies, or commit violent acts such as animal cruelty, arson, and sexual offending. Many of these children become perpetrators after years of victimization.

Pediatric health care professionals need information on forensics. Children rarely present in health care settings with a chief complaint of victimization or offending. Instead they may manifest the signs of stress disorders or somatization, or present with no symptom at all, warranting advanced assessment skills on the part of health care providers. However, most providers lack these needed skills. While health care providers do learn the basics of child abuse, they rarely learn how to conduct a forensic assessment, collect evidence, and testify as an expert witness. Concepts such as filicide, abductions, sexual exploitation, delinquency, school violence, gangs, and death investigation are rarely, if ever, mentioned in pediatric texts.

This book provides pediatric health care providers with the tools they need to assess, manage, and prevent forensic pediatric problems within health care settings. The authors, Drs. Muscari and Brown, bring their years of experience to this book in a way that makes these challenging and often disturbing topics accessible to those providers on the front lines of violence recognition and management.

Drs. Muscari and Brown have synthesized the key information on forensic pediatrics and produced a "must read" text that needs to be on every pediatric health care provider's bookshelf.

Ann Wolbert Burgess, DNSc., APRN, BC
Professor of Psychiatric Nursing
Boston College
Chestnut Hill, MA

Preface: The Forensic Aspects of Pediatrics

Forensic means "pertaining to the law" or "that which is legal." The word is derived from the Latin term *for ensis,* which means "open forum." Forensic health is the application of the health care sciences to public or legal proceedings; the application of the forensic aspects of health care combined with the bio-psycho-social education of the health care professional in the scientific investigation and treatment of trauma and/or death of victims and perpetrators of abuse, violence, and criminal activity.

Health care practitioners frequently—and sometimes unknowingly—work with victims of child abuse, sexual assault, and unnatural deaths, as well as juvenile offenders. Emergency practitioners encounter the specialty of forensic science with increasing regularity, as many are now expected to know how to gather and preserve evidence from victims of gunshot or stab wounds and from those who have been victimized by sexual violence or other forms of abuse.

Violence is a health problem. The Centers for Disease Control and Prevention (CDC) note that physical abuse can cause anything from minor injuries to permanent disabilities to death. Emotional trauma could result in posttraumatic stress disorder (PTSD) and depression. Violence touches the lives of children with alarming frequency. A recent survey confirmed that most of our society's children are exposed to violence in their daily lives. More than half were exposed to violence within the past year, either directly or indirectly, and nearly half were assaulted at least once in the past year. Juveniles of all ages are the victims of violent crime. Some of their offenders are family members, as is often the case for very young victims. Research has shown that child victimization and abuse are linked to problem behaviors that become evident later in life.

So an understanding of childhood victimization and its trends may lead to a better understanding of juvenile offending.

Children and adolescents become victims of neglect, physical abuse, sexual assault, prostitution, pornography, and abductions, and, many of these children complete the cycle of violence by becoming offenders, committing acts of bullying, cruelty, arson, rape, and even homicide. Health care professionals work with both victims and perpetrators, yet they have little education and resources for dealing with the everyday forensic issues of pediatric practice.

This guide helps fill the forensic void by providing current, concise, and easy-to-use information that assists pediatric practitioners with the prevention, identification, and management of pediatric victims and offenders. The book is designed to be integrated into advanced pediatric curriculums as a supplemental text, and to be utilized in primary, community, and acute care pediatric settings as an ongoing reference.

The book begins with a general principles section that defines the term forensics ("that which pertains to legal") and its implications in pediatric practice; describes the cycle, continuum, and cultural aspects of violence; and discusses the mechanisms of forensic assessment and documentation, evidence collection, the criminal and family justice systems, expert witness testimony, and working with the multidisciplinary team. It also describes the role of the pediatric provider in working with children who witness violence at home, in the community, and in the media, and gives practitioners an overview of the criminal and civil justice systems, child custody, and emancipation. Finally, it provides information on how professionals can manage their own mental health when working with these challenging issues.

The second section is devoted to children as victims. The child abuse chapters detail how to detect abusive parents as well as abused children and cover all aspects of intrafamiliar child abuse. Other chapters provide information on bullying, abductions, sexual molestation, pornography, and prostitution. Each chapter contains an overview of the problem, methods of victimization, the effects of victimization on children, recognition and problem management, and prevention techniques to provide to parents and children. The final chapters are devoted to instructing providers on working with abusive parents and to working with incarcerated parents and their children.

The third section focuses on children as offenders. The first chapter briefly explains delinquency and juvenile justice, as well as the pediatric provider's role in the interdisciplinary team. The next chapter is devoted to the occurrence, recognition, and management of delinquency, and the following two chapters concentrate on the special issues of female and child offenders. The next chapters deal with the description, assessment, management, and prevention of bullying, school violence, juvenile animal cruelty, arson, gang membership, juvenile sex offending, and dating violence. These issues were singled out because of the body of research that supports their relatively frequent incidence, specific management strategies, and preventative techniques (both primary and recidivism prevention).

The final section concentrates on unnatural pediatric deaths—sudden unexpected infant and child death, accidents, homicides, and suicides. The section explains the pediatric provider's role in child death review teams and in death investigations. There are also brief chapters on autoerotic fatalities, neonaticide/infanticide and filicide, which focus on prevention and early detection, and a chapter on working with grieving families who lost a child to homicide.

Whenever possible, chapters are organized as follows:

- *Definitions:* This section provides definitions of pertinent terms, as well as more in-depth information on the subject matter of the chapter. Example: *Parental kidnapping* describes the wrongful removal or retention of a child by a parent; however, since child kidnappings are frequently committed by other family members, the term *family abduction* is more accurate.
- *Prevalence:* This section provides statistics and relevant epidemiologic information. Example: A child is reported missing about every 40 seconds, and research shows that family abductions are the most prevalent child abduction type. More than 350,000 family abductions occur each year, accounting for about 1,000 per day.
- *Etiology:* This section addresses the cause or origin of the problem, as well as the factors that produce or predispose persons toward the problem, and/or issues found to correlate with the problem. Some chapters discuss typologies. Studies have revealed several reasons for parental abductions. Some are motivated by an effort to force reconciliation or to continue interaction with the left-behind parent. Others have a desire to blame, spite, or punish the other parent.
- *Assessment:* This section guides health care providers to assessment issues relevant to the specific problem. Health care providers can then incorporate this information into their daily assessments as needed.

■ *General Principles:* This section provides information that helps guide assessments. Example: Relationships among the perpetrator, child, and health care provider may be long-term and complex. This involvement may hinder the health care provider from considering Münchausen Syndrome by Proxy (MSBP) as a differential diagnosis.

■ *History and Physical Assessment:* This section provides suggestions for problem-specific subjective and objective data collection that can be incorporated into comprehensive, episodic, or interval assessments. Example: While the actual diagnosis of MSBP is for the perpetrator, the child remains a critical focus in making the diagnosis. There is no typical presentation. The literature notes more than 100 reported symptoms with the most common including lethargy, weight loss, fevers, abdominal pain, vomiting, diarrhea, seizures, apnea, infections, and bleeding.

■ *Diagnostic Testing/Screening Tools:* When applicable, this section suggests testing that can help confirm specific diagnoses, or, in most cases, provides a brief overview and access information for screening tools appropriate for settings such as primary care and emergency departments. Common tools, such as those used to screen for alcohol abuse and domestic violence, are included in the chapter or appendix. This section also provides overview and access information on more advanced instruments, such as those used for assessing violence recidivism risk. These tools require specific educational backgrounds and training. However, it does benefit health care providers to have an understanding of these instruments since they relate to some of their clients.

■ *Intervention:* This section provides information on therapeutic interventions and referrals.

■ *Prevention/Patient Teaching:* This section is structured using the public health model of prevention. Patient teaching information is given when applicable.

■ *Primary Prevention* is concerned with health promotion activities that prevent the actual occurrence of a specific illness or disease. Primary prevention attempts to serve those individuals who are not yet part of the problem, and strives to build skills and resiliency so that the problem will not develop.

■ *Secondary Prevention* promotes early detection or screening and treatment of disease and limitation of disability. By targeting individuals at high risk for the problem or who have displayed some form of antisocial or delinquent behavior, secondary prevention aims to keep these individuals from engaging in violent activity. Secondary prevention is also aimed at those who are at risk for becoming victims of violence to prevent the violence from occurring.

■ *Tertiary Prevention* is directed toward recovery or rehabilitation of condition after the condition has been developed. Tertiary prevention is designed to serve those individuals who have already become violent or chronic offenders and emphasizes punishment and rehabilitation through the justice system. The objective is to help prevent future violent activity. Tertiary prevention for victims focuses on prevention of further damage from the victimization, as well as prevention of future victimization.

■ *Resources:* This section provides readers with appropriate Web sites for further information.
■ *References:* This section provides references used for that chapter.

To better allow health care providers to perform comprehensive assessments, Appendix D includes the following assessment questionnaires from the KySS^{SM} (Keep your children/yourself Safe and Secure) Guide to Child and Adolescent Mental Health Screening, Early Intervention and Health Promotion:

■ KySS Assessment Questions for Parents of Older Infants and Toddlers
■ KySS Assessment Questions for Parents of Preschool Children
■ KySS Assessment Questions for Parents of School-age Children and Teens
■ KySS Assessment Questions for a Specific Emotional or Behavioral Problem

The information in this guide comes from health care and criminal justice literature, as well as credible professional organizations. Many of the issues in this book have yet to be well researched, and some topics do not lend themselves to the rigor of random controlled trials. Readers will find rich information for their practices, as well as ideas for future research.

Acknowledgments

We would like to acknowledge all the forensic health students whose classroom contributions help to stimulate ideas for this book, as well as those students who assisted in the literature review:

Lauren Conaboy (University of Scranton)

Essie Lee (Binghamton University)

Carlotta Mendez (University of Scranton)

Jolynn Sannicandro (Binghamton University)

We would also like to extend thanks to Peter Rocheleau, Makeda Alexander, and Pam Amri at Springer Publishing, and to Laura Stewart.

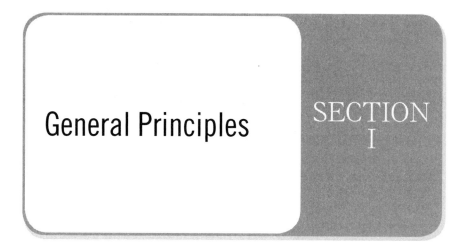

General Principles

SECTION
I

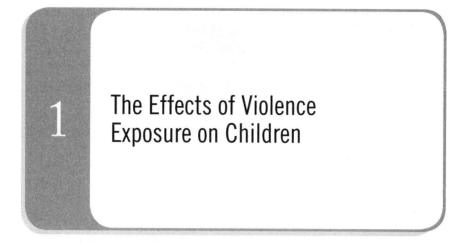

1

The Effects of Violence
Exposure on Children

Forensic means "pertaining to the law" or "that which is legal." The word is derived from the Latin term *for ensis,* which means open forum. Child and adolescent forensics is the application of pediatric heath care sciences to public or legal proceedings; the application of the forensic aspects of health care combined with the bio-psycho-social education of the health care professional in the scientific investigation and treatment of trauma and/or death of victims and perpetrators of abuse, violence, and criminal activity.

Violence is a health problem. The Centers for Disease Control and Prevention (CDC) note that physical abuse can cause anything from minor injuries to permanent disabilities to death. Emotional trauma could result in posttraumatic stress disorder (PTSD) and depression. Violence touches the lives of children with alarming frequency. According to the U.S. Department of Health and Human Services, Administration on Children, Youth and Families (2009), in 2007, state and local child protective services (CPS) investigated 3.2 million reports of child abuse and neglect, classifying 794,000 (10.6 per 1,000) of these children as victims. Fifty-nine percent of the children were classified as victims of neglect, 4% as victims of emotional abuse, 8% as victims of sexual abuse, and 11% as victims of physical abuse. Approximately three-quarters of all the abused and neglected children had no history of prior victimization.

According to the Centers for Disease Control and Prevention (CDC, 2009), 5,958 young people ages 10 to 24 were murdered in 2006—an average of 16 each day. Homicide was the second leading cause of death for young people ages 10 to 24 years old. The CDC (2008) also noted that in a 2007 nationally representative sample of youth in Grades 9–12:

- 35.5% reported being in a physical fight in the 12 months preceding the survey; the prevalence was higher among males (44.4%) than females (26.5%).
- 18.0% reported carrying a weapon (gun, knife, or club) on one or more days in the 30 days preceding the survey.
- 5.2% carried a gun on one or more days in the 30 days preceding the survey.
- Males were more likely than females to carry a weapon (28.5% versus 7.5%) on one or more days in the 30 days preceding the survey.
- Males were also more likely than females to carry a gun on one or more days in the 30 days preceding the survey (9.0% versus 1.2%).

Health care practitioners frequently—and sometimes unknowingly—work with victims of child abuse, sexual assault, and unnatural deaths, as well as juvenile offenders. Emergency practitioners encounter the specialty of forensic science with increasing regularity, as many are now expected to know how to gather and preserve evidence from victims of gunshot or stab wounds and from those who have been victimized by sexual violence or other forms of abuse. Primary care and other providers often see clients who present with vague symptoms that may indicate the hidden agenda of abuse. Therefore it is critical that forensic issues become a component in the education of health care providers.

THE EFFECTS OF VIOLENCE EXPOSURE ON CHILDREN

Children in the United States are more likely to be exposed to violence than are adults, and millions of children and adolescents in the United States are exposed to violence in their homes, schools, and communities as both victims and witnesses. The recent Comprehensive National Survey (Finkelhor, Turner, Ormrod, Hamby, & Kracke, 2009) on children's exposure to violence confirms that most of the children in the United States are exposed to violence on a daily basis. More than 60% of the children surveyed were exposed to violence within the past year, either directly or indirectly; and 46.3% were assaulted at least once in the past year. A little more than 25% witnessed a violent act and 9.8% saw one family member assault another.

Violence exposure can have significant effects on children as they develop and as they form their own intimate relationships throughout childhood and adulthood. Some children experience chronic community violence and are exposed to guns, knives, drugs, and random violence in their neighborhoods; some are exposed to witnessing violence against their mother perpetrated by their father or her paramour on a regular basis; some children are exposed to a plethora of violent acts on the screens of televisions, computers, video games, and other media. Many children are exposed to all of these. Risk factors are cumulative, and thus the risk of negative outcomes multiplies for children who are in "double jeopardy," such as those who are exposed to domestic and/or community violence. Children who are direct victims of assault and who witness repeated violence are more likely to have significant negative outcomes than children who are exposed to a single instance.

VIOLENCE IN THE HOME

Parents may think that their children are shielded from exposure to intimate partner violence; however, research findings indicate otherwise. Kennedy and colleagues (2009) noted that children frequently observe or hear the abuse as well as its aftermath (e.g., crying or injuries). In a sizable percentage of cases, the children are actually physically involved in their parent's partner violence and may be injured themselves.

Children who are exposed to intimate partner violence also are at risk of exposure to traumatic events, the risk of neglect, the risk of being abused, and the risk of losing one or both of their parents. These traumas can lead to negative outcomes for children and may affect their well-being, safety, and stability. Childhood problems associated with exposure to domestic violence fall into three primary categories:

Psychological: Fear, anxiety, low self-esteem, withdrawal, and depression; problematic relationships; higher levels of aggression, anger, hostility, oppositional behavior, and disobedience.

Cognitive: Lower cognitive functioning, poor school performance, lack of conflict resolution skills, limited problem-solving skills, proviolence attitudes, and belief in rigid gender stereotypes and male dominance.

Long-term: Higher levels of depression and trauma symptoms, increased tolerance for and use of violence in relationships during adulthood.

Reaction and risk exist on a continuum. Some children demonstrate resiliency, while others show signs of maladaptive adjustment. Protective factors can help protect children from the adverse effects of exposure to domestic violence. These include social competence, intelligence, high self-esteem, outgoing temperament, strong sibling and peer relationships, and a supportive relationship with an adult.

VIOLENCE IN THE COMMUNITY

Children's witnessing violence in urban communities is prevalent in the United States. Cooley-Quille, Boyd, Frantz, and Walsh (2001) found that inner-city youth with high levels of community violence exposure reported more fears, anxiety, internalizing behavior, and negative life experiences than those with low exposure.

The majority of these children report witnessing relatively less severe forms of violence such as seeing someone arrested or assaulted. There have been fewer studies relating to the effect of children's exposure to community violence within suburban or rural communities.

Community violence, with its associated mental health problems, may impact a child's ability to function effectively at school. Research demonstrates that increased levels of community violence are associated with decreased academic performance, as measured by grades, standardized test scores, and attendance. Psychological distress secondary to community violence exposure may be one explanation for these findings. However, few studies have examined mental health symptoms as a mechanism through which community violence exposure impacts functioning at school.

VIOLENCE IN THE MEDIA

Media violence (television, cinema, Internet) touches virtually every child. The average child spends about 5.5 hours every day watching electronic media. Children will see 200,000 acts of violence before graduation, including thousands of murders. Preschoolers witness almost 10,000 violent episodes every year just by watching 2 hours of cartoons each day.

According to the American Psychiatric Association, the typical American child watches 28 hours of television a week, and by the age of 18 will have seen 16,000 simulated murders and 200,000 acts of violence. Commercial television for children is 50 to 60 times more violent than primetime programs for adults, and some cartoons average more than 80 violent acts per hour. With the advent of videocassette sales and rentals of movies, pay-per-view TV, cable TV, video games, and online interactive computer games, many more children and adolescents are exposed to media with violent content than ever before.

Variances in population sampling, measuring criteria, and even the types of media have resulted in different outcomes in studies that addressed the relationship between violent media and human violence. Much of the literature on media violence was written in the post-Columbine era, and suggested both immediate and long-term effects on children. More recently, Ferguson and Kilburn (2009) conducted a meta-analytic review of studies that examine the impact of violent media on aggressive behavior to determine whether this effect could be explained through methodological problems inherent in this research field. The results from their analysis did not support the conclusion that media violence leads to aggressive behavior, and they noted that it cannot be concluded at this time that media violence presents a significant public health risk. Thus, the effects of media violence remain under debate.

DEVELOPMENTAL REACTIONS TO VIOLENCE EXPOSURE

Early Childhood

Young children who witness domestic or community violence show increased irritability, immature behavior, developmental regression, increased fears, temper tantrums, clinging, and difficulty separating from parents. They may even exhibit symptoms of posttraumatic stress disorder (PTSD). When exposed to violence, children as young as 2 can experience sleep disturbances, withdrawn or aggressive behaviors, developmental regression, and disruptions in the parent-child relationship.

Exposure to domestic violence has a negative impact on neurocognitive development, leading to lower intelligence scores in young children. There is also an overlap between domestic violence and child abuse. In families where one form of violence exists, it is likely that the other forms will also exit, and young children are at higher risk for child abuse than older children. Community violence exposure is associated with negative outcomes for children, including reduced behavioral and social competence.

Middle Childhood

Like preschoolers, school-aged children exposed to violence are more likely to have sleep disturbances, and less likely to explore and play freely or to show motivation in mastering their environment. They often have difficulty with attention and concentration because they are distracted by intrusive thoughts. School-aged children are likely to understand more about the intentionality of the violence and worry about what they could have done to prevent or stop it. School-aged children with extreme exposure to chronic community violence may also exhibit symptoms of posttraumatic stress disorder.

School-aged children who are exposed to family violence are affected similarly to those exposed to community violence. They often experience a greater frequency of internalizing (withdrawal, anxiety) and externalizing (aggressiveness, delinquency) behavior problems in comparison to children from nonviolent families. Overall functioning, attitudes, social competence, and school performance are often affected negatively.

School-aged children watch more television and thus maybe more exposed to television violence than other children. Studies of school-aged children exposed to media violence have also identified adverse effects over time. Exposure to media violence may increase negative behaviors because of the potential for social learning and modeling of inappropriate behaviors by youths. Fictionalized violence is likely to have negative impacts on children and increase their propensity for violence when the violence is dramatically portrayed and glamorized. However, real-life events shown in a sensationalized manner may overwhelm or numb the senses.

Adolescence

There is a considerable body of research that suggests adolescents exposed to violence, especially ongoing chronic community violence, tend to show high levels of aggression and acting out, accompanied by anxiety, behavioral problems, school problems, truancy, and revenge seeking. Adolescents may have more severe effects of violence exposure than younger children because they are exposed to more violence overall.

Adolescents who witness community violence can overcome the experience; however, many are affected. Some report giving up hope because they expect that they may not live through adolescence or early adulthood. These chronically traumatized youths often appear numb to feelings and pain, and show restricted emotional development. Some of these youths may attach themselves to gangs as substitute family and incorporate violence as a method of dealing with disputes or frustration.

Media violence comes in multiple forms for adolescents, including television, movies, the Internet, music lyrics, music videos, and electronic games. Playing electronic games has become one of the most popular leisure activities of children and adolescents in the United States and Europe. Boys and girls play regularly, but boys outnumber girls in terms of frequency and duration of game-playing sessions, especially for games with violent content. Electronic games are played throughout the lifespan, but early adolescence is the peak time for exposure in most Western cultures, and adolescents show a particular interest in violent games. Trait aggression increases during adolescence, and violent media fits into this developmental theme. Adolescents also show an increased need for novelty, risk-taking behavior, and a heightened level of physiological arousal. Action-oriented games, especially those with violence, satisfy those needs. At the same time, they provide a safe environment because all the risks happen in a virtual reality and do not lead to physical harm.

ASSESSMENT

Assess all families for the presence of domestic violence. Several health care organizations have issued position statements regarding routine screening of patients and their families for domestic violence, including the American Academy of Pediatrics (AAP), which classified the abuse of women as a pediatric problem. Children also should be questioned regarding their knowledge of the domestic violence, since they often are much more aware of the violence than adults may think. Monitor children for signs of PTSD and for child abuse as noted elsewhere in this book.

Comprehensive assessment of domestic and other violence exposure can inform decision making regarding the types of interventions needed for children living with violence. Factors that influence the impact of violence exposure on children include the nature and frequency of the violence, elapsed time since exposure, the age and gender of the child, the child's coping skills, and whether the child has been abused.

Age-Specific Indicators of Reactions to Domestic Violence

Observe for the following age-specific indicators of reactions to domestic violence, as suggested by the Alabama Coalition Against Domestic Violence (ACADV, n.d.):

Infants

> Basic need for attachment is disrupted
>
> Routines around feeding/sleeping are disturbed
>
> Injuries while "caught in the crossfire"
>
> Irritability or inconsolable crying
>
> Frequent illness
>
> Difficulty sleeping
>
> Diarrhea
>
> Developmental delays
>
> Lack of responsiveness

Preschool Child

> Somatic or psychosomatic complaints
>
> Regression
>
> Irritability
>
> Fearful of being alone
>
> Extreme separation anxiety
>
> Developmental delays
>
> Sympathetic toward mother

School-Aged Child

  Vacillate between being eager to please and being hostile

  Verbal about home life

  Developmental delays

  Externalized behavior problems

  Inadequate social skill development

  Gender role modeling creates conflict/confusion

Preadolescent Child

  Behavior problems become more serious

  Increased internalized behavior difficulties: depression, isolation, withdrawal

  Emotional difficulties: shame, fear, confusion, rage

  Poor social skills

  Developmental delays

  Protection of mother, sees her as "weak"

  Guarded/secretive about family

Adolescent

  Internalized and externalized behavior problems can become extreme and dangerous: drug/alcohol, truancy, gangs, sexual acting out, pregnancy, runaway, suicidal

  Dating relationships may reflect violence learned or witnessed in the home.

INTERVENTIONS

If child abuse is suspected, report to child protective services according to state laws. Not all children exposed to domestic violence will need therapy. However, all children should be referred to a therapist with expertise in working with children who have witnessed domestic violence so that they may receive a comprehensive evaluation. Children may also warrant treatment for PTSD, which is discussed in Chapter 14, "Psychological Effects of Victimization."

Provide the domestic violence victim, typically the mother, with local domestic violence crisis numbers and counseling resources. Listen to what the victim has to say and do not judge if the person is unable to leave the relationship or accept counseling. Discuss the possibility of a protective order and help the family to develop a safety plan.

Orders of Protection

Domestic violence cases may warrant that the adult victim obtain an order of protection. An order of protection is a legally binding court order that restrains an individual who has committed an act of violence against a person from further acts against that person. Protective orders vary state by state and are called by various names (restraining orders, Protection From Abuse orders [PFAs], etc.). Most are used to protect against family/intimate partner violence; some jurisdictions use them for strangers.

There are different types of protective orders, demonstrated by the three stages of Protection From Abuse (PFA) orders issued in Pennsylvania:

- Emergency Orders issued by District Justice when Court of Common Pleas is closed. It is in effect until the next business day at the Court of Common Pleas.
- Temporary Order issued on a daily basis by Court of Common Pleas in Media and is in effect until the hearing for a Permanent PFA is held.
- Permanent Order issued for up to 18 months at a hearing before Court of Common Pleas. The hearing date is scheduled when the temporary PFA is received.

Health care providers can contact the police, district attorney's office, or victim advocate center to learn how victims may obtain protective orders in their areas. However, it is best they do this before a situation occurs and keep the information readily available for emergent purposes.

The protection order can prohibit the abuser from committing acts of violence; exclude the abuser from the residence shared by the petitioner and abuser; prohibit the abuser from harassing or contacting the petitioner by mail, telephone, or in person; award temporary custody of minor children; establish temporary visitation and restrain the abuser from interfering with custody; prohibit the abuser from removing the children from the jurisdiction of the court; and order the abuser to participate in treatment or counseling. Some states, including New York, include pets in the protective orders. Although seemingly powerful, protective orders are nothing more than pieces of paper—they are not bullet proof. They seem to work best on those offenders who have something to lose if they disobey them, and in some cases, may aggravate the situation. Therefore, victims still need to take precautions to keep themselves safe.

VICTIM'S COMPENSATION

Crime victim compensation programs offer crucial financial assistance to victims of violence. According to the National Association of Crime Victim Compensation Boards, recovering from violence is difficult enough without having to worry about the costs of medical care and counseling. Every state has a crime victim compensation program that can provide substantial financial assistance to crime victims and their families. While money cannot erase the trauma and grief victims suffer, it can be crucial in the recovery process. By paying for care that restores victims' physical and mental health, compensation programs are helping victims regain their lives.

Compensation needs are more common in adult victimization; however, there are many cases where child victims qualify. Conviction of the offender is not required, and victims of crime under state, federal, military, and tribal jurisdiction are eligible to apply for compensation. Eligible crime victims include those who have been physically injured and/or who suffer emotional injury as a result of violence or attempted violence, even though no physical injury resulted. Some states also include family members of deceased victims and other individuals who pay for expenses resulting from a victim's injury or death.

According to the National Association of Crime Victim Compensation Boards, each state's eligibility requirements vary slightly, but victims are generally required to report the crime promptly to law enforcement, usually within 72 hours; file a timely application with the compensation program in the state where the crime occurred, and provide any information requested; cooperate in the investigation and prosecution of the crime; and be innocent of any criminal activity or misconduct leading to the victim's injury or death. Many states require that the application be filed within 1 year from the date of the crime, but some states have shorter or longer periods. Applications can be obtained from the state compensation program, police, prosecutors, or victim service agencies. Most state programs have brochures describing their benefits, requirements, and procedures. Health care providers can refer victims to victim service programs for assistance in completing the application. The application should be submitted to the compensation program as soon as possible, where it will be reviewed to determine eligibility and to decide what costs can be paid. The program will notify the applicant of its decision.

Depending on the state, expenses may be covered if they are not paid for by insurance or by another public benefit program, and if they result directly from the crime. These include medical and hospital care, and dental work to repair injury to teeth; mental health counseling; lost earnings due to crime-related injuries; loss of support for dependents of a deceased victim; and funeral and burial expenses. Expenses that are not covered usually include property loss, theft and damage (unless damage is to eyeglasses, hearing aids, or other medically necessary devices), and expenses paid by other sources, such as any type of public or private health insurance, automobile insurance, disability insurance, or workers compensation. A few states may pay limited amounts for the loss of essential personal property during a violent crime and for cleaning up the crime scene.

PREVENTION

Health care providers can prevent the circle of violence by assuring that violence-exposed children get the treatment they need. They can also discuss safe dating practices with preteen and teenage clients, instruct families on health media usage, and work with their communities to improve safety and decrease violence.

RESOURCES

Appendix C: Crime Victim Compensation Programs
Healing the Invisible Wounds: Children's Exposure to Violence: A Guide for Families: www.safestartcenter.org/pdf/caregiver.pdf
Helping Young Children Affected by Domestic Violence: The Role of Pediatric Health Settings: www.uiowa.edu/~socialwk/pape_1.pdf
National Association of Crime Victim Compensation Boards: www.nacvcb.org

REFERENCES

The Alabama Coalition Against Domestic Violence. (n.d.). *Effects of DV on children.* Retrieved from www.acadv.org/children.html#ageinfo

Centers for Disease Control and Prevention. (2008). Youth risk behavioral surveillance— United States, 2007. MMWR, 57 (No. SS–4).

Centers for Disease Control and Prevention. (2009, May 13). Web-based Injury Statistics Query and Reporting System (WISQARS). [Online]. (2006). National Center for Injury Prevention and Control, Centers for Disease Control and Prevention (producer). Retrieved from www.cdc.gov/injury

Child Welfare Information Gateway. (2003). *Children and domestic violence: Scope of the problem.* U.S. Department of Health and Human Services, Administration for Children and Families, Administration on Children, Youth and Families Children's Bureau. Retrieved from www.childwelfare.gov/pubs/factsheets/domesticviolence.pdf

Cooley-Quille, M., Boyd, R., Frantz, E., & Walsh, J. (2001). Emotional and behavioral impact of exposure to community violence in inner-city adolescents. *Journal of Clinical Child Psychology, 30*(2), 199–206.

Ferguson, C., & Kilburn, J. (2009). The public health risks of media violence: A meta-analytic review. *Journal of Pediatrics, 154,* 759–763.

Finkelhor, D., Turner, H., Ormrod, R., Hamby, S., & Kracke, K. (2009). *Children's Exposure to Violence: A Comprehensive National Survey.* U.S. Department of Justice, Office of Justice Programs, Office of Juvenile Justice and Delinquency Prevention, NCJ 227744. Retrieved from www.ncjrs.gov/pdffiles1/ojjdp/227744.pdf

Horner, G. (2005). Domestic violence and children. *Journal of Pediatric Health Care, 19,* 206–212.

Kennedy, A., Bybee, D., Sullivan, C., & Greeson, M. (2009). The effects of community and family violence exposure on anxiety trajectories during middle childhood: The role of family social support as a moderator. *Journal of Clinical Child & Adolescent Psychology, 38*(3), 365–379.

Koenen, K., Moffitt, T., Caspi, A., Taylor, A., & Purcell, S. (2003). Domestic violence is associated with environmental suppression of IQ in young children. *Development and Psychopathology, 15*(2), 297–311.

Mathews, T., Dempsey, M., & Overstreet, S. (2009). Effects of exposure to community violence on school functioning: The mediating role of posttraumatic stress symptoms. *Behaviour Research and Therapy, 47,* 586–591.

Moller, I., & Krahe, B. (2009). Exposure to violent video games and aggression in German adolescents: A longitudinal analysis. *Aggressive Behavior, 35,* 75–89.

Osofsky, J. (1999). The impact of violence on children. *The Future of Children: Domestic Violence and Children, 9*(3), 35–49.

Osofsky, J. (2004). *Young children and trauma: Intervention and treatment.* New York: Guilford Press.

U.S. Department of Health and Human Services, Administration on Children, Youth and Families. (2009). *Child maltreatment 2007.* Washington, DC: U.S. Government Printing Office. Retrieved from www.childwelfare.gov

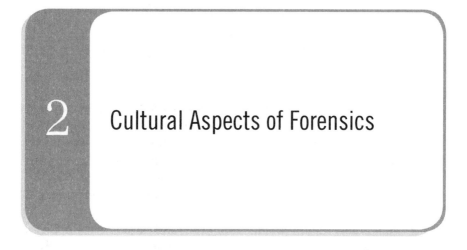

2   Cultural Aspects of Forensics

DEFINITIONS

Twenty-five percent of the U.S. population identifies themselves as belonging to one of the federally defined minority groups, and almost 20% of the American population speaks a language other than English as their primary language. And the American population is becoming even more diverse. It is predicted that shortly after 2050, no single racial-ethnic group will hold a majority population position.

The increasing diversity of Western society adds an important dimension to forensic practice. The understanding of cultural differences can aid health care providers in managing the cycle of violence, and the utilization of culturally competent health care can facilitate recovery from trauma. An example would be interpreting the meaning of a man disallowing his wife to answer questions. Western cultural may lead the health care provider to interpret this as controlling behavior. However, this behavior may be acceptable in some cultures to the point where the woman is comfortable with it and not comfortable with answering the questions.

The Merriam-Webster Dictionary (http://www.merriam-webster.com) defines *culture* as the integrated pattern of human knowledge, beliefs, and behaviors that depend on transmission to succeeding generations, and the traditional beliefs, social manner, and material traits of a racial, religious, or social group. Culture extends beyond ethnicity and religion to include elements such as gender identity (e.g., lesbian, gay, bisexual, transgender) and location (e.g., rural or urban), and it encompasses an array of values, beliefs, and customs.

- Values act as the foundation for culture. Values are acquired through socialization in early childhood and guide people's goals, aspirations, and behaviors. For example, people value time differently. Some are present-oriented, accepting each day as it comes with little regard for the past and future; others are past-oriented, maintaining traditions and worshiping ancestors. Still others are future-oriented, with a high value for change.
- Beliefs include knowledge, opinions, and faith about the world. Witchcraft and the "evil eye" are two personalistic folk beliefs.
- Customs are learned behaviors that are easily assessed through questioning and observation. Problems can develop if professionals do not validate the meaning of observed behaviors. For example, most health care providers consider lack of eye contact abnormal behavior; however, some cultures consider eye contact a sign of disrespect or even hostility.

Race is a social and political construct rather than a biological one. Ethnicity is a term used to describe a common heritage, history, and worldview. The U.S. Census Bureau combines race and ethnicity into the following categories: American Indian, Alaskan Native, Asian, Black or African American, Hispanic or Latino, Native Hawaiian or Pacific Islander, and White. The purpose of this categorization is to help the government understand the needs of its citizens, including mental health care. However, this classification can be confusing and inadequate. There are more than 40 Asian and Pacific Island Countries, and over 560 Native American and Alaskan Native tribes. African Americans whose ancestors lived in the United States centuries ago have different cultural norms than those from Africa or the Caribbean today. Latinos may be from different racial groups, and the White group includes a very diverse population of Americans of European descent, as well as people from the Middle East. Biracial persons have no unique category.

Culture also includes immigration status, an issue critical in forensics since foreign-born women are over-represented among intimate partner female homicide victims when compared to the general population.

- Permanent residents or immigrants are persons who come to the United States to remain permanently or for an indefinite period of time. The United States is their primary place of residence, and their permanent resident status is shown by possession of an identification card (green card).
- Refugees are those persons living outside of their country of nationality and who are unable or unwilling to return because of persecution or fear of persecution on account of race, religion, nationality, membership in a particular social group, or political opinion.
- Refugees make an application to U.S. authorities outside the United States and are approved for such status before coming to the United States. They are eligible to apply for permanent resident status after one year of continuous stay in the United States.
- Asylees must meet the definition for a refugee but differ because they make an application for asylum (protection) after arriving in the United States.
- Naturalization is the process of becoming a U.S. citizen. Lawful permanent residents may apply for U.S. citizenship by filing an application with the U.S. Citizenship and Immigration Services. It usually takes six months to two years to become naturalized.
- Undocumented immigrants are those who entered the country without valid documents, as well as those who entered with valid visas but overstayed their visas' expiration or otherwise violated the terms of their admission.

CULTURE AND FORENSICS

Certain cultural beliefs and customs have implications in the legal system, and health care professionals can assist law enforcement by performing detailed assessments to ascertain whether beliefs and behaviors are related to culture, mental health issues, or other factors. This may be important in cases where family violence is suspected or other violence has taken place.

Culture-Bound Syndromes

Culture-bound syndromes (culture-related syndromes) are folk illnesses with prominent alterations of behavior and experience. They usually do not conform to conventional diagnostic syndromes; however, they have cultural validity in the societies in which they occur. Some culture-bound syndromes involve somatic symptoms (pain or disturbed function of a body part), while others are purely behavioral. The ones noted here are those that may have legal implications:

- *Amok* or *mata elap* (Malaysia) is probably the most known in this category and is a dissociative episode characterized by an outburst of violent, aggressive, or homicidal behavior directed at people and objects. The episode is usually triggered by a perceived insult or slight and seems to be prevalent among males. Persons who "run amok" usually experience persecutory ideas, automatism, and amnesia during the episode, and a return to premorbid state following the episode. A similar behavior pattern is found in Laos, the Philippines, Polynesia (*cafard* or *cathard*); New Guinea and Puerto Rico (*mal de pelea*); and among the Navajos (*iich'aa*).
- *Ataquque de nervios* (Latinos from the Caribbean, and other Latino groups) manifests in symptoms of uncontrollable shouting, crying, trembling, and verbal or physical aggression. The individual may also experience dissociative experiences, seizure-like or fainting episodes, and suicidal gestures. These symptoms frequently occur after a stressful event relating to the family, such as separation, divorce, or an accident.
- *Boufée deliriante* (West Africa and Haiti) is a sudden outburst of agitated and aggressive behavior, marked confusion, and psychomotor excitement. *Boufée deliriante* may sometimes be accompanied by visual and auditory hallucinations or paranoid ideation.
- *Hi-Wa itck* (Mohave American Indians) is associated with the unwanted separation from a loved one, resulting in insomnia, depression, loss of appetite, and sometimes suicide.
- *Latah* (Malaysia and Indonesia) is characterized by hypersensitivity to sudden fright, often with echopraxia, echolalia, command obedience, and dissociative or trancelike behavior. The Malaysian syndrome is more common in middle-aged women. Similar syndromes are found in Siberian groups (*amurakh, irkunii, ikota, olan, myriachit,* and *menkeiti*); Thailand (*bah-tschi, bah-tsi,* and *baah-ji*); Japan (*imu*); and Philippines (*mali-mali* and *silok*).
- *Locura* (Latin America) is a severe form of chronic psychosis that is attributed to an inherited vulnerability, the effect of multiple life difficulties, or a combination of the two. Manifestations include incoherence, agitation, auditory and visual hallucinations, inability to follow social interaction rules, unpredictability, and possible violence.

- *Pibloktoq* or Arctic hysteria (Greenland Eskimos) is an abrupt dissociative episode accompanied by extreme excitement lasting up to 30 minutes and frequently followed by seizures and coma lasting up to 12 hours. The affected individual may be withdrawn or slightly irritable for a period of hours or days before the attack and typically reports complete amnesia for the attack. During the attack, the individual may shout obscenities, eat feces, flee from protective shelters, tear off his or her clothing, break furniture, or perform other irrational or dangerous acts.

- Qi-gong psychotic reaction (China) is an acute, time-limited episode characterized by dissociative, paranoid, or other symptoms that occur after participating in the Chinese folk health-enhancing practice of qi-gong. Individuals who become overly involved in the practice are especially vulnerable.

- *Shenkui* (China) is characterized by marked anxiety or panic symptoms with accompanying somatic complaints without obvious physical cause. Symptoms include dizziness, backache, fatigability, general weakness, insomnia, frequent dreams, and complaints of sexual dysfunction (such as premature ejaculation and impotence). Symptoms are attributed to excessive semen loss from frequent intercourse, masturbation, nocturnal emission, or passing of "white turbid urine" believed to contain semen. Similar symptoms are found in India (*dhat* and *jiryan*); and Sri Lanka (*sukra prameha*).

- *Tabanka* (Trinidad) is characterized by depression associated with a high rate of suicide and is usually seen in men who have been abandoned by their wives.

- *Zar* (North Africa and the Middle East) is an experience of spirit possession with symptoms that include dissociative episodes with laughing, shouting, hitting the head against a wall, singing, or weeping. Individuals may show apathy and withdrawal, refusing to eat or carry out daily tasks, or may develop a long-term relationship with the possessing spirit.

Cultural Customs Related to Female Reproduction

Female Genital Mutilation (May Mimic Intimate Partner Violence)

Female genital mutilation (FGM) refers to procedures that intentionally alter or injure female genital organs for nonmedical reasons. FGM is usually performed when a girl is between 4 and 8 years old. It is practiced in about 28 African countries, Asia, the Middle East, and increasingly in Europe, Australia, Canada, and the United States. The World Health Organization (WHO), which promotes the elimination of FGM, has estimated that between 100 and 140 million women have undergone FGM, and that two million more undergo some form of FGM every year.

The WHO has identified four types of FGM.

- Type I is a clitoridectomy, which is the only type that can accurately be referred to as female circumcision and involves the removal of the prepuce and all or parts of the clitoris. This procedure typically does not result in long-term complications.
- Type II involves removal of the clitoris and inner labia, possibly resulting in pain during intercourse and other long-term problems.
- Type III is an extreme form of circumcision that involves removal of the clitoris, at least two-thirds of the labia majora, and the entire labia minora. Incisions are made in the labia majora to create raw surfaces, which are then stitched or held together (sometimes by tying the woman's legs together), until a hood of skin grows to cover the urethra and vagina. Afterward, a tiny hole is made to allow for menstrual flow and urination.
- Type IV involves piercing or incising the clitoris and/or labia, and cauterization by burning of the clitoris and surrounding tissue.

Health care providers are likely to encounter women who have had FGM in their clinical practice, possibly for one of the adverse effects, which include: cysts, abscesses, and scar tissue; sexual dysfunction; dysmenorrhea; chronic pelvic infections; damage to the urethra; incontinence; chronic pelvic and back pain; chronic urinary tract infections; and difficulties with childbirth. It is important that health care providers not assume that all these women want this condition reversed. Women who have undergone FGM have been taught to believe that this rite of passage is normal. Their culture may believe that reversal of circumcision makes a woman unsuitable for marriage, liable for divorce, and virtually an outcast in their communities. Instead, providers should ask how this alteration has affected the woman's life, urination, and menstruation. Health care professionals can also refer these women to a counselor from the same cultural background to discuss deinfibulation or other possible treatments, if needed.

Practices Around Menstruation

Beliefs about the cause and purpose of menstruation vary among cultures. For example, Navajo culture views menarche as a symbol for passage into adulthood, whereas both Iranian and Orthodox Jewish cultures view menstruation as a period of uncleanness. Extremely Orthodox Jewish women separate themselves from all men during menses, and no man is allowed to touch or even sit where a menstruating woman has sat. Women are considered to be in a state of impurity for at least 12 days (5 days from the onset of the menstrual cycle and 7 clean days following it). They then must attend a *mikvah* (ritual bath) before engaging in sexual intercourse with their husbands.

Practices Related to Illness Treatment (May Mimic Child or Elder Abuse)

Coining, or *CaoGio* (Southeast Asia) is one of the most commonly practiced cultural folk remedies. Coining is rubbing or scratching with a coin on the skin of the back, neck, upper chest, and arms. Before or during rubbing, Tiger Balm (a mentholated ointment), Ben-Gay, an herbal liquid medicine or water is applied on the skin. The skin is then rubbed in a downward, linear fashion with the edge of the copper coin or a silver spoon until dark lines appear. These marks can persist for several days and have the appearance of being struck with a stick or whip.

Cupping (Hmong, Vietnamese, ethnic Chinese) or *bahnkes* (Russians, Koreans, and others) is performed on the chest, back, abdomen, and/or back of legs for pain, and the forehead and temples for headaches. A glass is held upside down, and a lit match, candle, or lighter is held under it in order to burn off the oxygen, creating a vacuum. The cup is quickly placed on the skin and the vacuum effect pulls the skin up, creating a mark that looks like a bruise and that may last for several days.

Stick burns and moxibustion, also called *poua*, are remedies used in certain cultures to relieve a variety of illness symptoms. These remedies are related to acupuncture; however, they cause a circular, cigarette-tip-size burn. The procedure calls for an incense-like stick to be lit and placed on the palms of the hands, soles of the feet, and genital area. Moxa herbs, usually mugwort (*Artemisia vulgaris*), or yarn are rolled into a pea-sized ball, placed on the skin, lit, and allowed to burn to the point of pain.

Pinching, or *bat gio* (Southeast Asia) is used to treat pain and a variety of conditions. For example, the area between the eyebrows, upper nose, and temples is pinched to relieve headaches. Tiger balm may be massaged into the area before pinching. The pressure from the pinching leaves a reddened area that may give the appearance of having been struck.

Air suctioning (Southeast Asia) is used to relieve headaches. The cut end of a bull or goat horn is placed on the patient's forehead and/or temples, and the practitioner sucks the air out of the other end. The horn sticks to the application site and is then plugged with wax and left on the forehead for 10 to 15 minutes. Blood drawn to the surface of the skin leaves a round, bruiselike mark after the horn is removed. The marks may persist for several days.

Fallen fontanel or *caida de la mollera* (Latino populations), a challenging and potentially fatal pediatric folk illness, may develop from any severe illness (such as gastroenteritis) resulting in a 10% body weight loss in an infant. Children with *caida* are believed to be neglected, creating a high degree of maternal guilt. The cause is believed to be mechanical, such as the soft palate pulling down the fontanel when the feeding nipple is suddenly pulled out of the infant's mouth. Folk remedies include: pressing upward on the soft palate with thumbs or fingers, sucking the anterior fontanel, holding the baby upside down over water with or without shaking or hitting the feet. Poultices may be applied to the fontanel with raw egg, oil, or liniment and the hair is pulled up (so that the roots will raise the skin back up).

Culture and Intimate Partner Violence

Intimate partner violence (IPV) seems to be more prevalent and more lethal among immigrant women than among U.S. citizens. The Office for Victims of Crime notes that there are several factors that may make this type of victimization more likely, as well increase the difficulty immigrant victims face in seeking safety and using the justice system effectively:

- Cultural barriers: Cultural beliefs and practices may make it difficult for a victim to leave an abusive relationship and may even reinforce the idea that violence against a spouse is acceptable.
- Fear of deportation: Immigrants may fear being deported and losing custody of their children. Perpetrators of domestic violence and other crimes may use the fear of deportation to thwart the victim from reporting the crime. Lack of proper legal documentation (social security number, green card, or employment authorization)

to work or live in the United States can contribute to immigrants staying with abusive partners and not seeking outside help.

- Language barriers: Lack of or limited English proficiency keeps victimized immigrants from seeking protection with the police, the court system, social service agencies, and shelters.
- Misinformation about the legal system: Many immigrants come from countries where women cannot receive justice. Immigrant victims may be wary of seeking assistance from official institutions based on real or imagined experiences.
- Fear of the police: Immigrants may come from countries where police repress citizens, respond only to bribes, or believe women should be subordinate to men.
- Economic barriers: An abusive spouse may be a woman's only means of support, and her immigrant status may make it impossible for her to legally obtain work or find child care.

The Violence Against Women Act (VAWA) of 1994 addresses the needs of immigrant women who are victimized by their spouses. This law created two ways for women who are married to U.S. citizens or lawful permanent residents to get their residency without having to rely on their abusive spouse: (a) Self-petitions allow a victim of IPV to file for and obtain permanent resident status without the knowledge, cooperation, or participation of the perpetrator. These petitions are applicable to victims of IPV who would have lawful immigration status through their spouses. These women should first consult a shelter worker, immigration attorney, or domestic violence or immigration agency for assistance. (b) Undocumented immigrant victims of IPV may be able to obtain U.S. residency through VAWA cancellation of deportation, if they are currently in or can be placed into deportation proceedings. Victims who qualify for cancellation may have their deportation waived by the court and may be granted residency. These women should consult an immigration attorney before proceeding.

Culture and Human Trafficking

The United Nations defines human trafficking as

> The recruitment, transportation, transfer, harbouring or receipt of persons, by means of the threat or use of force or other forms of coercion, of abduction, of fraud, of deception, of the abuse of power or of a

position of vulnerability or of the giving or receiving of payments or benefits to achieve the consent of a person having control over another person, for the purpose of exploitation. (United Nations, n.d.)

Many victims have language barriers and are isolated and unable to communicate with service providers, law enforcement, and others who might help them. They are often subjected to debt-bondage, usually in the context of paying off transportation fees into the destination countries, and are often threatened with injury or death or threats to the safety of their family back home. Please see chapter 12 for more on human trafficking.

Immigration Consultant Fraud

Scam artists prey upon immigrants seeking assistance in obtaining legal residence, work authorization, or citizenship. Many claim that they are attorneys or that they have close connections to the Immigration and Naturalization Service (INS). Others use titles such as notary public to deceive people into believing that they are lawyers. Typical scams include: charging excessive fees for immigration services and then failing to file any documents; filing false asylum claims; and charging fees to prepare applications for nonexistent immigration programs or for legitimate programs for which the client does not qualify.

CULTURAL COMPETENCY

Cultural competence goes beyond cultural sensitivity. It implies moving beyond awareness about different cultures to in-depth knowledge, and from sensitivity to issues to commitment to change situations of oppression. Culturally competent providers move beyond awareness about different cultures to an in-depth knowledge of them.

To provide culturally competent care, health care providers should:

- Develop knowledge about the norms of the ethnic and cultural groups they are likely to encounter in everyday practice
- Have the ability to perform a cultural assessment
- Make a commitment to spend time with diverse groups outside the health care setting

- Understand the political and social issues that affect these groups
- Understand how various groups react to stress

To provide culturally competent care:

- Become aware of your own professional and personal values about cultural practices. Ethnocentrism is common in all cultural and social groups, but health care professionals must transcend this bias. Health care professionals do not need to abandon personal values, beliefs, and cultural practices; however, they do need to understand how their personal perspectives may impact on their responses and assessments of diverse patients.
- Identify cultural nuances when assessing behaviors considered abnormal by Western society, such as lack of eye contact or an unresponsive or flat affect. These signs are often associated with mental illness or deceptiveness, yet in some cultures these are normal behaviors. Be sure to compare the patient's behavior with normative standards of his or her cultural group, not only with the Westernized diagnostic system.
- Try to understand patients and their situations within the context of their cultural group. Ask questions about beliefs, perceptions about the cause of a problem, and how this type of problem is usually addressed in their culture. Ask about religious and spiritual beliefs and experiences.
- Realize that not all members of a particular cultural group are the same. Information about cultural trends should not overshadow the understanding of the individual person. Avoid stereotyping.
- Empathy can bridge cultural differences. Convey a caring attitude toward patients, and show interest in cultural differences and acknowledge these with the patient.

The U.S. Department of Justice's Office of Victims of Crime presents five core tenets to providing high-quality multicultural victim assistance services:

- Develop the cultural awareness and competency
- Acknowledge the different and valid cultural customs of recovery from traumatic events
- Support cultural pathways to mental health and incorporate these into victim services and referrals

- Rely on multiethnic and multilingual teamwork to implement and monitor effective victim services
- Develop a cross-cultural perspective

RESOURCES

National Center for Cultural Competence: http://www.11.georgetown.edu/research/guc chd/nccc

Office for Minority Health Cultural Competency Section: http://www.omhrc.gov/tem plates/browse.aspx?lvl=&lvlID=3

Program for Multicultural Health: http://www.med.umich.edu/Multicultural/ccp/in dex.htm

Think Cultural Health (U.S. Department of Health & Human Services): http://www.thinkculturalhealth.org/

REFERENCES

Administration for Children's Services, U.S. Department of Health and Human Services. Human trafficking fact sheet. Retrieved from http://www.acf.hhs.gov/traffick ing/about/factsheets.html

American Psychiatric Association. (2000). *Diagnostic and statistical manual of mental disorders* (4th ed.). Washington, DC: Author.

Child Abuse Prevention Council of Sacramento, Inc. (n.d.). *Cultural customs.* Retrieved from http://www.capcsac.org/cultural-customs

Femicide in New York City: 1995–2002. New York City Department of Health and Mental Hygiene, October 2004. Retrieved from http://www.nyc.gov/html/doh/downloads/pdf/ip/femicide1995–2002_report.pdf

Gerace, L., & Salimene, S. (2009). *Cultural competence for today's nurses, part two: Culture and mental health.* Retrieved from http://www.nurse.com/ce/CE399-60/Course Page/2009

Salimene, S., & Gerace, L. (2009). *Cultural competence for today's nurses, part one: Culture and women's health.* Retrieved from http://www.nurse.com/ce/CE398-60/Course Page

Simons, R. (2001). Introduction to culture-bound syndromes. *Psychiatric Times, 18*(11). Retrieved from http://www.psychiatrictimes.com/display/article/10168/54246

United Nations. (n.d.). *Gender and human trafficking.* Retrieved from http://www.unes cap.org/esid/Gad/Issues/Trafficking/index.asp

U.S. Census Bureau. (2004). *U.S. interim projections by age, sex, race, and Hispanic origin.* Retrieved from http://www.census.gov/ipc/www/usinterimproj

U.S. Citizenship and Immigration Services. (n.d.). Glossary and acronyms. Retrieved from http://www.uscis.gov/graphics/glossary4.cfm#U

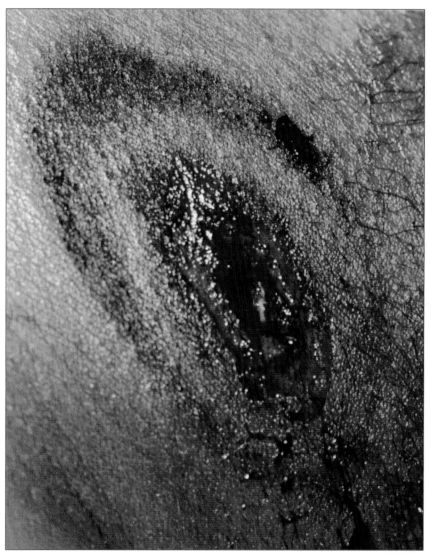

Figure 3.1 Gunshot wound. Notice the pattern of discoloration around the wound, probably from the gun muzzle.

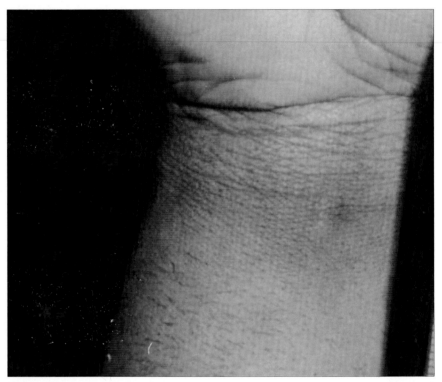

Figure 3.2 Bruising of the wrist. This bruising pattern is commonly seen as a result of forceful restraint.

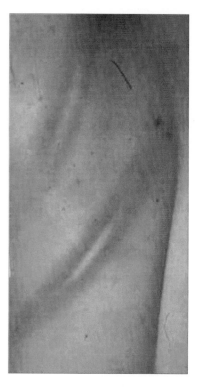

Figure 3.3 Patterned injury. Note the area of central clearing on the inside of the pattern.

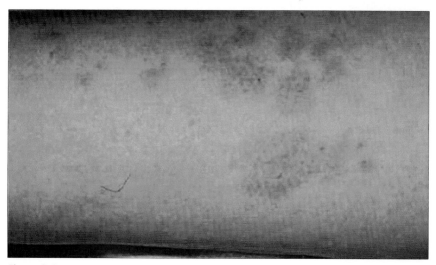

Figure 3.4 Bruising. Multiple bruises related to blunt force trauma that created bleeding under the skin.

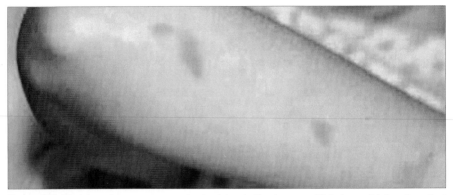

Figure 3.5 Bruising. A common area for bruising is the forearm. This type of injury is called a defensive injury.

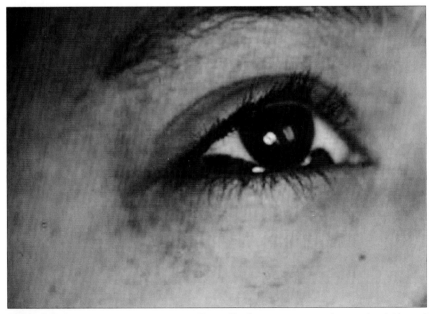

Figure 3.6 Petechiae and hemorrhage. These findings are commonly seen in victims of strangulation.

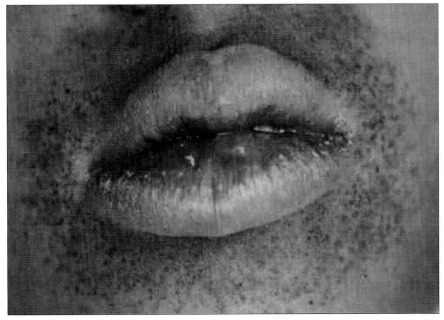

Figure 3.7 Abrasion. Note the removal of the most superficial tissue on the lips. Note the lack of bleeding.

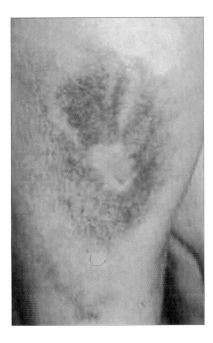

Figure 3.8 Patterned injury. Note that the area of central clearing in this photo resembles an open hand.

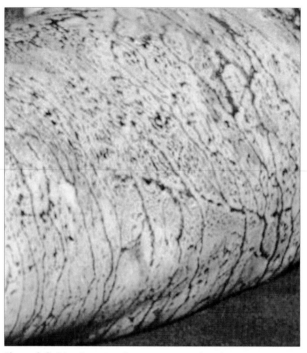

Figure 3.9 Blood spatter. Spatter, as seen in this photo, can and does occur on the body of the victim or the offender.

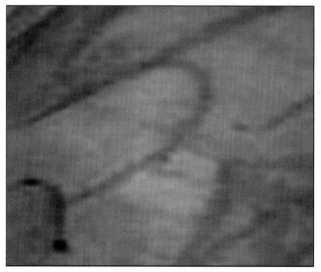

Figure 3.10 Pattern of injury. Note that the pattern of injury in this photo resembles the weapon used.

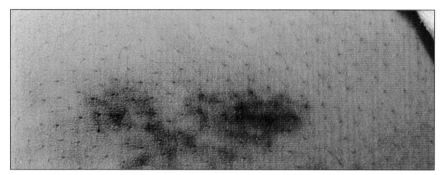

Figure 3.11 Bruising. This pattern of bruising is commonly seen as a result of a bite.

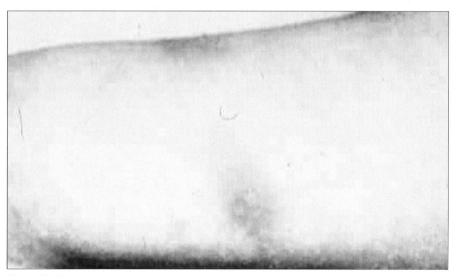

Figure 3.12 Bruising. This is a photo of fingertip bruising on a child victim.

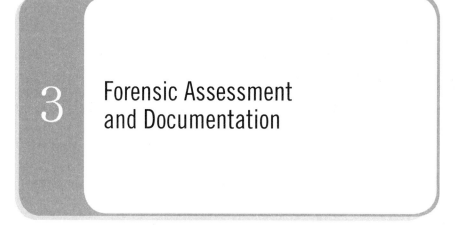

3

Forensic Assessment and Documentation

DEFINITION

Forensic assessments are those assessments performed for legal purposes. Health care providers who perform these assessments may be evaluating victims (as in sexual assault evaluations) or offenders (as in criminal competency evaluations). Forensic assessment differs from clinical assessment. Clinical assessments are confidential. Forensic assessments have limited confidentiality, because the assessment information may be used in court or for other purposes (such as parole evaluation). Thus, the forensic assessment requires that the client and collateral sources be informed of the limitations on confidentiality.

When performing clinical assessments, the health care provider listens empathetically to the subject in a nonjudgmental attitude, focuses on the subject's needs, facilitates the subject's ability to verbalize distressing feelings, and assists the subject with problem solving. When performing a forensic assessment, the health care provider must remain unbiased, objective, and void of emotional attachment to the subject. The focus is on gathering information in a methodical and purposeful manner. When conducting the forensic assessment, the subject is not the health care professional's client; the client is usually the state (if assessing for the prosecution), the plaintiff attorney (in civil cases), or the defense attorney (in civil and criminal cases).

ETIOLOGY

Health care providers frequently encounter clients whose clinical situation includes a legal component. Victims of crime, accident victims, and perpetrators of crime are frequently seen in health care settings. The role in forensic assessment is to help ensure that the legal aspects of their cases are appropriately addressed.

ASSESSMENT

General Principles

The purpose of a forensic assessment depends on the legal situation. If the subject warrants assessment for issues such as competency or risk, the purpose is usually to collect pertinent information from the subject and collateral sources (persons and documents relevant to the case) and perform specific psychological testing. For example, forensic assessment of a sex offender may warrant an interview with the subject, interviews with the victims and family, assessment of all past and present juvenile and adult criminal records, and performance of risk assessments such as the Static 2002.

These assessments are usually carried out by professionals with advanced psychological/psychiatric education and experience. The purpose of forensic assessment of crime victims is to gain facts for the legal investigation. This is achieved though obtaining the victim's account of the incident and identifying and collecting evidence that has transferred from the perpetrator and/or crime scene to the victim. For example, the forensic assessment of an elder-abuse victim would include an interview of the elder (if possible), a review of the elder's medical records, a physical examination to determine the extent and type of injuries, and pertinent diagnostic tests that would be used in this case to further diagnose elder abuse. This chapter focuses on forensic assessment of the crime victim.

The Forensic Interview

Whenever possible, health care providers interview the victim with a law enforcement professional present to avoid subjecting the victim to an additional interview process. The victim account of what occurred during the commission of the crime, in as much detail as possible, is most helpful for evidence collection and preservation. For example, in a sexual assault case, knowing where the suspect placed his mouth on the victim is likely to enhance the accuracy of the search for saliva. In cases of dating violence, knowing exactly what areas of the body may be injured makes the search for early bruising and patterns of bruising more likely to be successful. Knowing that the victim was restrained in any way during an assault, allows the examiner to carefully search for signs of restraint, such as bruising and tape marks.

Health care providers should record what the client/victim recalls in his or her own words as often as possible. An ideal victim interview is recorded in a series of quotes, in quotation marks, about what the victim recalls. Statements made by the victim to the health care provider can be used in court. The forensic role in interviewing is not to analyze or place judgment on the words of the victim, but simply to record them, in writing, exactly as stated, such as "He shoved his penis in my mouth," "He burned me with the curling iron," or "I was beat up by John." The victim's description should not be sanitized or interpreted, just recorded with as many exact quotes as possible.

An interview conducted with law enforcement present prevents the client/victim from the need to retell the account multiple times. Law enforcement must determine what crime or crimes were committed, gather information related to the crime scene, and obtain as much information as possible about the suspect(s) from the victim. Health care providers are seeking information about possible injury and possible evidence transfer from the suspect to the victim. Information desired by law enforcement and by health care personnel can be derived from the victim's description of the events preceding his or her entry into the health care system.

Because health care concerns are always a priority, the interview may be delayed until the victim is medically stable; but examination, evaluation, and treatment may proceed without the interview. The interview may also be delayed if the victim is unconscious or semiconscious, and/or under the influence of alcohol or drugs. Evaluation, treatment, and testing should proceed in these situations without an interview. The interview can be conducted at a later time. When the victim cannot speak for himself or herself, as in the case of confused elders, careful documentation of any and all observations of the victim by health care personnel becomes crucial.

Consent to collect forensic evidence and submit the evidence to law enforcement should be obtained. This consent is different from consent for medical treatment. Consent for photography should also be obtained.

The Forensic Physical Examination

The forensic examination is performed to gain facts for the investigation, specifically evidentiary information. A general assessment should be conducted, noting the physical and emotional state of the victim, as well as hygiene and appropriateness of the clothing. For nonfamilial abuse cases (e.g., sexual assault cases), the examiner should focus on the areas appropriate to the interviewing information about the incident. For elder abuse cases, a complete physical examination should be conducted, including nutritional assessment measurements. (More specific information on different aspects of elder abuse can be found in their appropriate chapters.) One of the critical aspects of the forensic physical examination is the differentiation of wounds.

Types of Body Injury

Injury or tissue damage occurs when some quantity or quality of force is applied to the body. Force can be applied to tissue either by a moving object impacting the body or by the body contacting an object. Blunt force trauma is the term associated with injury created by force applied with a blunt object. Blunt force trauma is divided into four types: contusions, lacerations, abrasions, and fractures.

The amount of force applied influences the trauma. Also, identical applications of force do not result in the identical injury in every person. The quality of the tissue subjected to blunt force trauma influences the injury. Several factors may contribute to increase bruising in older adults, including: fragility of capillary walls, thinning skin with loss of the protective fatty layer, and consumption of certain medications, including anticoagulants. Any disease of the skin and or any systemic disease may alter the body's response to blunt force trauma.

Patterned Injury. A patterned injury is a representation of the shape of the object that caused the injury. It is important to recognize and document patterns. The pattern can resemble the exact shape of the object that impacted the skin. The pattern can be represented by abrasions, contusions, or lacerations, or all of these.

The different types of injuries are defined by the layer of tissue they affect. The anatomy of the skin includes three layers of tissue: the epidermis, which includes the stratum corneum (keratinized cells) and the basal cell layer; the dermis, which forms the greater part of the skin and contains blood vessels, hair follicles, cutaneous glands, and nerve fibers; and the subcutaneous or fatty layer. Deep fascia or connective tissue and muscle lie beneath the three layers of the skin. The mouth and vaginal vault are lined with mucosal tissue. These areas do not have the same protective layers as the epidermis (keratinized cells) or fatty tissue; therefore, mucosa is more vulnerable to injury. (See the figures just prior to the start of this chapter for examples of injuries.)

Abrasions. Abrasions are superficial injuries to the skin, limited to the epidermis and superficial dermis. An abrasion is scraping and removal of the superficial layers of the skin. Small flaps of the uppermost layer of skin may remain attached to the area. These small flaps may indicate the direction in which the scraping occurred. Abrasions may also be called scratches when the injury is caused by a fingernail. Abrasions may also be called brush burns if the injury is caused by frictional force against a rough surface or by dragging along coarse carpet. Rope burns are abrasions caused by friction of rope against the skin. Abrasions can be caused by handcuffs and by tying and binding. Such abrasions are usually found on wrists and ankles. Abrasions can have patterns that reflect abrasive clothing or a textured object.

Some materials used to restrain the victim are more likely to create abrasions than others. For example, abrasive clothing is more likely to cause an abrasion than a towel or smooth articles of clothing. Bleeding does not usually occur with an abrasion. The superficial nature of the abrasion precludes bleeding. Abrasions begin to heal within several hours of injury. A fresh abrasion usually oozes fluid from the tissues for a day or two. Gradually the abrasion is covered with a crust or scab under which the healing proceeds until it is complete. The duration of healing is dependent upon factors such as the extent of the injury and repeated trauma in the same area. Infection can also alter the healing of an abrasion.

Contusions and Bruises. Bruises lie below the intact epidermis and consist of an extravascular collection of blood that has leaked from ruptured capillaries or blood vessels. A contusion or bruise is hemorrhage into the skin and the tissues under the skin or both. The bruise usually comes from a blow or a squeeze that crushes the tissue and ruptures the blood vessels. The quantity and quality of the force applied dictates the extent of the contusion. A contusion can occur in any tissue—skin, brain, or lungs. The following discussion will concern contusions of the skin. In contusions of the skin, the blood is trapped under the skin because the skin does not break.

Bruises can resemble the object that created the bruise, such as whips, shoes, boots, fists, hands, pipes, and gun handles. The forensic examiner should note any patterns within a bruise that may be indicative of the object used to create the bruise. Parallel tracklike lines of hemorrhage result from a blow with a rod or a stick or an object with a similar shape. The skin between the lines looks pale, because the force of the blow displaces the blood sideways.

Bruises do not occur immediately but may take hours or longer to develop. Several factors can influence the size, color, and appearance of a bruise: available space for blood to collect, weight of the force, vascularity of the area, fragility of the blood vessels, and the location of the bruise. Areas that do not have a hard structure such as a bone beneath may result in less trauma.

The color of a bruise changes over time. Fresh injury ranges in color from light bluish red to purple. In time the bruise changes to green and yellow and brown. This change proceeds from the periphery of the bruise toward the center. Light red usually becomes noticeable within a few hours. The change to purple occurs over time. The color of a bruise is affected by time, size and extent of the bruise, its depth, and the victim's circulatory efficiency and local circulation. No solid studies to date provide an accurate analysis related to age and color of bruising. Research has identified other factors influencing the color of bruising, such as impaired blood clotting, immunosuppression, certain diseases, diabetes, alcoholism, malnutrition, and age. Even the temperature of the environment has been noted to influence the appearance of a bruise.

Bruising occurs when blunt force trauma is applied to an area of the body. However, a contusion or bruise does not necessarily indicate the exact point of force. Blood can shift under the skin due to gravity. For example, if the victim is in a recumbent position, the blood can gravitate to the posterior. Petechiae are tiny red or purple spots on skin or other tissue. Petechiae less than 3 millimeters in diameter are pinpoint-sized hemorrhages of small capillaries in the skin or mucous membranes. In all situations, petechiae, ecchymosis, and bruises do not blanch when pressed.

Superficial face and scalp wounds generally bleed more profusely than similar injuries elsewhere. Also, people often get superficial hemorrhages in the skin following minor injury, due to age-linked fragility of the small blood vessels. Kicking can create minimal bruising on the skin, but deep organ damage may be under the bruises. Nurses must carefully appraise bruising in the abdomen, back, and chest related to kicking.

Erythema. Erythema, or redness of the skin, should not be mistaken for bleeding under the skin. Erythema blanches with gentle pressure. Erythema is usually diffuse and does not have a pattern. The cause of redness can be a forceful slap or pressure to the skin. With sudden pressure, the blood is momentarily forced out of the capillaries in the area of contact. When the pressure is withdrawn, the blood returns to the capillaries, which may then dilate. The result is redness or flushing of the skin.

Lacerations. A laceration occurs when the continuity of the skin is broken or disrupted by blunt force. It is a tear created by blunt trauma. Tissue opens due to force applied. The amount of force and its direction create the appearance of the laceration. The impact creates crushing and tearing of tissue. Lacerations can occur in any tissue, but the following discussion is confined to the skin. Between the sides of a laceration run multiple threads of tissue called tissues bridges. Theses bridges are tissue that remains connected after the blow. The bridges are made up of fiber and blood vessels. The wound edges of a laceration are usually abraded. The abraded area may resemble what made contact with the impacting surface. Lacerations are not cut injuries; rather, they are breaks in tissue from blunt force trauma applied to tissue with enough force to overcome the strength of the tissue. Lacerations sustained by falling are generally located on protuberant parts such as knees and cheekbones and jaws. Thus, in a fall, the eyes are typically spared and the rims of the eye socket are commonly abraded or torn.

A blow with a blunt object can produce a tear with finely abraded edges. Lacerations can indicate the point of force on the skin. Therefore, it is important to carefully examine and document all lacerations. Trace evidence from the crime scene such as dirt and fibers may be found in lacerations.

Cut Wounds. A cut wound occurs whenever a sharp object is drawn over the skin with sufficient pressure to produce an injury. The wound edges can be straight or jagged depending upon the shape of the cutting instrument. The edges of a cut wound are not abraded, and tissue bridging is not present in the wound. Cut wounds of the upper extremities, especially on the forearm and hands, are referred to as defensive wounds. These occur when the victim raises his or her arms in an effort to protect the face and chest. Defensive wounds can also be found on the legs of a victim if she or he was on the ground during the assault and was using the legs for defense.

If the examiner notes interruptions in cutting patterns, movement of the victim usually causes these. Fingernails can create breaks or cuts in the skin. Fingernails marks are usually superficial, semicircular, and irregularly shaped. These breaks in tissue are superficial. However, gouges corresponding to fingernails can be noted. Bruising may accompany fingernail cuts.

Stabbing. A stab wound results from penetration by an instrument into the body. A stab wound is deeper than it is long. The thrust of a weapon such as a knife produces the injury; however, any object that can be thrust into the body can create a stabbing injury. The edges of a stab wound are sharp, and the wound is deeper than the length on the skin. The edges of the wound may be abraded from the hilt of a knife. The amount of blood at the crime scene may be minimal because most of the bleeding is internal.

Bite Marks. Human bites seldom cause tears in the skin. Most often biting injuries result in semicircular or crescentic patterned abrasions. Bite marks create underlying hemorrhages. In cases of sexual assault, biting is generally located on breasts and on or near genitalia. Health care providers should note that the skin could become twisted or distorted during the act of biting, thus distorting the pattern. Expert dental consultation is advised in cases in which the victim experiences biting.

Strangulation. The hallmarks of manual strangulation are fingertip bruising and fingernail marks on the neck. In some cases there is extensive external injury and in other cases the external injury is minimal. Fingertip bruising is circular and oval, produced by pressure from the fingertips on the skin of the neck. Underlying muscles are usually bruised. Fingernail marks are thin linear or crescentic marks.

Strangulation by ligature creates a ligature mark resembling the ligature itself. Pinpoint and larger areas of hemorrhage are often noted on the face of the strangled victim. These areas of hemorrhage are often noted in the conjunctiva and on the eyelids. The offender may employ the use of a chokehold. In this form of restraint a forearm is placed across the front of the neck while the other hand pulls the forearm back. The chokehold causes airway compression. Chokeholds can cause serious damage and death. Petechial hemorrhage can be found in the eyes and face after application of the chokehold. Injury to the skin is usually absent.

Blockage of the nose and mouth can create asphyxia. This can occur by gagging the victim, holding a pillow over the victim's mouth and nose, or placing a hand over the mouth and nose.

Gunshot Wounds. Firearms are classified as either small arms or artillery, depending on the size of the projectile that they fire. Handguns, the most common firearm in gunshot injuries, are usually low-energy weapons with muzzle velocities less than 1,400 feet per second. There are three basic types of handgun: single-shot pistols, revolvers, or semiautomatics. Rifles are named for their rifle barrel and are grouped as single-barrel sporting, double-barrel sporting, or high-powered military assault-type rifles. Common types include the single-shot automatic and the lever, bolt, and pump action. Shotguns look like rifles; however, they lack rifling inside the barrel. Shotguns fire a missile that consists of a fuse of hundreds of pellets with muzzle velocities of 1,000 to 1,500 feet per second. Even though they are technically considered low-velocity weapons, they are definitely the most destructive of all small arms at close range. Common types include the single-shot, double-barrel, and also the automatic and pump action.

Range of fire is essentially the distance from the barrel or muzzle of the firearm to the target. In contact or near-contact range, the firearm is very close to or touching the victim's skin or clothing. Wound features would be the bullet hole, tearing of soft tissue from gases that escape behind the bullet under pressure, and powder or soot. They may also exhibit the barrel of the weapon in skin-contact injuries. Short or close-range shots are a few inches away from the victim. The wound would exhibit the bullet hole, powder grains or powder markings (fouling), and powder soot. Medium-range shots come from within a few feet of the victim. The wound contains the bullet hole and stippling or tattooing made by gunpowder residue. In distant or long-range shots, which are fired from more than a few feet away from the victim, only the bullet reaches the target. The type of weapon and ammunition also play a role in the wound appearance. When documenting the appearance of gunshot wounds, do not attempt to differentiate entrance and exit wounds.

DOCUMENTATION

Documentation consists of the narrative report, diagrams, and photographs.

The Narrative Report

The narrative report begins with a carefully documented history. Remember to use the subject's own words as often as possible and to document these with quotation marks. Accurately describe each injury and be sure to use the proper medical terminology. Measure all wounds in centimeters and describe wound size, shape, appearance, and location using readily recognized anatomic landmarks.

Diagrams

Each injury should be placed on a trauma diagram. Each injury should be drawn on the diagram and described in writing next to the drawing. Multiple front and back blank drawings are required for documentation. Utilize age-appropriate diagrams whenever possible. (See Appendix A for adult body diagrams.)

Photographs

It is difficult to document injury related to assault in words alone. Photography is required. Injuries to the body, including the genitalia, are photographed with a digital camera. Photo documentation is an important function; however, health care providers need not be professional photographers.

The purposes of forensic photography are to record injury, and to provide photographic evidence. Trauma to the body is of importance to legal proceedings, making it critical that evidence of injury be documented via photography. Injury to the body should be documented in color photographs.

If the victim is suffering from injury that will heal in time, injuries must be accurately preserved photographically. It takes months or years until any evidence is presented in a court of law, and injuries may be minimal or completely healed by that time. Photographs are all that will remain of the victim's injuries.

Digital photography is advantageous in forensic work. Images are recorded on a removable disk or memory card or memory stick. There is no film to be processed. Chain of custody can be simplified. Images can be transmitted instantly. The camera and computers process the pictures. Federal Rules of Evidence allow the admission of digital photography.

Authenticity of color in digital photographs can be assured with the use of a gray scale. Digital photographs should include a gray scale to ensure color accuracy. Scales that include reassurance of 90-degree angle are also recommended.

Consent for Photography

Consent for photography must be obtained by the client or guardian. In urgent cases where a signature is unobtainable, consent is implied. "Client consents to treatment and documentation of injury with photographs" is a typical statement found on a consent form given to sexual assault victims.

Taking Photographs

There are two kinds of light important to photography: ambient and artificial. Indoor artificial light must be added to the natural or ambient light in the room in order to get clear photographs of injury. Fluorescent light commonly found in hospitals tends to give photos a washed out or yellow or green hue. This can be eliminated by adding more artificial nonfluorescent light and by using a flash.

A full-body photograph should be taken first, ensuring that the face is included. This full-body photo will identify the victim and demonstrate the presence or absence of any overall injury. The overall photo often may also serve as photo documentation of "demeanor of the victim." Modesty must be considered in taking this first photo. Providing the victim with something to cover may be necessary.

After the overall photo, a far-away, midrange, and close-up photo of each injury should be taken. For example, injury on the back should be documented with first an overall photo of the entire back of the victim. Then a midrange picture is taken of the injury in a context of other body parts such as buttock or shoulder or waist. A close-up photograph is then taken of each injury. One close-up photo of each injury is taken with a scale and one is taken without the scale.

Recommended background for forensic photos of a person is non-cluttered and of a soothing color. The color white tends to be stark and does not demonstrate injury well. The colors back and red are also not good background colors for photographing injury. The colors light blue and light green make excellent backgrounds for photographing injury.

Flat surfaces as opposed to shiny surfaces make better backgrounds for photographing injury. Shiny surfaces reflect back light. A blue pad with the shiny side down and the dull side under the victim makes a good background for photographing injury.

Health care providers should be aware of the clutter in the workspace when taking photographs of injury. Covering or removing clutter will enhance photographs by placing emphasis on the injury and not on the clutter.

A 90-degree angle is recommended for photographing injury. Using a 90-degree angle eliminates distortion of size of the injury. Angling a photograph off 90 degrees can distort size. The scale placed in the photographs of injury should include a gray scale to ensure accurate color and symbols to ensure 90-degree angle.

Photo Log

The set of photographs represents a record of the event experienced by the victim. The full-body photo is the introduction to the photo log. This photo is listed as the number one photograph. Each photo of every injury is then listed, including all midrange and close-up photos.

Chain of Custody

Chain of custody or chain of evidence must be followed for photographs, as it is followed for all evidence. Photographs should be turned over to law enforcement, along with all other evidence collected. If photographs are saved to a computer, they must be encrypted so that only the medical team has access to the photographs. Law enforcement must sign the chain of custody forms, including the photo log.

Photography Review

Take photographs before and after cleaning up the victim. This is most important in cases with bleeding, blood spatter, gunshot residue, and excessive dirt. Take a full-length photo of the person that captures the person's face and overall injuries. Respect the client's privacy and allow her or him to cover up for this photograph. Take a far-away, midrange, and close-up photograph of each injury. Close-up photos should be taken with and without a scale. Label each photograph with date and time, medical record number or case number, name of the hospital, and the photographer's name.

Follow-Up Photographs

Follow-up photographs of injury may be required to document the progress of an injury. Photographs of healing may be desired. Injury that may heal without scarring may be photographed over time. Sexual assault examinations may be performed within hours of the event. At times, injury is not identified at early intervals because it is not yet evident. For example, fingertip bruising of the neck may not be evident in the first few hours after an assault. Dependent upon the amount of pressure applied to the neck, the bleeding from the ruptured vessels may be slow and take time to be obvious.

RESOURCES

American College of Forensic Examiners: http://www.acfei.com/programs.php
American Forensic Nursing (AFN): http://www.amrn.com
The Differences Between Forensic Interviews & Clinical Interviews: http://www.icctc.org/Resources/forensic.pdf
Duma, S., & Ogunbanjo, G. A. (2004). Forensic documentation of intimate partner violence in primary health care. *South African Family Practice, 46*(4), 37–39. http://www.safpj.co.za/index.php/safpj/article/viewFile/64/64
Patterns of Tissue Injury: http://library.med.utah.edu/WebPath/TUTORIAL/GUNS/GUNINJ.html

REFERENCES

Evans, M. (2004). *Gunshot wound ballistics.* Baylor College of Medicine. Retrieved from http://www.bcm.edu/oto/grand/02_12_04.htm
Hazelwood, R., & Burgess, A. (2001). *Practical aspects of rape investigation.* New York: Elsevier.
McCans, J. (2009). Forensic evidence: Preserving the clinical picture. *RN, 69,* 28–44.
Olshaker J., Jackson, M., & Smock W. (2001). *Forensic emergency medicine.* Philadelphia: Lippincott Williams & Wilkins.

Porteous, J. (2005). Don't tip the scales! Care for clients involved in police investigation. *Canadian Operating Room Nursing Journal, 23*(3), 12–144.

Ribaux, O., Walsh, S., & Margot P. (2006). The contribution of forensic science for crime scene analysis and investigation. *Forensic Science International, 156*(2–3), 171–181.

Saferstein, R. (2008). *Criminalistics: An introduction to forensic science* (9th ed.). Englewood Cliffs, NJ: Prentice Hall.

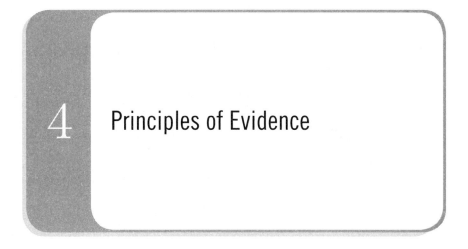

4   Principles of Evidence

DEFINITIONS

Forensic evidence is physical or trace evidence that is scientifically matched with a known individual or item. Crime laboratories analyze specimens retrieved from a suspect or a crime scene and compare the specimens with control specimens retrieved from the suspect in order to determine whether or not they have a common origin.

> *Individual evidence* is defined as evidence that can be associated with a common source with an extremely high degree of probability. This evidence is analyzed at a crime laboratory and used by law enforcement to identify a suspect. Individual scientific evidence includes fingerprints, DNA, tool marks, tire marks, and footprints.
>
> *Class evidence* is evidence that is associated only with a group and never with a single course. This evidence is analyzed at a crime laboratory and used by law enforcement to associate a suspect with a crime or crimes. Class scientific evidence includes paint, blood, hairs, and fibers.

Crime laboratories also determine the identity of a physical or chemical substance with as near absolute certainty as analytic techniques permit.

Types of Evidence

Circumstantial. Facts of circumstances that tend to implicate a person in a crime are called circumstantial. Forensic science results do not enter into circumstantial evidence. Examples of circumstantial evidence are a person owns a vehicle similar to one used in the crime; the suspect has made threats to the victim; the suspect has been known to engage in similar behavior. Circumstantial evidence has been described as the person has the motive, means, and opportunity to commit the crime.

Eyewitness testimony. Interviewing a witness to a crime is eyewitness testimony. In recent history, the credibility of eyewitness evidence is questioned. Criticism is particularly focused on the ability to identify a suspect via an eyewitness encounter. Witnesses have been known to make false identifications. False identification may be related to an eyewitness telling an untruth in a purposeful manner, but in most cases, misidentification occurs via an eyewitness without specific intent. The psychological trauma of witnessing appears to be related to misidentification. In other words, the eyewitness, due to the trauma of witnessing, is not able to accurately identify the suspect.

Direct evidence. Evidence found in the suspect's possession that was taken from the victim or taken from the crime scene is called direct evidence. This type of evidence is commonly called "fruits of the crime." This evidence may be items stolen from the victim(s) that have monetary value. It may also be a token or trophy taken from the victim by the suspect that has little monetary value. This trophy or token has value only to the suspect and serves as a reminder of the criminal activity. Direct evidence indicates a direct connection between the suspect and the victim or the suspect and the crime scene.

Collateral evidence. Evidence obtained about the suspect via investigation is collateral evidence. Forensic science is not a component of collateral evidence, which is commonly called "intelligence." A portion of any investigation is interviewing people who know the suspect about the suspect. Any information obtained about the suspect is collateral. Interviews are collateral information, but information found on computers, in books and journals is also collateral information. Finding information about the planning of crimes is considered collateral evidence.

PRINCIPLES OF EVIDENCE

Health care providers collect what the crime lab calls *trace evidence.* Trace evidence means a small amount. Health care providers collect trace evidence from a person's body. Law enforcement collects from the crime scene and from the suspect's residence. Law enforcement collects trace evidence and also collects large pieces of evidence such as computers, furniture, and automobiles. All forensic evidence is submitted to the crime laboratory via law enforcement.

The most important health care forensic skill associated with collection of evidence is observation—health care professionals need to be able to recognize potential evidence. Evidence can be anything on a client, but the most common types of evidence are clothing, bullets, bloodstains, hairs, fibers, and small pieces of material such as fragments of metal, glass, paint, and wood.

When evidence is identified, it should be collected and preserved. Submit all evidence to the crime laboratory reasonably dry. Trace evidence collected on swabs dries quickly. Specimens that are wet by nature such as urine for a toxicological screening must be handed to law enforcement identifying verbally and in writing that the specimen is wet. Any trace evidence collected by health care professionals must be clearly identified. On each specimen, a label must be attached that gives the name of the patient, the date and time, and who collected the specimen. The specimen should be labeled indirectly, meaning do not write on the evidence itself. Rather, put the evidence in an envelope or a container and add a label to the envelope. Noting on the label the body part from which the evidence was retrieved is necessary.

Chain of Custody

Each item that may be evidentiary in nature must be held in the presence of the person who collected the evidence until that evidence is given to law enforcement. If law enforcement is not present when evidence is collected, evidence must be held in a locked location until law enforcement arrives to retrieve the evidence.

- The chain begins with the person who collects the evidence, who may be the health care provider. The links in the chain are individuals having control or custody over evidentiary or potentially evidentiary material or personal property.
- This chain of custody should be defined in forensic protocol and generally requires a form of written documentation.
- Rules of evidence require a chain of custody for each item recovered from the patient, including trace and physical evidence, laboratory specimens of blood/body fluids, clothing, and personal articles.

- The integrity of every piece of evidence seized must be ensured to protect the admissibility in a court of law.
- Failure to maintain the chain of custody renders potentially important evidence worthless if lost, damaged, or unaccountable from the hands of the nurse to the police officer.

The examiner should remain in control of the collected evidence at all times. Nothing can be left unattended. All evidence must be in plain view of the collector. Evidence that is to be used in court must be appropriately packaged and given to law enforcement to maintain a continuity or chain of custody. In an ideal situation, the examiner maintains custody of all evidence until it is collected by law enforcement. All personnel who handle or examine evidence must be acknowledged to establish its integrity for presentation in a court of law. If evidence cannot be maintained in the sight of the examiner, it must be locked in a secure area at room temperature away from anyone not in the chain of custody.

Locard's Exchange Principle

Locard's principle essentially states that whenever two objects come into contact, a mutual exchange of matter takes place. This principle is used to link the suspect to the victim, the suspect to the crime scene, and the victim to the crime scene through forensic evidence. Most forensic scientists accept the Locard Exchange Principle, which was enunciated early in the 20th century by Edmund Locard, the director of the first crime laboratory, in Lyon, France. Every contact leaves a trace.

EVIDENCE COLLECTION

Forensic evidence collection is a methodical process that follows state and federal requirements. Evidence collection kits usually contain instructions for use, but evidence collection procedures should be written and readily available in health care settings for reference when needed. Health care providers must wear gloves during handling of all physical evidence, and they should change gloves often during evidence collection. All packages used to collect evidence must be sealed and labeled with the client's name, date and time of collection, description and source of the material (including anatomic location), name of the health care provider, and names and initials of everyone who handled the material.

Clothing

Health care professionals should be taught to recognize and preserve vital fragments of trace evidence by careful handling of the patient's clothing and personal property. Clothing worn at the time of the incident may contain trace evidence useful in linking the victim with the assailant or crime scene, which is consistent with Locard's Principle of Exchange.

- Check clothing for defects. Defects in clothes can be compared to wounds of the victim, and often clothes provide insight as to the type of weapon or wounding instrument used.
- Check clothing for blood, semen, gunshot residue, or trace materials such as hair or fibers: document, diagram, photograph, collect, and preserve. The clothing may contain fragments from the assailant. If the assailant was injured, his or her blood may be on the victim's clothing.
- Treat clothing from accidents the same as you would those from possible crime.
- Garments from automobile/pedestrian accidents may display tire impressions or conceal trace evidence such as paint chips or broken glass that could identify the vehicle that struck the victim.
- Check for laundry marks (which are not very common these days). Laundry markings may offer a clue to identification or origin of an unknown, unconscious, near-death, or deceased individual.
- Give special attention to the examination and security of clothing from a gunshot victim. Gunshot residues surrounding bullet holes in the clothes may determine the distance of the firearm from the victim at the time of firing (range of fire).
- Carefully remove clothing to protect any foreign fragments adhering to them. Do not shake clothes.
- Clothing is frequently cut away for emergency treatment, sometimes losing the article itself and/or evidentiary materials. When this happens, try to avoid cutting through tears, rips, and holes that may have resulted from the weapon or the assault.
- Do not discard clothing or throw it on the floor, which can result in cross-contamination of trace evidence with debris from the treatment environment.
- A clean, white sheet can be placed on an empty trauma table, mayo stand, or on the floor in the corner of the room for clothing to be placed until time permits for effective packaging.

- If possible, allow the victim to remove his or her clothes, while standing on a clean sheet or a large sheet of paper. This will collect any microscopic evidence that may become dislodged during removal. The sheet must be placed in a separate paper bag for transfer to the crime laboratory.
- If possible, hang up moist clothing to dry in a secure area. Tell police if clothing they are to retrieve is in a damp condition.
- Place clean, white paper over stains to avoid cross-contamination.
- Store each item of clothing in separate paper, not plastic, bags.

Plastic bags are *inappropriate* because there is a tendency for condensation to accumulate, resulting in a degradation of the integrity of the evidence.

- Seal each bag and clearly mark with the date, time, and signature or initials of the individual doing the sealing. Fortunately, a hospital is an excellent place to find all manner of containers (bags, bottles, boxes, and tubes) for properly storing evidence.
- Document, document, document!

Hair, Fiber, Debris, and Solid Objects

Health care professionals should be taught to recognize and preserve vital fragments of trace evidence by careful handling of the victim's hair, and fiber or other debris from the victim's body. Recommended procedure includes the following:

- Carefully comb the victim's hair to remove evidence that may not be visible. Place in plastic bag, label, and seal.
- Use forceps with plastic-coated tips to carefully remove hairs, fibers, or other debris from the client's body and place each item into paper envelopes.
- Dry surface debris can be gently scraped onto a glass slide.
- Place sharp objects found on the victim or in the victim's clothing (needles, blades, knives, glass fragments) in double peel-packs (heavy-gauge polyethylene pouch with tamper-evident adhesive closures) or in plastic, glass, or cardboard containers.
- Preserve evidence on the victim's hands until collected by securing paper bags over each hand (follow this procedure on deceased victims' hands).

Exhibit 4.1

PROCEDURE FOR CREATING A "DRUGGIST-STYLE" ENVELOPE

1. Place evidence in the center of the paper.
2. Fold paper in thirds.
3. Turn 90 degrees and fold in thirds again.
4. Tuck one edge into the other to form a closed package.

- Scrape or swab beneath fingernails, or clip off fingernails, package in an envelope, and label as right or left hand. If envelopes are unavailable, place fingernails, scrapings, and the orange stick or swab used to collect them in the center of a clean piece of paper, which is then folded "druggist style" and sealed (see Exhibit 4.1).
- Wrap bullets in gauze to preserve trace evidence and place in a peel-pack, cup, or envelope. Do not touch bullets with metal instruments, and do not write on them.
- Collect gunpowder residue with tape that is then applied to a glass slide, labeled, and placed in an evidence envelope.

Body Fluids

Health care professionals should be taught to recognize and preserve vital fragments of trace evidence by careful handling of the victim's body fluids. Use the following procedure for careful collection of forensic evidence:

- Use a high-intensity lamp to visualize stains or biological secretions (saliva, semen, urine, blood, etc.), especially on areas determined significant through the history (e.g., if the child states the perpetrator licked her abdomen, use the lamp on the child's abdomen).
- Collect dried secretions or fluids with a slightly moistened sterile swab, and air dry the specimen before packaging.
- Swab bite marks (after photographing) for biological specimens.
- In sexual assault cases, swab body orifices for biological specimens, and collect as much as possible. Biological samples should be

collected before further contamination by drinking, eating, smoking, or voiding.
■ Collect laboratory specimens for toxicology screens and control, or reference, samples to be used in DNA analysis.

RESOURCES

DNA: What Every Law Enforcement Officer Should Know: www.ncjrs.gov/pdffiles1/jr000249c.pdf

Evidence Collection and Care of the Sexual Assault Survivor: The SANE-SART Response: www.mincava.umn.edu/documents/commissioned/2forensicevidence/2forensicevidence.pdf

Hairs, Fibers, Crime, and Evidence: www.fbi.gov/hq/lab/fsc/backissu/july2000/deedric4.htm

REFERENCES

Gardner, R. (2004). *Practical crime scene processing and investigation (practical aspects of criminal & forensic investigations)*. Boca Raton, FL: CRC Press.

McCans, J. (2006). Forensic evidence: Preserving the clinical picture. *RN, 69*(9), 28–44.

Olshaker, J., Jackson, M., & Smock, W. (2001). *Forensic emergency medicine*. Philadelphia: Lippincott Williams & Wilkins.

Porteous, J. (2005). Don't tip the scales! Care for patients involved in police investigation. *Canadian Operating Room Nursing Journal, 23*(3), 12–22.

Ribaux, O., Walsh, S., & Margot, P. (2006). The contribution of forensic science for crime scene analysis and investigation. *Forensic Science International, 156*(2–3), 171–181.

Saferstein, R. (2008). *Criminalistics: An introduction to forensic science* (9th ed.). Englewood Cliffs, NJ: Prentice Hall.

Stokowski, L. (2008). Forensic nursing: Part 1. Evidence collection for nurses. *Medscape Nurses: Nursing Perspectives*, 03/06/2008. Retrieved from http://cme.medscape.com/viewarticle/571057

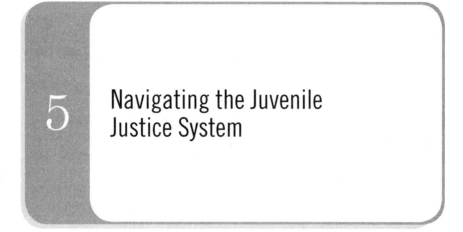

5 Navigating the Juvenile Justice System

JUVENILE JUSTICE SYSTEM OVERVIEW

A *juvenile* is defined as an individual who has not reached the age at which one should be treated as an adult by the criminal justice system. In most states, the age is 18, but as of 2005, youth aged 16 in 3 states (Connecticut, New York, and North Carolina) were under the original jurisdiction of the criminal court, as were youth aged 17 in an additional 10 states (Georgia, Illinois, Louisiana, Massachusetts, Michigan, Missouri, New Hampshire, South Carolina, Texas, and Wisconsin). Most states have extended juvenile jurisdiction over youth who have been adjudicated delinquent on offenses committed while under juvenile jurisdiction. The purpose of extended jurisdiction, which is typically to age 21, is to enable continued correctional commitment or supervision beyond the upper age of jurisdiction. (See Appendix B, "State Age Parameters in the Juvenile Justice System.")

As of 2004, several states had statutes that defined the lowest age of juvenile court delinquency jurisdiction, while other states rely on case law (law found in the collection of reported cases that form the body of the law within a given jurisdiction) or common law (the body of knowledge derived from judicial decisions). North Carolina has the lowest minimum age for juvenile jurisdiction at 6 years of age, followed by Maryland,

Massachusetts, and New York at 7 years of age. The minimum age for juvenile jurisdiction is 8 years of age in Arizona and 10 years of age in Arkansas, Colorado, Kansas, Louisiana, Minnesota, Mississippi, Pennsylvania, South Dakota, Texas, Vermont, and Wisconsin. However, few children under the age of 10 actually appear before the juvenile court for delinquency charges.

BRIEF HISTORY OF THE JUVENILE JUSTICE SYSTEM

Juvenile justice is a relatively new concept in the law. In the early development of the United States, children who broke the law were treated the same as adult criminals. Children below the age of 7 were presumed incapable of criminal intent and were not prosecuted and punished; however, children as young as 7 could stand trial in criminal court, and, if found guilty, faced prison and even the death sentence.

The juvenile justice system began a little more than 100 years ago in 1899 when Illinois enacted the Juvenile Court Act. This Act was the first legislation to establish a truly separate court with original and exclusive jurisdiction over all law violations by youth. This concept proved so popular that all but two states established juvenile courts by 1925. The British doctrine of *parens patriae* (the state as parent) was employed as the rationale for the right of the state to intervene differently with children than with adults. Because children were now viewed as not having full legal capacity, British doctrine was interpreted to mean that the state had the power and responsibility to provide protection for children whose natural parents were not providing appropriate care or supervision. The welfare of the child became paramount and thus delinquent children were seen as in need of the court's benevolent intervention.

The "juvenile crime epidemic" in the early 1990s (which peaked in 1993) fueled the public to scrutinize the system's ability to effectively control violent juvenile offenders. As a result, states adopted numerous legislative changes in an effort to crack down on juvenile crime. Although some differences between the criminal and juvenile justice systems have diminished in recent years, the juvenile justice system remains unique, guided by its own philosophy and legislation and implemented by its own set of agencies.

Today's model is one of balanced and restorative justice. This system is based on three concepts: competence development, community protection, and accountability, and it stresses that "community protection" or public safety is the primary responsibility of the court system. This typically translates into physical control (containment) or knowledge (electronic monitoring) of the juvenile's whereabouts.

JUVENILE JUSTICE PROCEDURE

According to the *Juvenile Offenders and Victims 2006 Report* by the Office of Juvenile Justice and Delinquency Prevention (Snyder & Sickmund, 2006), juveniles are processed in the juvenile system accordingly:

1. Each state's processing law of juveniles is unique, and within states case processing varies from community to community depending on local practice and tradition.
2. A decision is made at the time of arrest to either send the matter through the juvenile system or divert the case out of the system, often to alternative programs. Law enforcement often makes this decision after talking to the juvenile, the victim, and the parents, and after reviewing the juvenile's prior contacts with the juvenile justice system. In 2003, 20% of all juvenile arrests resulted in release of the youth; in 7 of 10 arrests, the cases were referred to juvenile court, while the remaining arrests were referred for criminal prosecution or to other agencies.
3. Most juvenile court cases are referred by law enforcement. The remaining referrals come from parents, victims, schools, probation officers, and others. The juvenile probation department and/or the prosecutor's office are typically responsible for the court intake function. At this point, intake must determine whether to dismiss the case, handle the matter informally, or request formal intervention by the juvenile court. The intake officer first reviews the case to determine if there is sufficient evidence to prove the allegation. If the evidence is insufficient, the case is dismissed. If the evidence is sufficient, intake then decides if formal intervention is necessary.

   Approximately half of all juvenile cases are handled informally, and most informally processed cases are dismissed. In the other informally processed cases, juveniles voluntarily agree to specific conditions for a specified period of time. Conditions, which may include school attendance, victim restitution, drug counseling, curfews, and other specifications, are frequently outlined in a written agreement usually termed a "consent decree." Most jurisdictions offer informal dispositions only if the juvenile admits to committing the act.

The juvenile's compliance with the consent decree is typically monitored by a probation officer, and this process is labeled "informal probation." If the juvenile successfully complies with the informal disposition, the case is dismissed. However, if the juvenile fails to comply, the intake decision may be to formally prosecute the case, and the case proceeds as if the initial decision had been to refer the case for an adjudicatory hearing.

If the case is handled in juvenile court, intake files one of two types of petitions: a delinquency petition requesting an adjudicatory hearing (trial) or a petition requesting a waiver hearing to transfer the case to criminal court. The delinquency petition states the allegations and requests the juvenile court to adjudicate (judge) the youth delinquent, making the juvenile a ward of the court. This language is different from that used in criminal court, where offenders are convicted and sentenced.

An adjudicatory hearing is scheduled in response to the delinquency petition. Witnesses are called and the facts of the case presented. In nearly all hearings, the judge determines whether the juvenile is responsible for the offense(s). Some states, however, give juveniles the right to a jury trial.

4. Juveniles may be held in a secure detention facility during the processing of a case if the court believes it is in the best interest of the juvenile or the community. Law enforcement often brings the juvenile to the local detention center after arrest. Juvenile detention or probation officers review the case and decide if the juvenile should be held pending a hearing by a judge.

   All states require that a detention hearing be held within a time period defined by statute, usually within 24 hours. The judge reviews the case and determines if continued detention is warranted at the hearing. In 2000, juveniles were detained in 20% of delinquency cases processed by juvenile courts. In some cases, detention may extend beyond the adjudicatory and dispositional hearings. If residential placement is ordered, and no beds are available, a juvenile may remain in detention until a residential bed becomes available.

5. Juveniles may be processed in the adult criminal justice system. Prosecutors and intake officers file a waiver petition when they believe that a juvenile case would be handled more appropriately

in the criminal court. Once the petition is filed, the juvenile court judge reviews the facts of the case and determines whether there is probable cause to believe the juvenile committed the act and whether juvenile court jurisdiction should be waived and the case transferred to criminal court. The judge's decision usually centers on whether the juvenile is amenable to treatment in the juvenile justice system.

The prosecutor may argue that the juvenile has been adjudicated several times and that the juvenile justice system has been unable to keep him or her from committing subsequent crimes or that the crime is so serious that the juvenile system is unlikely to be able to intervene for the time period necessary to rehabilitate the youth. If the judge decides that the juvenile's case should be transferred to criminal court, juvenile jurisdiction is waived and the case is filed in criminal court. In 2000, juvenile courts waived less than 1% of all formally processed delinquency cases. More than half of the 50 states allow for certain cases (serious ones) to be tried in criminal court. These cases are legally excluded from juvenile court, and prosecutors must file them in criminal court.

6. After a juvenile is adjudicated delinquent in juvenile court, the probation staff develops a disposition plan. They assess the youth and the available support systems and programs. In addition, the court may order psychological evaluations, diagnostic tests, or a period of confinement in a diagnostics facility.

    Probation staff may present dispositional recommendations to the judge at the disposition hearing, as may the prosecutor and the juvenile. The judge orders a disposition after considering the recommendations.

7. Most dispositions are multifaceted and involve some type of supervised probation. In 2000, formal probation was the most severe disposition ordered in 63% of the cases in which the youth was adjudicated delinquent. Probation orders often include additional requirements, such as drug counseling, weekend confinement in the detention center, or restitution to the victim and/or community. The length of probation may be for a specified period or open-ended. Review hearings are held to monitor the juvenile's progress, and after the conditions of probation are met, the judge terminates the case.

8. Judges may order residential placement, which was the case in 24% of the cases in 2000. Residential placement may be for a specified period or an indeterminate amount of time. Residential

facilities may be public or private and range from secure, prisonlike environments to homelike atmospheres. In some states, when the judge commits a juvenile to the state department of corrections, that department decides where the juvenile will be placed and when that juvenile will be released. In other states, the judge controls this decision.

9. Once released from an institution, the juvenile is ordered into aftercare, which is similar to adult parole. During this time, the juvenile is under the supervision of the court or the juvenile corrections department and must meet certain conditions. If the youth does not follow these conditions, the juvenile may be recommitted to the same facility or another.

10. Status offenses are processed differently. These offenses include behaviors such as running away from home, truancy, alcohol possession/use, incorrigibility, and curfew violations, which are considered law violations only for juveniles because of their status. Many of these cases enter the juvenile justice system through child welfare agencies and indicate that the child is in need of supervision. The federal Juvenile Justice and Delinquency Prevention Act discourages holding status offenders in secure facilities for detention or placement unless said juvenile has violated a valid court order, such as a probation order that requires the youth to observe a curfew or attend school.

11. All states have at least one court with juvenile jurisdiction, but most states do not call it juvenile court. Instead they use other terms, such as district, superior, circuit, county, family, or probate court. Courts with juvenile jurisdiction usually have jurisdiction over delinquency, status offenses, and neglect/abuse issues, and many also have jurisdiction over other matters such as adoptions, emancipation, and termination of parental rights. Regardless of their name, courts with juvenile jurisdiction are typically referred to as juvenile courts.

Health care professionals can work with the juvenile justice system, particularly juvenile probation, to assure that juvenile offenders receive appropriate health care and mental health referrals. Health care professionals play an especially critical role in working with those juveniles who fall outside the jurisdiction of the juvenile justice system because they are too young by state law to enter the juvenile system or because by age or offense, they fall into the adult criminal justice system. These children require adequate intervention to minimize their chance of chronic, serious, and violent offending, and health care professionals may be the only providers to have contact with these children if they have not yet entered the mental health system.

RESOURCES

Delinquency Cases in Juvenile Court, 2005: www.ncjrs.gov/pdffiles1/ojjdp/224538.pdf

The Future of Children: Juvenile Justice: http://futureofchildren.org/futureofchildren/publications/journals/journal_details/index.xml?journalid=31

Juvenile Court Statistics 2005: www.ncjrs.gov/pdffiles1/ojjdp/224619.pdf

Juvenile Delinquency Guidelines: Improving Court Practice in Juvenile Delinquency Cases: www.ncjfcj.org/images/stories/dept/ppcd/pdf/JDG/juveniledelinquencyguide linescompressed.pdf

REFERENCES

McCrone, S., & Shelton, D. (2001). An overview of forensic psychiatric care of the adolescent. *Issues in Mental Health Nursing, 22*(2), 125–135.

Office of Juvenile Justice and Delinquency Prevention. (1995). *Guide for implementing the comprehensive strategy for serious, violent and chronic offenders.* Washington, DC: U.S. Department of Justice.

Panel on Juvenile Crime: Prevention, Treatment, and Control, Committee on Law and Justice, and Board on Children, Youth, and Families, National Research Council, and Institute of Medicine. (2001). *Juvenile crime, juvenile justice.* Washington, DC: National Academy of Sciences Press.

Sickmund, M. (2003, June). *Juveniles in court.* Juvenile Offenders and Victims National Report Series Bulletin. Retrieved from http://www.ncjrs.org/html/ojjdp/195420/con tents.html

Snyder, H., & Sickmund, M. (2006). *Juvenile offenders and victims 2006 report.* Office of Juvenile Justice and Delinquency Prevention. Retrieved from http://ojjdp.ncjrs.org/ojstatbb/nr2006/index.html

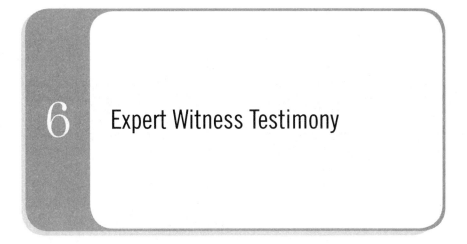

6 Expert Witness Testimony

OVERVIEW

Expert witness testimony is a method of enabling attorneys, judges, and juries to better understand the evidence presented in a case. An expert can also help get things into evidence that would otherwise be inadmissible. Expert witnesses differ from fact witnesses. Fact witnesses, also called eye witnesses or percipient witnesses, can give a firsthand account of something seen, heard, or experienced. Expert witnesses are allowed to do the one thing that all other types of witnesses cannot—offer opinions. These opinions must be reliable and not based on subjective belief or unsupported speculations.

Health care providers may be subpoenaed (a subpoena is a court order) as a fact witness to testify in court about an event that occurred in their presence. For example, a health care provider could be called to testify about the quality of a parent's parenting skills in a failure to thrive case. Another health care provider may be subpoenaed as an expert in that same case. This health care provider would be called to provide his or her expert opinion about the parent's parenting skills based on the expert's assessment of the case and the expert's knowledge of parenting.

EXPERT WITNESS QUALIFICATIONS

An expert is someone who knows something beyond common experience. Most expert witnesses are professionals, but there are also nondegreed experts whose background and experience qualifies them. Qualifications include technical and academic training, degrees, licenses, certificates, postgraduate training, membership in professional or industry organizations, titles, belonging to specific staff, writing and speaking professionally, positions held throughout one's career, and dealing with the same or similar issues as the one at hand.

Voir dire, French for "to speak the truth," is the term used in court proceedings for the questions to determine the competence of the expert witness. Health care providers may be asked for the following information to determine qualifications as an expert. These questions may be asked of a pediatric nurse in the following example to evaluate the competence as an expert witness:

1. Describe your current position and background as a pediatric nurse.
2. How long have you been a nurse and in what areas have you practiced?
3. How long have you been working as a pediatric nurse? What education prepared you for this specialty? Describe your work as a pediatric nurse.
4. What continuing education have you had in this specialty?
5. What professional organizations do you belong to?
6. Are you certified in your field?
7. Have you published any material in your field?
8. How does a forensic nurse conduct an examination (step-by-step)?
9. Pediatric sexual assault nurse examiners (PSANEs) may be asked to describe sexual assault response team (SART) members or examination of equipment.
10. How many cases have you done?
11. Have you qualified as an expert witness in court before? Which courts?

Health care providers should make sure their curriculum vitaes (CVs) are accurate, up to date, and error-free, as they need to present them to the court before testifying. The term *CV* is often used interchangeably with the term *résumé*. Sometimes these are differentiated by length (CV is comprehensive and long; résumé is pertinent and brief), and sometimes differentiated by style with the CV written in outline format and the résumé written as a narrative. Regardless, your CV should include the following information:

- Name and contact information
- Licenses and national/state certifications (include state, license/certification number, expiration date)
- Employment history (current employer, dates of employment; previous relevant employment, dates of employment)
- Education (name of school, location of school, name of degree, date of degree)
- Training and certificates (include conferences, workshops, training, in-services, seminars, etc., with the name of training, dates of training, type of certifications)
- Professional organization affiliations
- Research (include current and past project titles)
- Grants (include name of grant, granting organization, and whether or not funded)
- Publications (include articles for newspapers, newsletters, professional journals, brochures, academic publications, etc.; include name of article, name of publication, date of publication)
- Presentations (include in-service, community presentations, conferences, etc.; include name of presentation, name of conference, date of presentation)
- Awards (services related and community related; include name of award, presenting agency, date of award)
- Community service (volunteer activities)
- Prior testimony as an expert witness (name of the court, year of testimony, party for which you testified, type of case)

Do not underestimate opposing counsel, who may check into the background and representations of your CV.

RULES OF EVIDENCE

Health care providers should familiarize themselves with the Federal Rules of Evidence (2008). The Federal Rules of Evidence govern the introduction of evidence in proceedings, both civil and criminal, in federal courts. The rules of many states have been closely modeled on these provisions. These are the rules as they apply to expert witness testimony as of December 2008.

Rule 702. Testimony by Experts

If scientific, technical, or other specialized knowledge will assist the trier of fact to understand the evidence or to determine a fact in issue, a witness qualified as an expert by knowledge, skill, experience, training, or education, may testify thereto in the form of an opinion or otherwise, if (1) the testimony is based upon sufficient facts or data, (2) the testimony is the product of reliable principles and methods, and (3) the witness has applied the principles and methods reliably to the facts of the case.

Rule 703. Bases of Opinion Testimony by Experts

The facts or data in the particular case upon which an expert bases an opinion or inference may be those perceived by or made known to the expert at or before the hearing. If of a type reasonably relied upon by experts in the particular field in forming opinions or inferences upon the subject, the facts or data need not be admissible in evidence in order for the opinion or inference to be admitted. Facts or data that are otherwise inadmissible shall not be disclosed to the jury by the proponent of the opinion or inference unless the court determines that their probative value in assisting the jury to evaluate the expert's opinion substantially outweighs their prejudicial effect.

Rule 704. Opinion on Ultimate Issue

(a) Except as provided in subdivision (b), testimony in the form of an opinion or inference otherwise admissible is not objectionable because it embraces an ultimate issue to be decided by the trier of fact.

(b) No expert witness testifying with respect to the mental state or condition of a defendant in a criminal case may state an opinion or inference as to whether the defendant did or did not have the mental state or condition constituting an element of the crime charged or of a defense thereto. Such ultimate issues are matters for the trier of fact alone.

Rule 705. Disclosure of Facts or Data Underlying Expert Opinion

The expert may testify in terms of opinion or inference and give reasons therefore without first testifying to the underlying facts or data, unless the court requires otherwise. The expert may in any event be required to disclose the underlying facts or data on cross-examination.

Rule 706. Court Appointed Experts

(a) Appointment

The court may on its own motion or on the motion of any party enter an order to show cause why expert witnesses should not be appointed, and may request the parties to submit nominations. The court may appoint any expert witnesses agreed upon by the parties, and may appoint expert witnesses of its own selection. An expert witness shall not be appointed by the court unless the witness consents to act. A witness so appointed shall be informed of the witness' duties by the court in writing, a copy of which shall be filed with the clerk, or at a conference in which the parties shall have opportunity to participate. A witness so appointed shall advise the parties of the witness' findings, if any; the witness' deposition may be taken by any party; and the witness may be called to testify by the court or any party. The witness shall be subject to cross-examination by each party, including a party calling the witness.

(b) Compensation

Expert witnesses so appointed are entitled to reasonable compensation in whatever sum the court may allow. The compensation thus fixed is payable from funds which may be provided by law in criminal cases and civil actions and proceedings involving just compensation under the fifth amendment. In other civil actions and proceedings the compensation shall be paid by the parties in such proportion and at such time as the court directs, and thereafter charged in like manner as other costs.

(c) Disclosure of Appointment

In the exercise of its discretion, the court may authorize disclosure to the jury of the fact that the court appointed the expert witness.

(d) Parties' Experts of Own Selection

Nothing in this rule limits the parties in calling expert witnesses of their own selection.

ADMISSIBILITY OF SCIENTIFIC EVIDENCE

Admissibility is the legal concept that determines what evidence, both testimonial and physical, will be admitted by the court and what the jury will be permitted to hear. Admissibility is determined by statute, rules of evidence, and case law. This aspect of admissibility relates solely to the admissibility of the science/subject at issue and not to the qualifications of the individual. Three distinct "tests" or "standards" have evolved with respect to scientific evidence: Frye, Daubert, or hybrid. States opt for Daubert, Frye, or a method of their own, and the number of states that use either the Frye or the Daubert standard fluctuates over time.

1.   *Frye Rule (Kelly-Frye from US v Frye, 1923):* This case established, in the rules of evidence, that the results of scientific tests or procedures are admissible only when the tests or procedures have gained general acceptance in the particular field to which they belong. The *"Frye"* is also referred to as the "general acceptance" standard.
2.   *Daubert Test (Daubert v Merrell Dow Pharmaceuticals, 1993):* *"Daubert"* shifted the determining factor of admissibility away from the general acceptance of the relevant scientific community to the "gatekeeper" concept. Under *Daubert* the presiding judge would act as the gatekeeper and determine whether or not the proposed evidence was relevant, applicable to the case, and would be helpful to the jury. Expert opinion must be based on reliable methodology or analysis and not subjective belief or unsupported speculation. The reliability of the expert testimony is as important as the relevance of the expert testimony. All evidence can be challenged, but Daubert made criteria more rigorous.
3.   *Hybrid* states have adopted legislation or rules of evidence that modify or alter in some way either the *Frye* or *Daubert* standards.

EXPERT WITNESS PROCESS

While there is no specific expert witness process, there are suggestions for the pretrail, trial, and posttrial periods.

Pretrial

Trial preparation should be done relatively close to trial. If done too early, you may forget important details. Remember, as an expert witness, you are unbiased. Your role is to present scientific information and your opinion on a specific matter of the case. You are not there to "win" the case.

1. Obtain important documentations (reports, diagrams, photographs, etc.) relating to the case. What you get depends on the case.
2. Study all documents thoroughly to the point of memorization. Records may be accessed in the courtroom, but you will look more like an expert if you know all your details prior to testifying. Focus on significant information and be able to retrieve it from your memory promptly if questioned on it during testimony.
3. Take notes about the case. But remember that everything recorded, including your notes, may be discoverable (submitted as evidence in court). Write notes as if they may be used in court. You most likely will also be asked to prepare a report for the court. This will be admitted into evidence. You may refer to your report during the trial.
4. Never make notes on original documents. Make them on copies.
5. Prepare a series of questions for the attorney of record for your "side" to ask you. Attorneys do not have medical knowledge, and it is very helpful for you to prepare this list. You may also need to educate the attorney—and the judge and jury—as to your health care specialty.
6. As an expert witness, you assist the attorney in making testimony demonstrable and illustrative. Therefore, prepare "show and tell"—computerized slides, charts, or whatever is needed to illustrate your important testimony.
7. Meet with the attorney before the court date. This is not a rehearsal, but it gives you time to give the attorney your questions and to review your résumé/qualifications.
8. Ascertain the identity of the opposing expert witness and what that witness will be testifying about. Whenever possible, obtain a copy of the opposing expert's report and review it before the trial. The attorney may ask you to review the report for assistance with cross-examination questions. (The opposing attorney and expert will most likely do the same with your report.)

9. If possible, observe the courtroom before the trial. This is especially helpful for your first few cases as it will help decrease your anxiety.
10. Check out all your equipment ahead of time and make sure it works. Bring back-up equipment if you have it.

Depositions

You may be asked for a deposition. A deposition is the testimony of a witness taken outside the court where the witness is subject to both direct and cross-examination. It is usually reduced to writing and taken under oath and is a prediscovery method, whereby a witness statement concerning the case is taken under oath with all parties and their attorneys present.

Trial

Voir Dire

After you are called to the witness stand and are sworn in, you begin the voir dire process. You must qualify as an expert prior to giving testimony. The attorney you are working with will present your CV and ask questions that will demonstrate your expertise. The opposing counsel may ask questions to try to disqualify you. After questioning, the judge determines if you qualify as an expert. Once qualified, testimony begins as the attorney you are working with asks you questions.

Testimony

Direct Examination. Direct examination is what occurs as the attorney you are working with asks you questions. This is when you will present any material you have developed, including your report. The attorney may also ask you to describe evidence.

Cross-Examination. Cross-examination is when the opposing attorney questions you. This can be very stressful. Be aware of leading questions that suggest an answer, especially answers you would not otherwise give.

Redirect. The direct examiner asks questions after the cross-examiner. (This process can continue back and forth.)

Exhibit 6.1

HELPFUL HINTS FOR COURT APPEARANCES

Dress professionally.
Relax.
Walk into the courtroom with authority.
Sit up straight and look attentive.
Do not fidget.
Speak clearly.
Make eye contact with those you are speaking to, as well as the judge and jury.
Exude confidence.

Posttrial

Contact the attorney you worked with once the trial has concluded to find out the outcome. Juries are often interviewed to see how they reached their conclusions. Find out what the strongest and weakest evidence was; what helped the case most, least; where there any shortcomings that failed to support the evidence; if the defendant was found guilty, what was the most compelling evidence. If the defendant was found not guilty, what motivated the jury to acquit? (See Exhibit 6.1.)

REFERENCES

American Academy of Pediatrics Committee on Medical Liability. (2002). Guidelines for expert witness testimony in malpractice litigation. *Pediatrics, 109*(5), 974–979.
DiLuigi, K. (2004). What it takes to be an expert witness. *RN, 67*(2), 65–66.
Federal Rules of Evidence. (2008, December). Retrieved from www.uscourts.gov/rules/EV2008.pdf
National Institutes of Justice Firearm Examiner Training Court Room Testimony. (n.d.). Retrieved from www.ojp.usdoj.gov/nij/training/firearms-training/module14/fir_m14_t08.htm

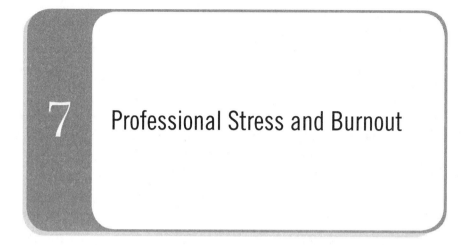

7   Professional Stress and Burnout

The work environment can significantly affect one's physical, psychological, and/or spiritual health, and professional job stress can be quite apparent among those working in health care professions. Health Care Professionals deal with life-threatening injuries and illnesses, complicated by overwork, understaffing, tight schedules, paperwork, intricate or malfunctioning equipment, complex authority hierarchies, dependent and demanding clients, and client deaths, all of which contribute to stress. Those who work with victims of violent crimes and/or offenders face the additional stressors that come from working with these challenging populations. The consequences of stress can be devastating to health care professionals and can result in decreased professional effectiveness, delivery of inadequate client care, the destruction of home life, and overall burnout.

TYPES OF PROFESSIONAL STRESSORS

Working with forensic clients exposes forensic health care professionals to specific types of stressors. All face the same stressors faced by other health care workers. However, they face the additional issues of compassion fatigue and vicarious trauma. While all of these issues affect overall job satisfaction and functioning, they are inherently different. Research on work life and the work environment has demonstrated that the professional/client relationship may not play a central role in the onset of burnout. On the other hand, trauma research suggests that interpersonal relationships, particularly the concept of empathy and emotional energy, may play a key role in the development of compassion fatigue or vicarious traumatization. When working with clients who are experiencing pain, suffering, or trauma, the health care professional may experience adverse effects similar to that of their clients, frequently resulting in professionals reassessing their reality and creating a new reality based upon what they have been exposed to.

Traditional Stress

According to the National Institute of Occupational Safety and Health, job stress results from a poor match between job demands and the capabilities, resources, or needs of workers. Job stress can also result from fear of job loss and unsafe working conditions. And even the best jobs have stress from performance evaluations, deadlines, and other responsibilities.

In addition, a poor economy can mean both downsizing and increased crime, adding to workload demands. Technological advances including smart phones and netbooks have made it possible to take work everywhere, and far too many jobs are expecting just that. Many health care professionals find that the only way to stay on top of things is to arrive at work early, stay late, work through lunch and on weekends, and bring work home. This leaves little time for self, family, and pleasurable pursuits, leaving professional lives seriously out of balance.

Images of acts of terrorism and mass shootings lurk in the back of most people's minds. Such images can contribute to the fear experienced by many health care professionals who work in places where the possibility of violence is a more common event, such as emergency departments and community centers. Violence in the health care workplace is a serious safety and health issue. The media tends to over-sensationalize some rare types of violent assaults, such as mass shootings by disgruntled employees, but less dramatic risk factors can be just as dangerous. One example is domestic violence that surfaces when angry spouses act out at the workplace. Other examples include:

■ Threats: Communications of intent to cause harm, including verbal threats, threatening body language, and written threats.

- Physical assaults: These may range from slapping to rape and homicide.
- Muggings: Aggravated assaults that are usually conducted by surprise and with intent to rob.

Compassion Fatigue

One can care too much. Compassion fatigue can result from helping or wanting to help a traumatized or suffering person. It tends to happen more suddenly than burnout. This phenomenon seems to be connected to the therapeutic relationship between the health care professional and the client, whereby the experience of the client triggers multiple responses in the health care provider. Factors such as poor collaborative work environments, lack of support, and the blur between work and home caring roles, as well as societal and organizational factors, may be associated with an increased risk. This concept is not new, and most of what is known comes from the hospice literature. However, providing effective victim intervention requires tremendous emotional energy and resilience, which can be a near-constant source of stress. Compassion fatigue is connected to posttraumatic stress disorder (PTSD), because it is a very intensive psychological assault on an individual that is almost immediately overwhelming.

Compassion fatigue creates a deep physical, emotional, and spiritual exhaustion accompanied by acute emotional pain. Health care providers with burnout tend to adapt to their exhaustion by becoming less empathetic and more withdrawn, while those with compassion fatigue continue to give themselves fully to their clients, finding it difficult to maintain a healthy balance of empathy and objectivity. They often describe this state as being sucked into a vortex that pulls them slowly downward, leaving them with no idea of how to stop the downward spiral, so they work harder and continue to give to others until they are completely drained.

Vicarious Traumatization

Vicarious traumatization refers to the negative transformation in the health care provider's inner experience, resulting from empathic engagement with clients' traumatic events. Continuous exposure to graphic accounts of human cruelty, trauma, and suffering, as well as the empathetic relationship between the client and health care provider, may leave the provider open to emotional and spiritual consequences. A number of factors contribute to the onset of vicarious traumatization: individual characteristics such as previous personal trauma, lack of coping strategies, and unrealistic self-expectations; social and community context; physical, organizational, structural, and contextual work environment; and work-related attitudes such as the need to fulfill all the needs of the clients.

The effects of vicarious traumatization resemble those of PTSD, including recurring feelings of horror, fear, and helplessness. These effects can disrupt and alter the health care provider's sense of self. While few studies have investigated this phenomenon and its associated symptoms with regard to nurses, it would seem reasonable to suggest that health care workers who provide continuous care for victims of violent crimes may experience similar effects, particularly if caring work is delivered in a work environment that is incongruent with the philosophy of their health care profession. Health care providers may experience intrusive images, alterations in the ability to trust, loss of independence, decreased capacity for intimacy, and loss of control, as well as increased arousal, including anxiety, unexplained anger, and irritability. The effects are argued to be cumulative and permanent, and these may overlap both the personal and professional life of an individual.

Burnout

Burnout occurs when a person is unable to relieve the physical and mental symptoms associated with unrelenting stress. Anyone can feel burnout, although certain commonalities occur. It is a psychological experience that manifests itself in individuals as part of their working practice. Burnout is a negative experience that results from interaction between environment and individual and is thus a response to chronic occupational stress. Some providers who work with forensic mental health clients (typically mentally ill offenders) have been identified as at risk of suffering from occupational stress and possibly developing burnout syndrome. The main stressors on these professionals are identified as interprofessional conflicts, workload, and lack of involvement in decision making.

SIGNS OF STRESS

Stress overload can challenge the health care provider's ability to provide effective services and maintain personal and professional therapeutic relationships. It can also cause stress-related disorders. Stress-related disorders encompass a broad array of conditions, including psychological disorders (depression, anxiety, PTSD), emotional distress (job dissatisfaction, fatigue, tension), maladaptive behaviors (aggression, substance abuse), and cognitive impairment (concentration and memory problems). These conditions can lead to poor work performance or even injury, as well as various biological reactions that may lead ultimately to compromised health, such as cardiovascular disease. Stress is also expensive. High levels of stress are associated with substantial increases in health service utilization, longer disability periods for occupational injuries and illnesses, and major turnover in organizations.

Chronic stress leads to feelings of being "stressed out" or "burned out." Stress may not be easy to recognize because it often affects the body, leading the stressed person to believe that they are ill rather than stressed. Signs of chronic stress include:

- Headaches, backaches, chest pain, stomachaches, indigestion, nausea or diarrhea
- Rashes
- Overeating or undereating
- Sleep disturbances (too much sleep, restless sleep, difficulty falling asleep, difficulty staying asleep, waking up early)
- Fatigue
- Disillusionment
- Sexual dysfunction
- Workaholic behavior and/or continuously thinking about work
- Twitching
- Having trouble concentrating or with school work
- Breakdown of personal relationships
- Feeling anxious or worried
- Feeling inadequate, frustrated, helpless, or overwhelmed
- Feeling bored or dissatisfied
- Feeling pressured, tense, irritable, angry, or hostile
- Aggressive behavior
- Substance abuse
- Excessive or inappropriate crying
- Avoiding others
- Mood swings
- Inability to organize or make decisions
- Blocked creativity or judgment

- Poor memory/forgetfulness
- Difficulty concentrating

MANAGING STRESS

The effects of stress disorders can be devastating; however, health care professionals can actively work to avoid these pitfalls, especially compassion fatigue, vicarious victimization, and burnout. Stress should be minimized at both the individual and institutional level, even if the "institution" is a small private practice.

Individual Stress Management

Stress overload can impair overall functioning. Do not make major life decisions (job changes, divorce, relocations) while stressed, and do not make major purchases, which may cause temporary relief but long-term stress if you cannot afford them. Do not blame others for job-related problems; instead, work together to find solutions.

- Practice what you preach.
- Maintain professional boundaries, including those between work and home lives.
- Take time for yourself with time-outs and leisure activities.
- Make time for family and friends.
- Use humor—laughter is the best medicine.
- Eat right, exercise regularly, and get enough sleep.
- Discontinue or minimize your use of caffeine.
- Use time management techniques.

  - Keep a calendar.
  - Do not overcommit yourself.
  - Prioritize.

- Try meditation or relaxation exercises.
- Delegate—rely on teamwork and do not do it all.
- Stop being a perfectionist.
- Debrief—develop a professional group to discuss your caseload.

The Center for Sex Offender Management (CSOM, n.d.) suggests an ABC approach to decreasing one's risk of secondary trauma: awareness, balance, and connection (with modifications for health care professionals):

Awareness

- Be aware of your own "trauma map." Acknowledge your past and be aware that it can affect how you view and perform with victims and offenders.
- Inventory your current lifestyle choices and make necessary changes—are you eating, sleeping, and exercising adequately?
- Take care of yourself. Make a self-care list and post it prominently in your home or office. Include some of the following:
  - Be creative.
  - Get away.
  - Get outside and appreciate the weather.
  - Enjoy other environments.
  - Have fun.
  - Socialize with people who aren't criminal!

Balance

- Allow yourself to fully experience emotional reactions. Do not keep your emotions bottled up.
- Avoid working overtime and do not spend all of your free time socializing only with coworkers, discussing the negative factors of your job.
- Know your limits and accept them. Set realistic goals.
- Practice time management skills to help achieve a sense of balance in both your professional and personal lives.
- Seek out a new leisure activity unrelated to your job.
- Recognize negative coping skills and avoid them, and substitute these coping skills with more positive coping skills.

Connection

- Listen to feedback from colleagues, friends, and family members, and encourage at least one of them to conduct periodic "pulse checks."
- Avoid professional isolation and remain connected with and supported by your coworkers on the job. Just don't spend all your time with them.

- Debrief after difficult cases.
- Develop support systems with an informal peer support group, or seek out or become a mentor.
- Obtain continuing education to improve job skills and capacity. Get certified in forensics if possible.
- Nurture your spiritual side.

Institutional Stress Management

Institutions benefit greatly when they keep stress levels to a minimum; employees are more productive and clients are more satisfied. Administrators can start by being positive role models, managing their own stress at home and work. Administrators can also:

- Educate health care professionals about job stress, compassion fatigue, and vicarious trauma.
- Minimize stressors, including work overload, inadequate work space, insufficient resources, and unsafe equipment and situations.
- Hold regular staff meetings; keep the lines of communication open and provide support.
- Provide regular debriefing meetings.
- Maintain an organized and efficient workplace.
- Take action on legitimate complaints.
- Provide readily available counseling.

Employers can also establish programs that address workplace stress, such as Employee Assistance Programs (EAP). EAPs can improve the ability of workers to cope with difficult work situations. Stress management programs teach workers about the nature and sources of stress, the effects of stress on health, and personal skills to reduce it.

RESOURCES

Compassion Fatigue Awareness Project: http://www.compassionfatigue.org
National Institute for Occupational Safety and Health: http://www.cdc.gov/niosh
Occupational Safety and Health Administration: http://www.osha.gov

REFERENCES

Center for Sex Offender Management (CSOM). (n.d.). *Secondary trauma and the management of sex offenders.* Retrieved from http://www.csom.org/train/index.html

Collins, S., & Long, A. (2003). Working with the psychological effects of trauma: Consequences for mental health-care workers—a literature review. *Journal of Psychiatric and Mental Health Nursing, 10,* 417–424.

National Institute of Occupational Safety and Health: Center for Disease Prevention and Control. (2008). *Workplace stress.* Retrieved from http://www.cdc.gov/niosh/blog/nsb120307_stress.html

Office for Victims of Crime. (n.d.). *Victim assistance training.* Retrieved from http://www.ovcttac.gov/VATOnline_Course

Pfifferling, J., & Gilley, K. (2000). Overcoming compassion fatigue. *Family Practice Management.* Retrieved from http://www.aafp.org/fpm/20000400/39over.html

Sabo, B. (2008). Adverse psychosocial consequences: Compassion fatigue, burnout and vicarious traumatization: Are nurses who provide palliative and hematological cancer care vulnerable? *Indian Journal of Palliative Care, 14*(1), 23–29.

Tehrani, N. (2007). The cost of caring—The impact of secondary trauma on assumptions, values and beliefs. *Counselling Psychology Quarterly, 20*(4), 325–339.

U.S. Department of Labor: Occupational Safety and Health Administration (OSHA). (n.d.). *Stress.* Retrieved from http://www.osha.gov/SLTC/etools/hospital/hazards/stress/stress.html

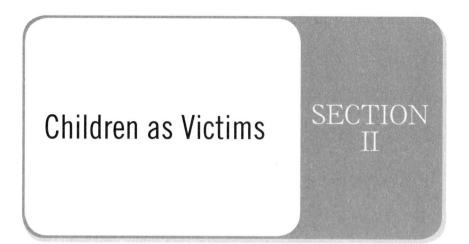

Children as Victims

SECTION II

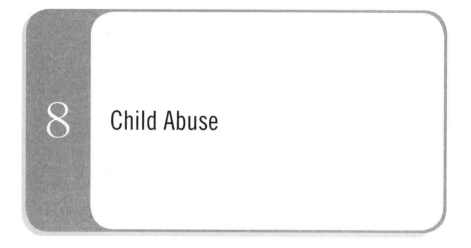

8   Child Abuse

DEFINITIONS

Physical abuse is the intentional infliction of injury to a child by a caretaker. It can result in bruising, burns, fractures, poisoning, and head or abdominal trauma. Shaken baby syndrome (SBS) is a form of physical abuse.

Münchausen syndrome by proxy (MSBP) is the fabrication or inducement of illness by one person onto another (usually mother to child). The child usually requires multiple medical procedures, and the perpetrator usually denies knowing the cause of the child's illness. Acute illness manifestations disappear when the child is separated from the perpetrator. MSBP is addressed in Chapter 10.

Emotional abuse is the deliberate attempt to destroy the child's self-esteem or competence by rejecting, ignoring, criticizing, isolating, or terrorizing the child.

Neglect is the failure of the child's parent or legal guardian to exercise a minimum degree of care in supplying the child with adequate food, clothing, shelter, or education or medical care:

- *Physical neglect* involves deprivation of necessities, such as food, clothing, and shelter.

■ *Emotional neglect* involves the conscious or unconscious failure to meet the child's need for attention, affection, and emotional nurturing.

■ *Medical neglect* involves the caretaker's withholding of medical care or treatment.

Sexual abuse is contact or interaction between a child and an adult when the child is used for sexual stimulation of an adult. Sexual abuse is addressed in Chapter 11. (Please also refer to Chapter 3, "Forensic Assessment and Documentation," and Chapter 4, "Principles of Evidence," for further information relevant to child sexual abuse.)

PREVALENCE OF ABUSE

During 2007, an estimated 794,000 children were victims of abuse or neglect:

Children from birth to 1 year had the highest rate of victimization at 21.9 per 1,000.

51.5% of the child victims were girls and 48.2 percent were boys.

46.6% of all victims were White; 21.7% were African American, and 20.8% were Hispanic.

59% of victims suffered neglect.

10.8% of the victims suffered physical abuse.

7.6% of the victims suffered sexual abuse.

4.2% of the victims suffered from psychological maltreatment.

The National Child Abuse and Neglect Data System (NCANDS) reported an estimated 1,760 child fatalities in 2007, which translates to a rate of 2.35 children per 100,000 children in the general population. Very young children (ages 3 and younger) are the most frequent victims of child fatalities. NCANDS data for 2007 demonstrated that children younger than 1 year accounted for 42.2% of fatalities, while children younger than 4 years accounted for 75.7% of fatalities.

The estimated number of child abuse victims is much higher. Physical abuse remains an underreported, and often undetected, problem for several reasons including individual and community variations in what is considered "abuse," inadequate knowledge and training among professionals in the recognition of abusive injuries, unwillingness to report suspected abuse, and professional bias. Children and infants with abusive head trauma are sometimes initially misdiagnosed, with these children more likely to be younger, White, have less severe symptoms, and live with both parents when compared with abused children who were not initially misdiagnosed. Practitioners must be vigilant to the possibility of abuse when evaluating children who have atypical accidental injuries or obscure symptoms that are suggestive of traumatic etiologies but who do not have a history of trauma.

ETIOLOGY

Child abuse is a complex phenomenon resulting from a combination of individual, family, and social factors.

Predisposing Factors

There are several predisposing factors that contribute to child abuse. These include caretaker factors, child factors, and environmental factors. Certain characteristics increase the risk of these factors contributing to the occurrence of child abuse. Although child factors may play a role in child abuse, these factors do not mean that the child is in any way responsible for that abuse.

Caretaker factors include the following characteristics:

- Severe punishment of caretakers themselves as children
- Poor impulse control
- Free expression of violence
- Social isolation
- Poor social-emotional support system
- Low self-esteem
- Substance abuse
- A history of cruelty to animals

Child factors include the following characteristics:

- Temperament "misfit"
- Illness, disability, and developmental delay
- Typically no other siblings abused
- Illegitimate or unwanted pregnancy
- Hyperkinesis
- Resemblance to someone the caretaker does not like
- Bonding failure
- Problem pregnancy, delivery, or prematurity

Environmental factors include the following characteristics among all socioeconomic groups:

- Chronic stress
- Poverty, poor housing, unemployment
- Divorce
- Frequent relocation

ASSESSMENT

General Principles

Most physical abuse injuries are likely to go unreported or undetected. Minor injuries may not require medical attention and may be obscure or hidden. Kellogg and the American Academy of Pediatrics Committee on Child Abuse and Neglect (2007) note that infants and children are reported as suspected victims of physical abuse when one or more of the following occurs:

- An individual (including a professional) sees and reports a suspicious injury.
- An individual witnesses an abusive event.
- A caregiver observes symptoms and brings the child in for medical care but is unaware that the child has sustained an injury.

■ An individual asks a child if he or she has been hurt in an abusive way.

■ The abuser thinks the inflicted injury is severe enough to require medical attention.

■ The child victim discloses abuse.

The presenting injury may not be the most serious. Life-threatening head and/abdominal trauma may present without visible external signs or history to suggest such an injury. Therefore, a rapid assessment for life-threatening injuries should commence before the more in-depth assessment.

Take photographs of all visible injuries as soon as possible. It is particularly important to obtain photographs of burns before a dressing is applied. (See Chapter 3, "Forensic Assessment and Documentation," for information on how to take photographs.)

History

A careful and well-documented history is the most critical element of the medical evaluation. If the child is verbal, obtain parental and child histories separately; interview adults separately, too. Use open-ended, nonleading questions, especially with younger children. Inquire about physical abuse, neglect, sexual abuse, domestic violence, and witnessed abuse.

Obtain the present history. Assess plausibility of the presenting problem. Assess if the problem is developmentally possible. Essentially, if they don't cruise, they don't bruise. Note whether the mechanism of the injury fits with the injury. For example, a 4-year-old is apt to fracture more than a jaw by falling from a five-story fire escape. Evaluate the consistency of the presenting problem. Note if caretakers give different histories, if the history changes over time, if the history is vague, or if the history is incomplete. Caretakers may blame each other or a third party for the injury. Note if caretaker neglects to state cause of the injury or if caretaker is "very good" at bringing the problem to the practitioner's attention, as in the case of MSBP. Note if caretaker minimizes or exaggerates symptoms or if caretaker is anxious about discussing injury. (Realize that minor discrepancies in the history are usually insignificant.)

Evaluate rationale if parent delays seeking treatment. Abusive caretakers hope that injury will clear on its own. Most normal caretakers seek immediate attention when a child has an accident. Inquire about a triggering incident. Many caretakers abuse children after such incidents as inconsolable crying, bowel or bladder soiling, sleep problems, or discipline problems. Ask about recent crises. Many abusive caretakers are in the midst of financial or other stressors. Assess for predisposing factors, including caretaker substance abuse. Assess for other factors that can suggest abuse: child states that caretaker caused injury and/or child or caretaker attempts to hide injury by using concealing clothing.

Obtain the developmental/psychosocial history. Question if caretakers associate with other families in the neighborhood and if they participate in school activities. Many abusers do neither of these. Ask if child fights with classmates, acts out in the classroom, or destroys things. Ask if child abuses animals.

Inquire about child's participation in bullying behaviors to ward off other children. Query about child's ability to make friends; abused children find it hard to make friends. Ask if child avoids doing things with other children or if child avoids doing things that are pleasurable. Ascertain if child is parentified; that is, child engages in falsely grown-up behaviors, such as caring for the adults in the household. Ask if child participates in self-abusive behaviors. Inquire about school performance and attendance. School failure and poor attendance may indicate abuse, as can arriving early at school or leaving school late. Inquire about suicidal ideation, eating disorders, and sleep disorders.

Obtain the past history. Ask about previous injuries. Abused children frequently have a history of many unusual or unexplained injuries. Inquire about health care history. Child may not have received adequate health care, or child may have been brought to multiple health care providers or emergency rooms in an attempt to cover up the abuse.

Physical Assessment

Growth measurements. Assess height, weight, head circumference (when applicable), and BMI (when applicable) for signs of neglect, especially failure to thrive. Plot all measurements on growth chart.

General behavioral assessment. Observe child for the following: sadness and crying, depression, tiredness, overcompliance, excessive tearfulness, indiscriminate attachment, apprehensiveness when other children cry, fear of going home, aggressiveness and destructive behavior, apathy and withdrawal, and attention-seeking behaviors.

Assess caretaker-child interaction for the following: clinginess of child to caretaker, fear of caretaker, overprotectiveness of caretaker, caretaker blaming child for illness or behavior problems, and dramatic behavior change in child when caretaker leaves.

Cutaneous injuries. Assess for cutaneous injuries. Note location of injury: The back of the body, from the neck to the knees, is the most common location for intentional injuries. Head injuries, especially in young children, may be abuse. Knee, elbow, and shin injuries are more likely to be associated with accidental injury. Multiplanar injuries, such as back and front together or right and left side together, suggest abuse.

Common sites of injuries and common injuries include the following:

- Head: head injuries, missing or broken hair

- Face: slap (handprint) marks

- Eyes: bilateral "black eyes," conjunctival hemorrhages

- Ears: pull marks and pinching

- Mouth: lacerations and bruises to lips and frenulum

- Neck: choke marks

- Torso, including buttocks: bite marks, burns, bruising, strap, or other object marks

- Extremities: burns, bruises, grab marks, tether marks, friction burns (from being tied up)

- Genitals: burns, pinch marks, signs of penis wrapping

- Bruises: Assess pattern or shape because it may indicate the mechanism of injury. Examples include adult handprints, belt marks, paddle marks, coat hanger marks, and pinch marks. Assess ages of injuries. Bruises cannot be reliably aged by examination of color or any other technique in a clinical examination, but yellowish bruises are likely to be older than purple ones. Injuries in different stages of healing suggest abuse. Note characteristics of injury.

- Bite marks: Assess the oval impression of a pair of crescentic bruises that follows a bite. The severity depends on location, degree of force, and movement of the jaw and the victim. Adult- and child-inflicted bites can be differentiated but warrant a forensic odontologist to make this assessment, as well as assist in documenting and preserving a bite mark.

■ Burns: Assess depth, and compare it to injury history. Burn depth is a function of temperature, exposure time, and thickness of the exposed skin. Water at 150°F can cause a second-degree burn faster than 120°F water. Discrepancies between injury and history suggest abuse. Observe for splash marks that occur when child attempts to pull himself or herself from the source of the burn injury, particularly hot liquids. Liquids normally flow downward, and they cool as they flow.

Therefore, proximal areas are more severely burned and broader, while distal areas are less severe and more narrow, creating an "arrow" appearance. Splash marks will be absent in children whose body part(s) are forcibly held in hot liquids. Observe for scalding injuries, which are the most common intentionally inflicted burn injuries in children. Infants and young children are usually immersed, and older children usually have hot liquid thrown or poured on them. Sharply demarcated areas, such as "glove marks" or "stocking/sock marks," indicate that the child was held in hot liquid. Inspect perineum and buttocks. Burns in these areas may have a "donut" pattern (circle of burned skin from hot liquid with the central area spared where child was pressed down against the cooler tub). Observe for "zebra burns" that result from child being held by the hands and feet under the hot water faucet. The creases in the abdomen and upper legs are spared, creating the striped pattern.

Assess for branding burns, which mirror the outline of the object that caused them (irons, curling irons, heaters, grills, hot plates, radiators, hot knives). Assess for cigarette burns (small round excoriations), which are usually found on the hands, soles, and diaper area. Inspect for friction burns on wrists and ankles that are typically caused by rope or cord used to bind child.

Central nervous system (CNS) injuries (most common cause of child abuse death). Assess for severe brain injury. Diffuse, severe brain injury usually requires that significant deceleration forces be applied to the head, with or without an impact to the head. Without such forces, unexplained, severe, diffuse brain trauma in infants could indicate abuse. Injuries most seen in intentional head trauma include subgaleal hematomas, skull fractures, subarachnoid hemorrhages, subdural hematomas, and parenchymal brain injuries.

Epidural hematomas may be inflicted but are most often caused by accidental falls. Asymptomatic subdural hematoma (SDH) is seen in neonates born vaginally as well as by cesarean deliveries that follow a trial of labor. This occurs even without obvious traumatic delivery. Birth-related subdural hematomas are limited in both their size and location, and they typically occur in the posterior fossa above and below the tentorium and in the occipital lobe.

Assess for injuries resulting from direct impact, asphyxia, or shaking. Assess for direct trauma from punching, slapping, or an object being thrown at child's head. Assess for head injury: Falls from heights of less than 4 feet by children younger than 2 years of age rarely result in simple or complex fractures. Suspect abuse if skull fracture is noted in any child with a history of a minor injury or in any child with retinal hemorrhages. "Raccoon eyes" may be noted in children with subgleal hematomas following traction on the hair and scalp. The following head injuries are typically inflicted: Subgleal hematomas and cephalhematomas (sudden and violent hair pulling or blunt impact trauma), scalp bruising and soft-tissue edema (direct blows), subdural hematomas, subarachnoid hemorrhages, and retinal hemorrhages (shaken baby syndrome, whiplash), and skull fractures and suture widening (blunt trauma). (See Chapter 9, "Shaken Baby Syndrome/Abusive Head Trauma.")

Assess for head injuries. Common presentations for the child with an abusive head injury include:

- Acute critical illness at the time of presentation (unresponsiveness, apnea, bradycardia, seizures, cardiopulmonary arrest)
- Subtle subacute or chronic symptoms (vomiting, lethargy, irritability, or increasing head circumference). There may be no visible head trauma.

Assess for choking injuries. Distinct bruising from attempted strangulation may be noted on the neck. Frequently there are minimal external signs when choking and suffocation result in asphyxial injury. Assess for shaken baby syndrome. (See Chapter 9.) Possible symptoms include poor feeding, vomiting, lethargy, or irritability that occur intermittently or for days or weeks prior to health visit. If the child is violently shaken into unconsciousness, the abuser may wait to seek help, hoping the child will awaken. The child is frequently brought in convulsing or comatose, not sucking or swallowing, unable to follow movements, and not smiling or vocalizing. Many of these infants have respiratory difficulty that can progress to apnea or bradycardia, resulting in cardiopulmonary arrest.

Skeletal trauma. Assess for fractures. Multiple fractures in various stages of healing are considered to be child abuse until proven otherwise.

Unexplained fractures in children under 2 years suggest abuse. Spiral, long bone fractures in young children who are not walking indicate abuse. Unexplained healing or healed fractures detected on X-rays may be child abuse. In young infants, fractured collarbones or simple linear skull fractures may result from a minor accidental fall from a height of 3–4 feet or less.

Assess location of fracture. In children under 2 years, fractures that involve the metaphyseal-epiphyseal plate, thoracic cage, scapula, and vertebrae suggest abuse. These fractures require significant force, which cannot come from a minor fall or everyday handling of a child. Metaphyseal-epiphyseal fractures, rib fractures, and sternum fractures suggest abuse. They are usually caused by violent compression of shaking of a young child. Clavicular, femoral, supracondylar humeral, and distal extremity fractures usually result from accidental injury unless accompanied by other stigmata.

Correlate age of fracture with history, even though this cannot be performed with great precision. Time frames are shorter in infants, and longer in children with malnutrition or chronic underlying disease. Fractures of flat bones (skull) cannot be aged. Soft-tissue swelling decreases in 2 to 5 days. Periosteal new bone appears on X-ray as early as 4 days after injury. Long bone callus appears 8 to 10 days after injury. Soft callus lasts about 3 to 4 weeks. Hard callus and bone remodeling occur over a few months.

A careful family history and an experienced radiologist can usually rule out rare inherited bone disorders, such as osteogenesis imperfecta. However, some cases will warrant a genetics consultation with or without skin biopsy and fibroblast collagen analysis.

Eye injuries. Assess for evidence of eye injury. Unilateral or bilateral retinal hemorrhages can go undetected unless examined by a pediatric ophthalmologist or a practitioner experienced with these hemorrhages. The size, number, and character of hemorrhages vary from case to case. Vitreous and retinal hemorrhages and nonhemorrhagic changes, including retinal folds and traumatic retinoschisis, can be characteristic of shaken baby syndrome.

Assess for signs of direct trauma, including abrasions, subconjunctival hemorrhages, globe fractures, and orbital edema. Globe fractures and orbital edema can lead to extraocular entrapment and altering of the visual axis and amblyopia. Anterior chamber injuries, including hyphema, signify severe blunt trauma.

Oral and facial injuries. Assess for oral and facial injuries. Consider abuse when children present with head, neck, and oral cavity injuries. If soft-tissue injuries to the maxillary lip or frenulum are observed, suspect forced feeding. However, young children can develop these injuries when they fall with a hard object in their mouth.

Assess for intraoral lacerations or mucosal injuries that may be caused by the forceful introduction of objects into a child's mouth, especially scalding or caustic substances. Evaluate child for "tin ear syndrome," which results from blunt trauma to the ear. This is manifested by subperichrondral hematoma and associated intracerebral injury as a result of the rotational acceleration of the head.

"Coffee table bruises," bruises to the forehead, nose, lower lip, and chin, are common in young children and should be differentiated from inflicted injuries. Dental trauma may be abuse and usually warrants evaluation by a dentist.

Visceral injuries (second most common cause of child abuse death). Assess for signs and symptoms of an acute abdomen because children with blunt trauma abdominal injuries rarely have external injuries. These manifestations may include the following: rigidity, guarding, diminished bowel sounds, vomiting, abdominal pain, and abdominal distention.

Consider child abuse in children who present with unexplained bilious vomiting in the absence of fever or peritoneal irritation (duodenal hematoma). Consider blunt trauma as part of the differential diagnosis in children who present with nonspecific abdominal complaints or acute abdomen symptoms. Injuries include hematomas of the bowel wall, perforations of the bowel, and trauma to organs (liver, spleen, pancreas, or kidneys).

Emotional abuse. Assess for possible emotional abuse by observing both behavioral indicators displayed by the child or by the caretaker and for physical indicators displayed by the child.

- *Child behaviors:* Habit disorders (rocking, biting, hair pulling), withdrawal, depression, apathy, unusual tearfulness, conduct problems, acting out, behavioral extremes (very passive or very aggressive; excessive rigidity), age-inappropriate behaviors, attempted suicide.

- *Caretaker behaviors:* Placing unrealistic demands or impossible expectations on child; using child to settle marital problems or satisfy their own; ego demands; referring to child as "it" or treating child as object.

Observe for physical indicators in the child: failure to thrive, developmental lags, feeding problems, enuresis, sleep problems.

Neglect. Physical neglect (deprivation of necessities, such as food and shelter) can be detected by observing the child for behavioral indicators, for physical indicators, for signs of inadequate medical or dental care, and by the presence of emotional behaviors.

Observe for behavioral indicators. the infant is dull, inactive; the child begs or steals food; school attendance problems (arrives early, leaves late) occur; child reports having no caretaker.

Assess for physical indicators. malnutrition, constant hunger or fatigue, poor hygiene, inappropriate clothing for weather, inadequate dental care, failure to thrive, developmental delays. (Note: Bald patches on back of infant's head are no longer considered a significant sign of neglect due to the Back to Sleep positioning.)

Assess for inadequate medical or dental care. Inquire about other factors: lack of adequate supervision, abandonment, inadequate health care, household problems (unsafe conditions, lack of heating or plumbing, inadequate food).

Emotional neglect involves failure to meet child's need for attention, affection, and emotional nurturance.

Observe for behavioral indicators: exaggerated fears, withdrawal, depression, apathy, sadness, unresponsiveness, delinquency, antisocial behaviors, attention-seeking behaviors, drug and alcohol abuse, school problems.

Differential Diagnoses

Health care providers should always consider abuse when children present with suspicious factors. However, they should also consider all possible differential diagnoses to minimize the chances of wrongful accusations. This includes evaluating the child for possible normal variations, such as Mongolian spots, as well as illness manifestations including the petechiae and ecchymosis of idiopathic thrombocytopenic purpura (ITP).

Physical Abuse

Bruising

Domestic violence

Bleeding disorders: purpura, hemophilia

Normal childhood injuries: as noted above

Allergic shiners: dark circles under eyes

Mongolian spots: over lower back and buttocks in dark-skinned children

Coining and cupping (cultural practices to treat illnesses): usually seen along the rib margins and spine

Phytophotodermatitis: photoxic reaction that occurs when the skin that has come into contact with certain plants is exposed to the sun

Hypersensitivity reactions

Erythema multiforme

Erythema nodosum

Lymphangiomas

Clothing dye, especially from blue jeans

Burns

Impetigo

Toxic epidermal necrolysis

Epidermolysis bullosa

Moxibustion (cultural practice of inducing cutaneous burns on areas of skin that correspond to afflicted organs)

Drug eruption

Diaper dermatitis

Skeletal Trauma

Osteogenesis imperfect

Rickets, scurvy

Renal osteodystrophy

Oosteomyelitis

Congenital syphilis

Neoplasia

Head Trauma

Noninflicted trauma

Spontaneous bleeds of vascular anomalies

Signs of ventricular injury

Hair Loss Disorders

Alopecia areata

Trichotillomania

Emotional Abuse: Psychiatric Disorders Not Caused by Child Abuse

Neglect

Poverty and homelessness

Parental mental retardation

Child mental retardation or psychiatric disorder

DIAGNOSTIC TESTING

Diagnostic testing depends on presentation and may include, per Ricci, Botash, and McKenney (2009):

- Complete blood count including hematocrit: Chronic anemia may be found in infants who are neglected and undernourished, but anemia in the setting of unexplained tachycardia or abdominal trauma may be indicative of internal hemorrhage.
- Urinalysis: Hematuria may indicate kidney or urethral trauma. Occult blood without red blood cells may indicate rhabdomyolysis.
- Urine toxicology screen: May be indicated in the infant with an altered level of consciousness.

■ Stool guaiac: For history of gastrointestinal bleeding or suspicion of occult abdominal trauma.

■ Prothrombin time, activated partial thromboplastin time, and platelet count: Child with suspicious bruising if exclusion of bleeding diatheses is needed. Other coagulation screens (factor tests) may require consultation with a hematologist.

■ Liver transaminases and amylase levels: For abdominal trauma, elevation should point to the need for abdominal CT scan with contrast as the next step.

■ Cardiac enzymes—troponin and creatine kinase with muscle and brain subunits (CK-MB): May be indicated if cardiac injury is suspected.

■ Radiographic bone survey: A full radiographic abuse survey (skeletal survey) is indicated in any child aged 2 years or younger with evidence or strong suspicion of physical abuse. This should include at a minimum two views of each extremity (individual long bones are highly recommended), anteroposterior (AP) and lateral skull, AP and lateral spine, chest, abdomen, pelvis, hands, and feet. Films should be reviewed carefully for classic metaphyseal lesions and healing fractures, particularly of the posterior ribs.

■ Abdominal CT scan: May be useful in the unconscious child or when abdominal trauma is suspected, especially if bleeding is present and source cannot be found.

■ Chest CT scan: Can be combined with the abdominal views to look for rib and lung injury.

■ Brain MRI may be more sensitive for detecting diffuse axonal injury and for detecting and dating subdural hematomas and parenchymal brain injury than CT scan for rapid identification of CNS injury. Three-dimensional reconstruction of CT imaging for rib and skull fractures has shown very good results in detecting these injuries.

■ Radionucleotide bone scan: May be useful to detect rib fractures prior to callous formation and to confirm the presence of fractures that are not well delineated on the skeletal survey.

■ Dilated fundoscopic examination by an ophthalmologist in the infant suspected of SBS.

■ Lumbar puncture (LP): A spinal or subdural tap may be diagnostic of a subarachnoid hemorrhage if blood is present in the cerebral spinal fluid (CSF). Xanthochromia should be noted, especially if the differential diagnosis is between a traumatic lumbar puncture and old subarachnoid blood. However, careful thought should be given before performing a LP because of the possibility of cerebellar herniation, and thus a CT scan prior to LP may be warranted.

Evaluating Failure to Thrive

In cases of neglect, especially potential failure to thrive, consider a work-up to rule out both an organic and nonorganic problem. The work-up to rule out an organic cause may include:

Urine culture and urinalysis

Stool sample for ova and parasites

Sweat test

Lead level

HIV testing

Tuberculin skin testing

Nonorganic failure to thrive is the more common form of this disorder, and is usually related to social and economic factors within the family. This diagnosis is best made during an inpatient stay with careful monitoring of the child and a comprehensive family assessment. Organic failure to thrive is less common, but causes include kidney disease, immune disorders/HIV/AIDS, leukemia/other malignancy, heart disease, cystic fibrosis, other malabsorption disorders, allergies/asthma, thyroid disorders, and diabetes mellitus.

INTERVENTION

The management of a possibly abused child is not significantly different from standard pediatric care. Severely injured children must be stabilized before further evaluation is undertaken. This initial evaluation may warrant a trauma response team and pediatric specialists in surgery, emergency medicine, and critical care. Careful documentation may not be possible initially and must always be secondary to resuscitation and stabilization of the patient. If the child has injuries to the genital area, the child should be evaluated for sexual abuse.

The treatment of the physically abused child is the same as that of the accidentally injured child, except that forensic data collection and analysis are of particular and pressing importance. Treatment of neglect should be targeted to the child's individualized needs. All abused children should be referred for counseling, including those who are emotionally abused. Chapter 11 provides information on sexually abused children.

All 50 states and the District of Columbia have statutes that mandate reporting of suspected child abuse and neglect. Health care providers are mandated to immediately report or see that a report is made to the appropriate authorities and state agency when abuse is suspected. It is usually appropriate to notify parents when a report to child protective authorities is being made; however, notification can be withheld if there is concern it may cause the caregiver to flee, harm the child, or cause significant disruption in the health care setting. Hospitalize the child if medically indicated or if there is a concern for the child's safety. The health care provider should also contact social services to assess the safety of the other children in the household, as well as the safety of the mother since domestic violence may also be occurring. When reporting laws allow and circumstances warrant it, contact animal control to assess the safety of family pets.

PREVENTION/PATIENT TEACHING

Primary Prevention

Primary prevention should aim at mitigating the risk factors of child abuse, including substance abuse, parenting difficulties, and poor impulse control. Health care providers can encourage positive parenting. Please see the American Academy of Pediatrics' Connected Kids Program at www.aap.org/connectedkids. Additional positive parenting support programs include parent education programs and support groups that focus on child development, age-appropriate expectations, and the roles and responsibilities of parenting; family support and family strengthening programs that enhance the ability of families to access existing services, and resources to support positive interactions among family members; and public awareness campaigns that provide information on how and where to report suspected child abuse and neglect. (See Table 8.1.)

Table 8.1

POSITIVE PARENTING RESOURCES

PROGRAM CATEGORY	DESCRIPTION	EXAMPLES
Public Awareness	Public Service Announcements (PSAs), posters, and brochures that promote healthy parenting, child safety, and how to report suspected abuse	Tips for Parents Sheets at Childwelfare.gov: www.childwelfare.gov/pubs/res_guide_2009/en_tips.pdf Brochures from the American Academy of Pediatrics' Connected Kids Program at www.aap.org/connectedkids
Skills-Based Curricula	Content includes child safety and protection skills; many of these programs focus on preventing sexual abuse	Anger Management Toolbox for Parents: www.joe.org/joe/2006december/tt4.php Darkness to Light—Child Sexual Abuse Prevention www.darkness2light.org
Parent Education	Help parents develop positive parenting skills and decrease behaviors associated with child abuse and neglect	The Nurturing Parents Program: www.nurturingparenting.com National Effective Parenting Initiative (NEPI): www.ciccparenting.org/cicc_effective.asp
Parent Support Groups	Parents work together to strengthen their families and build social networks	Parents Helping Parents: www.parentshelpingpar ents.org Circle of Parents: www.circleofparents.org
Home Visitation	Focuses on enhancing child safety by helping pregnant mothers and families with new babies or young children learn more about positive parenting and child development	Nurse Family Partnership: www.nursefamilypartnership.org National Healthy Start Association: www.healthy startassoc.org
Respite and Crisis Care	Offers temporary relief to caregivers in stressful situations by providing short-term care for their children	Local community-based agencies
Family Resource Centers	Works with community members to develop a variety of services to meet the specific needs of the people who live in surrounding neighborhoods	Local community-based agencies

This chart was adapted from the Child Welfare Information Gateway Factsheet on Child Abuse. Available online at www.childwelfare.gov/pubs/factsheets/preventingcan.cfm.

Secondary Prevention

Early detection of at-risk families, as well as children with less severe abuse, and appropriate intervention may prevent future abuse. Several strategies have been implemented to prevent child maltreatment. However, little data have supported the effectiveness of most prevention strategies. The most proven program that targets high-risk families is the Nurse-Family Partnership (NFP), which establishes a long-term professional relationship between a visiting nurse and an at-risk mother *prenatally*. This program has demonstrated, in repeated randomized control trials, efficacy in lowering maltreatment rates as measured by several outcomes.

Tertiary Prevention

The Child Welfare Information Gateway (2009) notes that tertiary prevention activities focus on families where maltreatment has already occurred, seek to reduce the negative consequences of the maltreatment, and prevent its recurrence. These prevention programs may include services such as intensive family preservation services with trained mental health counselors that are available to families 24 hours per day for 6 to 8 weeks; parent mentor programs with stable, nonabusive families acting as "role models" and providing support to families in crisis; parent support groups that help parents transform negative practices and beliefs into positive parenting behaviors and attitudes; and mental health services for children and families affected by maltreatment to improve family communication and functioning.

RESOURCES

Child Abuse State Reporting Phone Numbers: www.childwelfare.gov/pubs/reslist/rl_dsp.cfm?rs_id=5&rate_chno=11-11172
Child Abuse—Medline Plus: www.nlm.nih.gov/medlineplus/childabuse.html
Child Abuse—Office for Victims of Crime: http://www.ojp.usdoj.gov/ovc/help/ca.htm
Child Welfare Information Gateway: www.childwelfare.gov
Multi-Agency Identification and Investigation of Severe Nonfatal and Fatal Child Injury: Guidelines for Networking, Communication and Collaboration: http://ican-ncfr.org/trnCalEMAprotocol.asp
Nurse Family Partnership: www.nursefamilypartnership.org/index.cfm?fuseaction=home
Strengthening Families and Communities: www.childwelfare.gov/pubs/res_guide_2009/guide.pdf
Tips for Parents: www.childwelfare.gov/pubs/res_guide_2009/en_tips.pdf

REFERENCES

Child Welfare Information Gateway. (2009). *Child abuse and neglect fatalities: Statistics and interventions.* Retrieved from www.childwelfare.gov/pubs/factsheets/fatality.cfm

Kellogg, N., & the American Academy of Pediatrics Committee on Child Abuse and Neglect. (2007). Evaluation of suspected child physical abuse. *Pediatrics, 119,* 1232–1241.

Ricci, L., Botash, A., & McKenney, D. (2009). *Pediatrics, child abuse.* eMedicine. Retrieved from http://emedicine.medscape.com/article/800657-overview

U.S. Department of Health and Human Services, Administration on Children, Youth and Families. (2009). *Child maltreatment 2007.* Washington, DC: U.S. Government Printing Office.

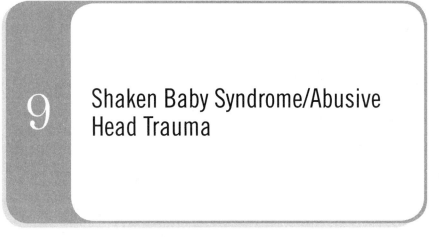

Shaken Baby Syndrome/Abusive Head Trauma

9

DEFINITION

Shaken baby syndrome (SBS), once referred to as shaken impact syndrome or whiplash-shaken infant syndrome and now referred to as abusive head trauma (AHT), refers to the signs, symptoms, clinical, radiographic, and sometimes autopsy findings that have resulted from the violent shaking of an infant or young child. It is a form of physical child abuse that can cause a myriad of neurological, cognitive, and other functional deficits. SBS is the most common cause of child abuse–related mortality, and it accounts for the most long-term disabilities in infants and young children due to physical child abuse. These disabilities include learning disorders, severe mental retardation, blindness, and paralysis.

Although the term "shaken baby syndrome" is well known and has been used for decades, advances in the understanding of the mechanisms and spectrum of injury associated with abusive head trauma compelled the American Academy of Pediatrics (AAP) to modify its terminology to keep pace with our understanding of pathologic mechanisms in May 2009. Shaking can cause neurologic injury, but so can blunt impact or the combination of shaking and blunt impact. The American Academy of Pediatrics recommends that pediatricians (and other health care providers) develop skills to recognize the manifestations of abusive head injury, including those caused by both shaking and blunt impact, consult with pediatric subspecialists when necessary, and embrace a less mechanistic term, "abusive head trauma," when describing an inflicted injury to the head and its contents.

The American Academy of Pediatrics further notes that the term "shaken baby syndrome" has become recognized, that prevention strategies for curtailing the incidence of AHT have been developed and researched, and that some states have mandated shaken baby syndrome education for parents of all newborns. The American Academy of Pediatrics recognizes the utility of maintaining the use of the term "shaken baby syndrome" for prevention efforts but recommends adoption of the term "abusive head trauma" as the diagnosis used in the medical chart to describe the constellation of cerebral, spinal, and cranial injuries that result from inflicted head injury to infants and young children. Health care providers are encouraged to use the term "abusive head trauma" (AHT); however, the term "shaken baby syndrome" will be used for the remainder of this chapter since it was derived from the SBS literature that focused on shaking as part of the abusive process.

PREVALENCE

There are no firm statistics on SBS because the challenges in detecting and reporting SBS have been difficult to overcome. However, the American Association of Neurological Surgeons (2000) notes there are an estimated 50,000 cases of SBS per year in the United States. Victims range from newborns to 4-year-olds, although the majority of cases occur before age 1year with an average age of 3 to 8 months. Most victims are male.

SBS can occur in any segment of society; however, involved infants and families may have unique demographic features that could be beneficial to screening and prevention efforts. Some possible characteristics include parents who are young, unmarried, not well-educated, and who did not seek prenatal care.

ETIOLOGY

The most common precipitating factor in SBS is inconsolable crying. The frustrated or angry caretaker loses control, grabs the baby by the chest, underarms, or arms, and violently shakes the infant. Most perpe-trators are male. The perpetrator is most often (in descending order): the father, the mother's boyfriend, a female babysitter, or the mother.

All models and theories have known limitations, and many clinicians and researchers acknowledge that precise mechanisms for all abusive in-juries remain incompletely understood. Shaking times vary, usually rang-ing from 5 seconds to 15 or 20 seconds, with an average of 2 to 4 shakes per second. During shaking, the head rotates on the cervical axis creat-ing multiple forces within the head. The child stops crying and breath-ing, causing decreased oxygenation, particularly to the brain. Lack of mylenization and the normally high water content of the infant brain make it softer than the adult brain, allowing the infant brain to become more easily distorted and compressed within the skull.

Shaking and the sudden deceleration of the head at the time of im-pact results in several problems:

- The veins that bridge from the brain to the dura are stretched and torn, creating the subdural hematoma or subarachnoid hemor-rhages that are characteristics of the syndrome.
- The brain strikes the inner surfaces of the skull, causing direct trauma to the brain itself.
- The axons can shear off during the commotion to the brain.
- Hypoxia causes further irreversible damage to the brain sub-stance.
- Damaged nerve cells release chemicals, which add to oxygen de-privation and cause direct further damage to the brain cells.

The combined effect of these problems creates massive traumatic destruction of the brain tissue, leading to immediate cerebral edema and increased intracranial pressure.

Associated injuries occur with the destruction of brain tissue. The most significant of these are *retinal hemorrhages*. The retinal hemor-rhages seen in SBS are variable, ranging from a few scattered hemor-rhages to extensive hemorrhages involving multiple layers of the retina. Retinal hemorrhages seen in other conditions are usually closer to the surface, so-called preretinal hemorrhages, and resolve quickly. A study by Odom et al. (1997) showed that retinal hemorrhages are rarely found af-ter chest compressions in pediatric patients with nontraumatic illnesses, and those that are found appear to be different from the hemorrhages found in SBS.

Other associated injuries include *skull fractures* resulting from the impact when the infant is thrown against a hard or soft surface; *fractures of the posterior arcs of the ribs* near the spine due to the levering of the fingers of the hands of the perpetrator while holding the baby during shaking; *clavicle fractures;* and *long bone fractures,* attributed to the flailing of the arms and legs during shaking; and bruising of the skin of the head, face, and body.

ASSESSMENT

General Principles

Health care professionals should keep the following principles in mind when examining children under age 2:

1. Incomplete or inaccurate assessment can result in serious or deadly consequences because further damage (retinal hemorrhage, cerebral edema, intracranial bleeding) may still be occurring after the attack has ended.
2. Detection is challenging due to perpetrator cover-up, inaccurate caregiver reporting, and the sometimes misleading physical findings, which can mimic problems such as mild viral illness, feeding dysfunction, or colic.
3. Signs and symptoms are variable, depending on the severity and length of the shaking and whether the infant was thrown onto a surface. SBS can be viewed as a continuum from a short duration of shaking with little or no impact, to severe, prolonged shaking with major impact.
4. The resulting signs and symptoms range from decreased responsiveness, irritability, lethargy and limpness, through vomiting from increased pressure within the skull, increased breathing rate, low body temperature and low heart rate, and convulsions, to coma with fixed and dilated pupils, and finally to death. These symptoms are due to generalized cerebral edema secondary to trauma, and they begin immediately after the shaking and reach their peak within 4–6 hours.
5. Possible symptoms include poor feeding, vomiting, lethargy, and/or irritability that occur intermittently or for days or weeks prior to health visit.

6. Frequently, if child is violently shaken into unconsciousness, the abuser will wait to seek help, hoping the child will awaken. The child is frequently brought in convulsing or comatose, not sucking or swallowing, unable to follow movements, and not smiling or vocalizing. Many of these infants have respiratory difficulty that can progress to apnea, as well as bradycardia, resulting in cardiopulmonary arrest.

7. The signs of SBS may suggest meningitis with a lumbar puncture that yields bloody cerebral spinal fluid (CSF). Centrifuged CSF that is xanthochromic (yellow-colored) should raise the suspicion of head trauma that is at least several hours old; it is not the result of a traumatic tap.

History and Physical Assessment

Interview all adults separately to minimize collaboration, and perform a psychosocial assessment. This may be accomplished by another qualified health professional if the child's condition requires your full attention. If the child is developmentally and physically capable of questioning, interview the child separately from the adults.

Be Aware of Red Flags

No explanation for the injury

No witnesses to the injury

Injury inconsistent with history

Injury inconsistent with physical findings

Injury inconsistent with child's developmental abilities

Delay in seeking care for the child

High-risk social situation

Previous suspicious injuries

One of the classic features of SBS is the lack of external injuries. When assessing infants and toddlers with nonspecific symptoms, such as fever, irritability, or vomiting, consider SBS in the differential diagnosis. Perform a complete physical examination, including assessment of head circumference and fontanels, and be alert to the minor and potentially misleading signs and symptoms of SBS: lethargy, irritability, excessive crying, feeding difficulty, vomiting, fever, apnea or respiratory difficulty, tremors, and developmental delay.

Assess for evidence of abdominal injuries and rib fractures (such as patterned bruising) due to the perpetrator grasping the child around the thorax. Observe for signs of long-bone fractures secondary to the flailing of the child's arms and legs. A fundoscopic exam should be performed by a pediatric ophthalmologist who is familiar with the retinal changes found in SBS. The diagnosis of child abuse should be seriously considered in children who present with apparent life-threatening events (ALTEs), and the evaluation of ALTEs should include fundoscopic examination since ALTEs and retinal hemorrhage (RH) are associated with child abuse (CA). In one study, Pitteti and associates (2002) found that RH was detected in 1 of 73 infants (under 24 months) with ALTE, and in 1of 3 infants who were victims of child abuse and presented with an ALTE. CA was detected in 2.3% of patients who presented with an ALTE.

Diagnostic Testing

Laboratory testing may reveal: *Mild to moderate anemia* (common in SBS); *clotting dysfunction* (coagulation study changes are common with brain trauma and are sometimes severe (disseminated intravascular coagulation [DIC]); *high amylase* levels may indicate pancreatic damage; *elevated transaminase* levels may indicate occult liver damage.

Chest roentgenograms may appear normal or show rib fractures. *Computed tomography (CT)* is the first line in imaging evaluation for a brain-injured child. CT is usually the method of choice for demonstrating subarachnoid hemorrhage, mass effect, and large extra-axial hemorrhages. The initial CT should be performed without contrast and should be assessed using soft-tissue and bone windows. CT should be repeated after a time interval or if the neurologic picture changes rapidly. However, CT often fails to show some aspects of the injury, and false-negative results occur, especially early in the evolution of cerebral edema.

Magnetic resonance imaging (MRI) is an excellent adjunct to CT in the evaluation of brain injury. It optimizes the detection and assessment of intracranial injury including intraparenchyymal hemorrhage, contusions, shearing injuries and edema, and it is sensitive for detecting significant spinal injury and previous parenchymal hemorrhage. But because of the lack of universal availability of technology, physical limitations of access to MRI when life-support is required for critically ill infants or children, and because of the relative insensitivity to subarachnoid blood and fractures, MRI is considered complementary to CT and should be obtained 2 to 3 days later if possible.

In the absence of significant accidental trauma, a posterior, intrahemispheric subdural hematoma noted on either CT or MRI is indicative of inflicted injury. CT and MRI can also assist in determining when the injuries occurred and in substantiating repeated injuries by documenting changes in the chemical states of hemoglobin in affected areas. Therefore, they provide evidence for intervention and criminal proceedings.

Once the infant's condition permits, obtain a *skeletal survey* of the hands, feet, long bones, skull, spine, and ribs to pinpoint orthopedic injuries. The survey should be performed with high-detail systems, as a single view of the entire infant ("babygram") is inadequate. Skeletal imaging should be repeated in 2 to 3 weeks as it may provide evidence of a healing injury that was not apparent on initial studies.

Scintigraphy, a nuclear medicine test that detects areas of increased or decreased bone metabolism, has demonstrated an increased sensitivity for detecting rib fractures. Some practitioners are utilizing this as a primary screening tool in suspected abuse cases.

INTERVENTION

Promptly report the suspected abuse to the proper authorities. Rapid reporting facilitates thorough investigation before the history becomes clouded by time or before the caregivers compare or invent explanations. Provide information regarding the chain of caretakers, as well as an interpretation of the likely scenario, timing, and nature of the involved injuries. Siblings and other children in the same environment may be in danger and/or have signs of inflicted trauma. Therefore, immediate medical and child protective assessments should be available to ensure the current and future safety of these children.

There is no difference in the actual treatment of unintentional versus intentional injuries in children. Detailed explanation of intensive treatment is beyond the scope of this book; however, the treatment team should consist of:

- A health care provider who can immediately resuscitate and stabilize the victim while diagnostic studies are performed.
- A diagnostic team, consisting of pediatric specialists in radiology, neurology, neurosurgery, and ophthalmology, and a pediatric specialist in child abuse. In areas where these specialists are not available, such as rural and medically underserved areas, utilize a regional consultation system.

This same team should conduct follow-up examinations to document and treat developmental, ocular, and neurological sequelae of trauma.

PREVENTION/PATIENT TEACHING

Primary Prevention

Some states have enacted legislation for hospital-based education programs to teach all parents about the dangers of shaking a child. For example, Pennsylvania law mandated the implementation of the Shaken Baby Syndrome Education Act (http://www.dsf.health.state.pa.us/health/cwp/view.asp?a=179&q=233012). This program replicates the Upstate New York SBS prevention program (http://www.wchob.org/shakenbaby/), which has demonstrated a near 50% reduction in the incidence of SBS in the regions where the education is offered.

During well-baby visits, assess parents for caretaker stress, discipline practices, response to crying, and substance abuse. Talk to parents about crying. Many parents become frustrated because they do not know what to expect, and have questions such as: "How much should a baby cry?" "Why won't the baby stop crying?" "Am I doing something wrong?" Educate them about the properties of early crying using the National Center for Shaken Baby Syndrome's *"Period of PURPLE Crying."*

P = peak

U = the unpredictability of crying bouts

R = resistance to soothing

P = painlike expression

L = long crying bouts

E = evening clustering

Some techniques to provide parents in managing their crying baby include:

When Your Baby Cries . . .

- Remember that the baby is not misbehaving; crying is a form of communication.
- Offer the baby a pacifier, toy, or other distraction.
- Make sure all of the baby's basic needs are met (food, clean diaper).
- Cuddle the baby close to you.
- Walk or console the baby.
- Sing to the baby or play soft music.
- Swaddle the baby.
- Take the baby for a ride in the car or use an infant swing.
- Call a friend, relative, or neighbor to give you support.
- Be patient; remember that the crying will come to an end.

If nothing else works, place the baby in his or her crib, making sure he or she is safe, close the door, and check on him or her about every 5 to 10 minutes.

- Take a break—exercise, listen to music.
- Call a crisis hotline if necessary.

No matter how angry you become, never shake your baby.

Talk to parents about the appropriate measures of choosing babysitters and other child care providers.

Secondary Prevention

The target populations who are at risk for SBS are parents with one or more risk factors. The risk factors include parents who are young, unmarried, less educated, and who had little or no prenatal care. Since most perpetrators of SBS are male, assure that at-risk fathers and boy-friends are targeted for teaching and counseling as needed.

Arrange for home visitation in the newborn and early infancy period for at-risk families. *Antenatal visits* are also helpful to assess parental coping, strengths and needs, and to screen for postpartum depression.

Assist in the development of community parent education programs and family resource centers in targeted neighborhoods or communities.

Tertiary Prevention

Prevention strategies focus on reducing the negative consequences associated with abuse, as well as preventing future episodes. Programs include intensive family preservation services, parent mentoring programs, and mental health services to improve family functioning.

RESOURCES

National Center on Shaken Baby Syndrome: www.dontshake.com
Shaken Baby Alliance: www.shakenbaby.com
Shaken Baby Syndrome: www.preventchildabuse.com/shaken.htm
Shaken Baby Syndrome Information Page of the National Institute of Neurological Disorders and Stroke: www.ninds.nih.gov/disorders/shakenbaby/shakenbaby.htm
Shaken Baby Syndrome: Rotational Cranial Injuries: www.aap.org/policy/t0039.html

REFERENCES

American Academy of Pediatrics Committee on Child Abuse and Neglect. (2001). Shaken baby syndrome: Rotational cranial injuries—technical report. *Pediatrics, 108*(1), 206–210.

American Association of Neurological Surgeons. (2000). *Shaken baby syndrome—a potentially deadly concern.* Retrieved from http://www.medem.com/MedLB/article_detaillb.cfm?article_ID=ZZZ9G8DUE8C&sub_cat=355

Christian, C., Block, R., & the American Academy of Pediatrics Committee on Child Abuse and Neglect. (2009). Abusive head trauma in infants and children. *Pediatrics, 123,* 1409–1411.

Gutierrez, F. (2004). Shaken baby syndrome: Assessment, intervention and prevention. *Journal of Psychosocial Nursing & Mental Health Services, 42*(12), 22–30.

Miehl, N. (2005). Shaken baby syndrome. *Journal of Forensic Nursing, 1*(3), 111–118.

Odom, A., et al. (1997). Prevalence of retinal hemorrhages in pediatric patients after in-hospital cardiopulmonary resuscitation: A prospective study. *Pediatrics, 99*(6), 3.

Pitteti, R., et al. (2002). Prevalence of retinal hemorrhages and child abuse in children who present with an apparent life-threatening event. *Pediatrics, 110*(3), 557–562.

Reese, R., & Kirschner, R. (n.d.). *Shaken baby syndrome/shaken impact syndrome.* Retrieved from http://www.dontshake.com/Audience.aspx?categoryID=8&PageName=SBS_SIS.htm

U.S. Department of Health and Human Services, Administration on Children, Youth and Families. (2006). *Child maltreatment 2004.* Washington, DC: U.S. Government Printing Office.

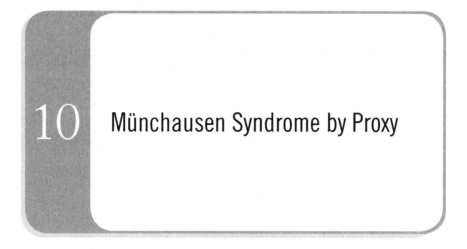

10   Münchausen Syndrome by Proxy

DEFINITION

Although a rare problem, Münchausen syndrome by proxy (MSBP, MSP) represents a form of physical and psychological child abuse, as well as neglect. It is difficult to diagnose and difficult to treat. Münchausen syndrome by proxy usually describes the deliberate production of, or feigning of, physical or psychological symptoms in another person who is under the individual's care. It usually involves a mother and young child; however, there are also cases of MSBP where persons produced or feigned illness in vulnerable adults and even pets.

The term "Münchausen syndrome by proxy" (MSBP) was first coined in 1977 by Roy Meadow when he published a report on a new form of child abuse. MSBP was named after 18th-century German dignitary Baron von Münchausen who was known for telling outlandish stories. MSBP has also been called Polle syndrome, named after Baron von Münchausen's only child. In 2002 the American Professional Society on the Abuse of Children (APSAC) suggested a new terminology, "pediatric condition falsification" (PCF).

MSBP is classified as factitious disorder by proxy in Appendix B ("Criteria Sets and Axes Provided for Further Study") of the *Diagnostic and Statistical Manual of Mental Disorders*, text revision (*DSM-IV-TR*; APA,

2000). The research criteria for MSBP include intentional production of, or feigning of, physical or psychological symptoms in a person under one's care; perpetrator motivated by assuming the sick role by proxy; external incentives (such as monetary gain) are absent; and the behavior is not better accounted for by another disorder (APA, 2000) Although the fabrication/induction of a pediatric illness is a mental health disorder, it is also a form of child abuse that carries the possibility of a fatal prognosis if the child is left in the home.

Subtypes of MSBP are characterized by frequency and intensity.

- *Chronic Münchausen by proxy* is distinguished by the constant pursuit of attention through inducing symptoms on another perpetrator. Perpetrators of this subtype are compulsive, and the disorder consumes most of their lives.
- *Episodic Münchausen by proxy* occurs in spurts with intervals when the perpetrator experiences symptoms of MSBP and intervals where the perpetrator lives a normal life.
- In *mild Münchausen by proxy,* perpetrators fabricate medical histories for their child and lie about their child being sick rather than actively causing sickness. These perpetrators crave the emotional gratification they receive from medical attention.
- In cases of *intense Münchausen syndrome by proxy,* the perpetrator resorts to measures such as inducing vomiting, poisoning, removing blood from the child, and suffocation. The perpetrator can induce severe illness in their own child, yet remain cooperative, concerned, and compassionate in the presence of health care providers.

PREVALENCE

The prevalence of MSPB is most likely more common than once estimated. The literature suggests rates from 200 to 625 per year, with some studies showing rates in specific populations, such as 1% of children with asthma and 5% of children with food allergies. However, these numbers are estimates, since they refer to those cases diagnosed and treated, usually in hospital settings.

ETIOLOGY

Research does not show a single cause for MSBP, but causes are thought to include the following: maternal history of abuse or reported abuse; rejection of the child; use of the child to maintain control; pathologic relationship with the child; and psychological reward received from the medical community because of the sick child. MSBP is also associated with psychiatric comorbidities, including Münchausen syndrome, somatoform disorder, factitious disorder, dissociative pseudologia phantastica (lies not totally improbable and often built on some truth), narcissistic and borderline personality disorders, sudden unexpected infant death syndrome, and pediatric condition falsification.

Perpetrators are usually the victim's biological mother (about 95% of cases), but may also be other caretakers such as fathers, stepparents, grandparents, and babysitters. Maternal perpetrators tend to be motivated by a psychological need to assume the sick role by proxy. External reasons for the behavior, such as financial gain, are absent and the behavior is not related to another psychiatric disorder. Life stressors and family dysfunction may also be present. Perpetrators of MSBP are often described as attentive and devoted caregivers. However, some are hostile, emotionally labile, and obviously dishonest. Perpetrators may have previous health care knowledge or training or may be fascinated with the medical field. Some try to establish close relationships with the health care staff, often becoming a source of support for staff members or the families of other patients. All can be deceiving and manipulative, and their ability to convince others should not be underestimated. These are not overanxious or overprotective caretakers; MSBP is premeditated, calculated, and unprovoked. They tend to be calm and collected when caught on camera inflicting harm on the child. The perpetrators rarely admit to their abusive behavior even when confronted with overwhelming evidence. They also know their behavior is wrong, demonstrated by the great care they take to conceal their actions. Perpetrators rarely have severe mental illness but may have personality disorders and a history of attention seeking, unusual family health problems, illness fabrication, and child abuse.

The maternal perpetrator's partner rarely plays an active role in the child's medical care and typically disengages from the family. Unsuspecting partners may support the perpetrators and unknowingly become passive accomplices of the ongoing abuse, while other partners may be abusive. Occasionally, abusive mothers may fabricate the child's illness to bring her partner back into her life.

Victims can be any age but are usually young children since this abuse generally starts early in life. Victims are equally male and female, but children most at risk are those aged 15 to 72 months. They frequently present with baffling symptoms and see multiple providers before a diagnosis of MSBP is made. Older victims may collude with their mothers by confirming the fabricated stories either out of fear of revenge or because of their mother's persuasion. Some may believe they have an illness that cannot be diagnosed; others may think that no one will believe them if they tell on the perpetrator.

ASSESSMENT

General Principles

When assessing children and their parents for possible diagnosis of MSBP, several characteristics may come into play, including the following:

- Relationships among the perpetrator, child, and health care provider may be long term and complex. This involvement may hinder the health care provider from considering MSBP as a differential diagnosis.
- There is no typical presentation of MSBP, and the range of symptoms is as variable as human imaginations. The biological mother is responsible for the event in 98% of the cases. Common characteristics of perpetrators include female, White, experiencing marital discord, having health care knowledge or training, friendly and cooperative with staff, very attentive to the child, and may have a history of abuse and/or psychiatric disorders.
- Perpetrators of MSBP may be help-seekers who search for medical attention for their children in order to communicate their own exhaustion, anxiety, or depression. Others may be active inducers who create their children's illnesses through dramatic measures. And finally, some may be "doctor addicts" who are obsessed with getting treatment for their children's nonexistent illnesses.
- Diagnosis of MSBP tends to be difficult because the signs and symptoms are undetectable (when exaggerated or imagined) or inconsistent (when induced or fabricated).

History and Physical Assessment

While the actual diagnosis of MSBP is for the perpetrator, the child remains a critical focus in making the diagnosis. There is no typical presentation. The literature notes more than 100 reported symptoms with the most common including lethargy, weight loss, fevers, abdominal pain, vomiting, diarrhea, seizures, apnea, infections, and bleeding. The American Academy of Pediatrics Committee on Child Abuse and Neglect suggests that providers ask themselves the following questions:

1. Are the history, signs, and symptoms of disease believable?
2. Is the child receiving unnecessary, harmful, or potentially dangerous testing and medical care?
3. If these are so, who is prompting the evaluations and treatment? The challenge is to connect the history and physical in a rational fashion.

Observe for warning signs:

- Illness that is multisystemic, prolonged, unusual, or rare
- Symptoms that are inappropriate or incongruent
- Multiple allergies to a wide variety of food and/or medications
- Symptoms that disappear when caretaker is absent
- One parent, usually the father, is absent during hospitalization
- History of seeking care at numerous other health care facilities ("medical wandering")
- Reluctance to let you contact previous health care providers or family and friends
- Parent angered by health care provider's inability to diagnose child
- History of sudden infant death syndrome (SIDS) in siblings
- Parent who is overly attached to the patient
- Parent who has medical knowledge/background ("medical sophistication")
- Normal or negative results on laboratory tests
- Blood in lab samples do not match the child's blood
- Chemicals in the child's blood, urine, or stool
- Child who has poor tolerance of treatment
- Parent who encourages medical staff to perform numerous tests and studies
- Parent who shows excessive concern for feelings of the medical staff

Consider MSBP in the differential diagnosis in the following presentations:

Complex pattern of illness and recurrent infections without physiologic explanation

Multiple infections with varied and unusual organisms

Seizure activity that does not respond to medication and that is only witnessed by the caretaker

Bleeding from anticoagulants, and poisons; use of caretaker's own blood or red colored substances to simulate bleeding

Vomiting from ipecac administration

Diarrhea induced from laxatives or salt administration

Hypoglycemia from insulin or hypoglycemic agents

Rashes from caustic substances, scratching or skin painting

Hematuria or rectal bleeding from trauma

Recurrent apparent life-threatening events (ALTE) from suffocation

Central nervous system depression, usually from drug administration

The American Academy of Pediatrics Committee on Child Abuse and Neglect notes that health care providers must substantiate the credibility of the signs and symptoms, determine the necessity and benefits of the medical care, and question who is the instigator of the evaluations and treatments. The presence of the following two factors are warranted to make the diagnosis of MSBP: a caregiver who is fabricating illness or pursuing unnecessary treatment, and harm or potential harm to the child from excessive intervention.

Diagnostic Testing

Health care providers may be tempted to order diagnostic tests that can be injurious, thus essentially adding to the abuse suffered by the child due to the factitious illness. Therefore, when facing an unusual presentation, health care providers should consider MSBP in the differential diagnosis, and investigate accordingly.

Diagnosis of MSBP cannot be made quickly; admission and consultation is usually necessary before the diagnosis can be proved. Admission allows for continuous observation by nursing and other supportive staff. Hospital rooms with covert video surveillance (CVS) have been recommended to capture a parent's misbehavior, as when a child is being physically abused in the hospital. The graphic evidence of abuse obtained through the use of CVS has been accepted by courts in many U.S. jurisdictions as evidence of MSBP. However, hidden cameras may also fail to confirm reported symptoms when they are being exaggerated or exonerate a suspected caregiver when disease does exist. These cameras may be used in highly suspicious cases, but require carefully developed protocols for their use. These protocols should involve child protective agencies, police, and hospital security to coordinate the use of these surveillance systems.

Evaluation should be based on symptoms and specific tests should be aimed at detecting the potential method by which factitious symptoms are being induced. Possible tests include urine toxicology screening, chemistry panels, electrocardiography (ECG), toxicology levels for suspected poisoning agents (medications and chemicals), cultures, coagulation studies, and head computed tomography (CT) scan.

INTERVENTION

MSBP requires mandatory reporting for child abuse and involvement of child protective services and most likely law enforcement. Treatment involves treating the perpetrator, the child (victim), and the family.

When confronting the offending parent, your suggestion to the mother that she is the cause of the child's illness may be met with denial and a focus on your diagnostic failure. Instead, be supportive and emphasize that recognizing the diagnosis is the first step toward returning the family to normalcy. The child must be separated from the perpetrator, which may be agreed to by parents who are intent on demonstrating their innocence, or may require court involvement. Visits must be restricted and closely observed by a person familiar with the syndrome who will directly observe every aspect of the visit, including intercepting any food or drink brought to the child.

The perpetrator requires referrals for evaluation and treatment. Assessment of the perpetrator should include physical examination, diagnostic testing, and psychological evaluations to determine if other problems exist. Psychotherapy will most likely focus on changing the thinking and behavior of the individual with the disorder (cognitive-behavioral therapy). Psychotherapy is also warranted to decrease anxiety, stressors, and other problems that perpetuate the illness. Parenting classes should be prescribed so that the perpetrator can learn to care for her children effectively while meeting her own needs.

Make sure the child is safe. Hospitalization may be warranted to keep the child safe from further abuse. Assure the safety of the siblings since they may be receiving the same type of abuse from the same parent. Medical interventions for the child victim of MSBP are aimed at relieving the symptoms and any injury made by the person who induced them.

The family will require therapy that should begin with education regarding MSBP and discussions about whether reunification of the perpetrator and child is possible. If there are other children at home, evaluate their health status and provide appropriate treatment as needed. All family members should receive therapy, and if the family is reunited, supervision is mandatory to ensure safety of the children.

PREVENTION/PATIENT TEACHING

Primary Prevention

Given that the cause of MSBP is unknown, methods of specific primary prevention are also unknown at this time.

Secondary Prevention

The best way to prevent MSBP from becoming a long-term disability is to diagnose it in its early stages. Therefore, health care providers need to know the warning signs of MSBP and should consider it in their differential diagnosis when faced with diagnostic dilemmas.

Tertiary Prevention

Children subjected to MSBP can develop serious long-term psychological and behavioral disorders, such as feeding disorders in infants; withdrawal, hyperactivity, and oppositional behaviors in preschoolers. Older children may display conversion symptoms, school problems, and signs of posttraumatic stress disorder (PTSD). All ages may demonstrate sleep problems. Therefore, it is critical that victims of MSBP begin psychological treatment as soon as possible to prevent or minimize long-term psychological effects.

RESOURCES

Mothers Against Münchausen Syndrome by Proxy Allegations (MAMA): www.msbp.com
Münchausen Syndrome by Proxy: www.medscape.com/viewarticle/430136_1

Münchausen Syndrome by Proxy: www.webmd.com/mental-health/tc/munchausen-syndrome-by-proxy-topic-overview
Münchausen Syndrome by Proxy: www.mayoclinic.com/health/munchausen-syndrome/DS00965

REFERENCES

American Psychiatric Association (APA). (2000). *Diagnostic and statistical manual of mental disorders* (4th ed., text rev.). Washington, DC: Author.

Cleveland Clinic. (2005). *Münchausen syndrome by proxy*. Retrieved from http://www.cleve landclinic.org/health/health-info/docs/2800/2822.asp?index=9834&src=news

Cyr, A. (2007). What is Münchausen syndrome by proxy? *Nursing, 17*(4), 30.

Lieder, H., Irving, S., Mauricio, R., & Graf, J. (2006). Münchausen syndrome by proxy: A case report. *AACN Clinical Issues, 16*(2), 176–184.

Maltack, J., Consolini, D., Mann, K., & Raab, C. (2006). Taking on the parent to save a child: Münchausen syndrome by proxy. *Contemporary Pediatrics, 23*(6), 50–59, 63.

Mason, J., & Poirier, M. (2007). *Münchausen syndrome by proxy*. eMedicine. Retrieved from www.emedicine.com/emerg/topic830.htm

Schreier, H., & Libow, J. (1993). *Hurting for love: Münchausen by proxy syndrome*. New York: Guilford Press.

Stirling, J., & the Committee on Child Abuse and Neglect. (2007). Beyond Münchausen syndrome by proxy: Identification and treatment of child abuse in a medical setting. *Pediatrics, 119*(5), 1026–1030.

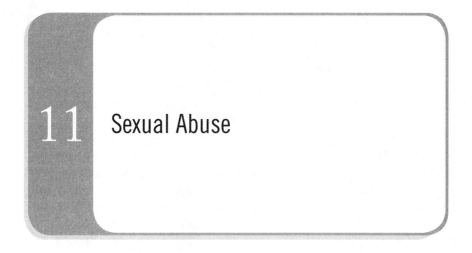

11   Sexual Abuse

All sexual assault victims need to be believed, taken seriously and supported, and all need to hear the words: "You can heal."

DEFINITION

Sexual abuse is contact or interaction between a child and an adult when the child is used for sexual stimulation by an adult. The American Academy of Pediatrics defines child sexual abuse as the engaging of a child in sexual activities that the child cannot comprehend, for which the child is developmentally unprepared and cannot give informed consent, and that violate the social taboos of society.

In the United States, minor children cannot consent to any sexual activity, but the legal age of consent may vary by state. Sexual activities involving a child may include activities intended for sexual stimulation, categorized as noncontact and contact abuse. *Noncontact sexual abuse,* which is common, includes exhibitionism, voyeurism, and the involvement of a child in verbal sexual propositions or the making of pornography. *Contact sexual abuse* ranges from *nonpenetrating* (sexual kissing and fondling) to *penetrating* (digital, penile, and object insertion into the vagina, mouth, or anus). *Rape* is a legal term used to define forced sexual intercourse that occurs because of physical force or psychological coercion. Legal terminology for sex crimes varies among jurisdictions.

All child health professionals should routinely identify those at high risk for or with a history of abuse, and primary pediatric health care providers will most likely encounter sexually abused children in their practices and may be asked for consultation.

Evaluations of sexual abuse require knowledge of normal and abnormal sexual behaviors, physical signs of sexual abuse, appropriate diagnostic tests for sexually transmitted infections, and the differential diagnosis of medical conditions confused with sexual abuse. However, because the evaluation of suspected victims of child sexual abuse often involves careful questioning, evidence-collection procedures, and specialized examination techniques and equipment, many health care providers do not feel prepared to conduct these assessments.

Health care providers should either complete education and practicum in sexual abuse evaluations or refer children to a Children's Advocacy Center (probably the best place for a child sexual assault examination because it uses a highly trained multidisciplinary team) or another child sexual assault forensic specialist. Many jurisdictions utilize trained examiners (generally Sexual Assault Nurse Examiners, or SANE teams) to perform evidence collection and to provide initial contact with the aftercare resources of the center.

In such cases, the health care provider can confidently defer the forensic examination to the SANE since studies have repeatedly demonstrated their accuracy. Health care providers should still be diligent and exacting in their general examination and in their documentation. Discrepancies between the health care provider record and the SANE report can sow doubt about the facts of the case in the minds of juries, and defense lawyers will not fail to exploit such discrepancies.

(Please also refer to Chapter 3, "Forensic Assessment and Documentation," and Chapter 4, "Principles of Evidence," for further information relevant to child sexual abuse.)

PREVALENCE

Child sexual abuse is reported up to 80,000 times a year. However, the number of unreported instances is far greater. Children and adolescents are afraid and/or ashamed to disclose the abuse, and the legal procedures for validating an episode are difficult. Research suggests that approximately 1% of children experience some form of sexual abuse each year, resulting in the sexual victimization of 12% to 25% of girls and 8% to 10% of boys by 18 years of age.

ETIOLOGY

The question of what causes an individual to become a sexual offender has attracted considerable scientific attention over the past several years. Theoretical models focus primarily on a single or small cluster of causal factors, including biological mechanisms in the onset of sexually deviant behavior; postulating that genetic determinants, hormone imbalances, or both are responsible for sexual aggression.

Other theorists point to brain abnormalities, as well as attachment disturbances with insecurely attached boys with emotionally unsupportive parents being more likely to become sexual predators later in life. Social learning theory notes that children learn from their social environments, and that if those childhood social environments include violence, abuse, and the degradation of women, the propensity to mimic those behaviors is strengthened. These reasons have led some theorists to suggest that the graphic violence on television, in conjunction with the portrayal of women as submissive and sexualized, desensitizes children to violence and promotes sexual aggression. Although these theories have supportive evidence, none of them can account for all instances of sexual violence. Etiological pathways to sexual offending are multiple and complex, and thus, more recent models have attempted to incorporate several, or all, of these individual factors.

Groth's Typology for Child Sexual Abusers (Groth & Birnbaum, 1978) is an older model, but it provides a framework for understanding into child abusers.

> *Fixated child sexual abusers* have sexual desires and preferences that center around children. They are unlikely to have healthy sexual contacts with age–appropriate partners, and they tend to be emotionally immature, and are preoccupied with children. These individuals usually go to great lengths to establish "relationships" with more vulnerable children, often using extensive grooming and premeditation.

Regressed child sexual abusers have "normal" sexual interests toward and encounters with appropriate partners. They do not tend to be interested sexually in children; however, they turn to sexual contact with children as a means of coping or as a substitute for an appropriate partner during times of considerable stress in their lives. Thus, their behaviors may be more situational, opportunistic, and impulsive.

RAPE TRAUMA SYNDROME

Rape trauma syndrome (RTS) is a form of posttraumatic stress disorder (PTSD) that often affects rape survivors. Not all rape survivors experience RTS, and those who do experience it have varied reactions than can range from severe to none at all. There are three main phases of RTS:

The acute phase. The acute phase of RTS usually occurs right after an assault and typically lasts for several weeks after the attack. Rape survivors may display "expressed" or "controlled" emotional responses during the acute phase. People with controlled response may seem withdrawn, resistant to talking, silent, distracted, numb, or disconnected from their feelings. Survivors may also experience changes in sleeping and eating habits and may also be extremely aware of their physical surroundings.

The reorganization phase. During this phase, the initial shock fades and survivors face the reality of the event. This can last for months or years and can be very painful. Survivors sometimes feel guilty or ashamed; some may hate their bodies and use unhealthy eating patterns or other behaviors to punish themselves. Some do other things that seem out of character, such as withdrawing from activities and people that they usually enjoy or engaging in self-destructive or risky behaviors such as substance abuse and cutting, as a way to block the feelings that they are experiencing.

The resolution phase. In this phase, survivors come to terms with their experiences. They may still feel the emotional experiences of the assault, but now begin to focus on recovering and moving forward with their lives. Survivors in the resolution phase can still experience flashbacks and nightmares about the assault, usually triggered by certain sounds, places, or smells that remind survivors of the assault.

ASSESSMENT

General Principles

Sexually abused children may present to medical settings with a variety of symptoms and signs. Since they are often coerced into secrecy by the perpetrator, the health care provider needs a high level of suspicion and may need to carefully and appropriately question the child to detect sexual abuse in these situations. Presenting symptoms may be so general or nonspecific (such as sleep disturbances, abdominal pain, enuresis, encopresis, or phobias) that caution must be exercised when the pediatrician considers sexual abuse because the symptoms may indicate physical or emotional abuse or other stressors unrelated to sexual abuse.

Certain equipment and supplies are essential to the exam process, even though they may not be used in every case. These include a copy of the most current exam protocol used by the jurisdiction, standard exam room equipment and supplies, comfort supplies for patients, sexual assault evidence collection kits, an evidence drying device/method, a camera, testing and treatment supplies, an alternate light source, and written materials for patients. A *colposcope* or other magnifying instrument is strongly suggested. Some jurisdictions are using telemedicine to allow examiners offsite consultation with medical experts by using computers, software programs, and the Internet. Telemedicine is especially helpful in rural areas.

HISTORY

When it is suspected that a child is being sexually abused, a behavioral, social, gynecologic, and general medical history is required. Health care providers need to obtain detailed information about the current incident of sexual abuse to ensure that all needed evidence is properly collected. Investigative interviews will most likely be conducted by social services and/or law enforcement agencies; however, health care providers still need to ask relevant questions to obtain a detailed pediatric history and a review of systems that includes the medical history, past incidents of abuse or suspicious injuries, and menstrual history (when appropriate). The history should also include information helpful in determining necessary diagnostic tests, how to interpret medical findings when present, and what medical and mental health services should be provided to the child and family.

Interview the child and parent separately and ascertain reason for visit:

1. Children may be seen for routine wellness examination or for an episodic illness visit that includes sexual abuse as part of the differential diagnosis.
2. Children have been or are thought to have been sexually abused and are brought in by a parent for evaluation.
3. Children are brought in by social service or law enforcement personnel for evaluation of possible abuse as part of an examination.
4. Children are brought to the emergency department after a suspected episode of abuse for evaluation, evidence collection, and crisis management.

Assess presenting symptoms. Symptoms may be vague: abdominal pain, headache, fatigue, enuresis, encopresis, sleep problems, phobias, decreased appetite, and hyperactivity; or specific: genital or rectal bleeding, sexually transmitted diseases, and developmentally unusual sexual behavior.

Obtain history of behavioral indicators.

- Under age 5: regression, feeding or toileting disturbances, temper tantrums, requests for frequent panty changes, and seductive behavior

- Ages 5 to 10: school problems, night terrors, sleep problems, anxieties, withdrawal, refusal of physical activity, and inappropriate behaviors

- Adolescence: school problems, running away, delinquency, promiscuity, drug and alcohol abuse, eating disorders, depression, and other significant psychological problems, such as suicide attempts

When assessing adolescent females, obtain the gynecologic history and include the following: date of last menstrual period, number of pregnancies, possible gynecologic surgery or traumatic injury to the genital area, date of the last consensual intercourse and use of contraceptives, prior sexually transmitted infections.

Obtain family and social histories to understand the environment in which the abuse occurred, and obtain a brief developmental history, which may be critical in legal aspects of a child's case.

Health care providers need to follow local statutes and protocols when evaluating sexual abuse cases. In many situations, the forensic (investigative) interview will be performed with the assistance of trained law enforcement officials and/or social workers from child protective services. The forensic interview differs from a good medical history, and thus, both are necessary. The forensic interview is essential to prosecution of a case and is often a critical aspect of the evaluation; is mostly concerned with detailed answers to who, what, where, and when the abuse occurred; should not replace the medical history obtained by the health care provider from the child.

Questions regarding the incident should be focused but not leading. For example, instead of asking, "What did Jake do to hurt you?" ask a series of questions that include, "What are some things that Jake does that you like?"; "What are some things that Jake does that you don't like?" Children with special communication needs, including children with developmental disabilities, may require sign language, use of assistive devices, or illustrations. The record should clearly document who was present when the child disclosed the information, what question or activity prompted the disclosure, and, if possible, the exact words spoken recorded in quotation marks.

Physical Assessment

The examination should not result in additional trauma for the child. Health care providers should explain the examination to the child before it is performed and should allow a supportive adult not suspected of involvement in the abuse to be present during the examination unless the child prefers otherwise. Children may be anxious about giving a history, being examined, or having procedures performed, and thus adequate time must be allotted to relieve the child's anxiety. This means that these examinations cannot be performed adequately by a primary care or emergent provider who has a waiting room full of patients in need of care.

Preparation of the child and family should include explaining the following in language that both the child and family can comprehend:

1. The fact that almost all prepubertal children do not need a speculum or internal examination;
2. Information on the use of cotton-tipped swabs to check for infections (if determined that these will be needed);
3. If a colposcope will be used for the examination, children should be allowed to see the equipment and look through the eyepieces or at the video screen;
4. Parents and older children should be informed about the use of equipment and given the opportunity to consent to the use of photographs for legal documentation. (Consent for photographs may not be warranted if the case is under investigation; however, it is still recommended that consent be obtained.)

Physical examination alone is not often diagnostic unless accompanied by history and laboratory findings. Physical findings are often absent even if the perpetrator admits to penetration. Many types of sexual abuse leave no physical evidence, and mucosal injuries heal quickly. Children suspected of being sexually abused may need an examination emergently, urgently, or electively scheduled for a later time.

Emergent examinations. Children with a history of sexual contact within 96 hours of presentation should be examined for evidence of sexual abuse. Utilize a sexual assault exam kit if the child presents for an examination within 96 hours of the sexual abuse. (*Do not refer to this kit as a "rape kit."* Rape kits are what rapists keep in the trunks of their cars.) Children with acute bleeding or injury should be examined immediately, as should children in severe emotional crisis. Children exposed to HIV-positive alleged perpetrators need to begin HIV postexposure prophylaxis within 36 hours of exposure, and adolescents who desire pregnancy prevention need to be evaluated within 120 hours.

Urgent examinations. Indications for an urgent examination include vaginal discharge, the possibility of STIs, and pregnancy in the pubertal child. These may take place within 2–3 days of an incident of sexual abuse.

Delayed examinations. These are the most common because children generally do not disclose abuse until they feel safe. Delayed exams may occur months or years after the incident of abuse, and many exams are warranted based on behavioral signs in children who have not disclosed.

Perform a complete assessment, unless otherwise indicated. Evaluate child for signs of physical and emotional abuse (see Chapter 8). Pay close attention to the areas involved in sexual activity: the mouth, breasts, genitals, perineal region, buttocks, and anus. In female children, the examination should include inspection of the medial aspects of the thighs, labia majora and minora, clitoris, urethra, periurethral tissue, hymen, hymenal opening, fossa navicularis, posterior fourchette, perineum, and perianal tissues. Male exams should focus on the thighs, penis, scrotum, perineum, and perianal tissues. Carefully document signs of trauma using detailed diagrams or photography.

Proper positioning of the prepubertal child for the genitalia examination enables better visualization. Common positions include the supine-frog-leg position, the knee-chest position, and use of the labial traction technique, but some health care providers use a technique with a Foley catheter to get a better view of the hymen or utilize water to "float" the hymen for better visualization. Examine male genitalia with the child supine or standing. Begin both examinations by assessing sexual maturity (Tanner Scale).

Physical signs of sexual abuse are rare. Most females have normal findings, possibly because of the elasticity of the hymenal tissue and genital mucosa and rapid healing of any injuries, but most likely because forced penetration is not common. Normal findings in prepubertal girls include a crescent-shaped hymen, midline avascular areas, periurethral bands, longitudinal intravaginal ridges, superior and lateral notches, and some bumps and hymenal tags. Other anatomical configurations of the hymen normally observed in prepubertal girls are annular hymen, fimbriated hymen, septate hymen, and microperforate hymen.

Findings consistent with sexual abuse in prepubertal girls may include lacerations and bleeding of the genital area or more subtle chronic findings. Hymenal findings should be documented by noting the location using the clock analogy, documented on a body diagram and photographed. A hymenal tear may result in a healed transection of the hymen; however, these may heal completely over time, leaving no signs of trauma or scarring. Absence of all or part of the hymen, particularly in the posterior portion of the hymenal ring, should be confirmed using different examination positions or techniques. Hymenal tissue may be adherent to part of the vaginal wall, and using a moist swab or drops of water to loosen the edge should clarify the finding.

It is not necessary to measure the vaginal introital diameter. If the diameter appears large, the hymenal rim should be observed for signs of narrowing and attenuation or absence of tissue. Superficial notches in the hymen may be a normal finding, but fresh lacerations or tears located in the genital area without a history of accidental trauma should be documented. Digital or speculum examinations should not be performed on the prepubertal child unless under anesthesia and then only when warranted (such as for suspected foreign body). Digital examinations of the rectum are not necessary.

Findings of abuse in boys may include injuries to the glans, shaft of the penis, or scrotum.

It is unusual to find anal changes in either gender. However, there may be scars, distorted or irregular folds, flattening of the anal folds, and poor anal tone. Adolescents warrant a speculum examination, which will also be utilized to obtain appropriate STI cultures.

Inspect other areas of the body for signs of injury, including the oral pharynx for bruises to the hard or soft palate. The extremities should be inspected for defensive wounds, as well as grasp, rope, or tie marks.

Differential Diagnosis

As with other forms of child abuse, certain conditions and disorders can mimic sexual abuse, and thus health care providers need to carefully consider the following as possible differential diagnoses:

- Some symptoms may be nonspecific, such as erythema of the vulva.
- Bruises that are widespread can be a sign of a bleeding disorder.
- Lichen sclerosis is a dermatologic condition that is manifested by genital soreness and subpendymal hemorrhages. It usually affects the vulva and perianal regions and has an hourglass appearance.

- Treptococcal infection can produce marked redness and vaginal discharge.
- Foul-smelling discharge may indicate a foreign body.
- Poor hygiene and pinworm infestation can cause redness and pruritus.
- Other nonsexually transmitted organisms, such as Candida, can cause discharge.
- The anal/rectal lesions of Crohn's disease may be mistaken for abuse.

Diagnostic Testing

Consider the following factors in deciding which STIs to test for, when to test, and which anatomic sites to test: age of the child, type(s) of sexual contact, time lapse from last sexual contact, signs or symptoms suggestive of an STD, family member or sibling with an STD, abuser with risk factors for an STD, request/concerns of child or family, prevalence of STDs in the community, presence of other examination findings, and patient/parent request for testing.

Universal screening of postpubertal patients is recommended—as is a pregnancy test for postpubertal females, but more selective criteria are often used for testing prepubertal patients. Vaginal, rather than cervical, samples are adequate for STI testing in prepubertal children. Given the prolonged incubation period for human papillomavirus (HPV) infections, a follow-up examination several weeks or months after the initial examination may be indicated. The family and patient should be informed about the potential for delayed presentation of lesions.

Testing before any prophylactic treatment is preferable to prophylaxis without testing. The identification of an STI in a child may have legal significance as well as implications for treatment, especially if there are other sexual contacts of the child or perpetrator. Cultures are considered the "gold standard" for diagnosing *Chlamydia trachomatis* (cell culture) and *Neisseria gonorrhoeae* (bacterial culture).

The colposcope is generally considered state of the art for most expert child sexual abuse evaluations. It is used to document normality and for comparison to cases in which children later return with abnormal findings and is useful for both clinical and legal purposes. The colposcope can be used to address altered body image, identify discrepancies in examinations, provide information to the nonoffending parent, and assist the forensic examiner by magnifying the image onto a video screen

or using optics. These images can provide legal evidence, possibly reduce the child's anxiety, and can be used as a teaching and research tool.
When a colposcope is not available, use an otoscope to enhance magni-
fication and photographs.

INTERVENTION

The most important intervention is the health care professional's gentle
reassurance that the child is now safe and that efforts will be made to
ensure continued safety. Reassure the child and family that there is no
permanent genital damage (in most cases), but take care to avoid promises that cannot be kept.

Initiate treatment for identified STI in prepubertal children. Prophylaxis is not usually indicated for STDs in prepubertal children but
may be considered in adolescents. Adolescents should also receive counseling on possible pregnancy. Prophylaxis for HIV should be considered
if the sexual contact was within 36 hours. Treatment depends on local
protocols, and in most cases, consultation with infectious disease experts
is needed.

Refer for mental health counseling in almost every case of child sexual abuse. A children's advocacy center or victim intervention program
can provide an advocate for the child and family. The advocate will assist
them through the legal process and help assure they get proper medical
follow-up.

PREVENTION/PATIENT TEACHING

Primary Prevention

Health care providers can provide parent teaching to help parents reduce their child's risk of being sexually abused.

Although you can never completely protect your child from sexual
abuse, you can do your best to drastically minimize her chances of being
abused:

Preschoolers

Teach her the proper name for body parts, including genitals and
breasts.

Tell her that no one—strangers, friends, or relatives—has the right to touch her private parts (parts coved by a bathing suit) or hurt her.

Tell her it's okay to say "NO" to people who make her feel scared, uncomfortable, or embarrassed.

Instruct her to tell you if adults ask her to keep secrets.

School-Aged Children

Give her straightforward information about sex.

Reinforce that her body belongs to her and that no one has the right to touch her private parts.

Explain that some grown-ups have problems and are confused about sex and that these adults may try to do things that make her feel uncomfortable.

Teach her personal safety and to get away from those adults who make her feel uncomfortable.

Tell her to come to you immediately if such an adult bothers her.

Teenagers

Explain that unwanted sex is an act of violence, not an act of love.

Discuss rape, date/acquaintance rape.

Reinforce her right to say "NO."

But remember, sexual abuse can occur under your own roof—family members, babysitters—so keep the lines of communication open at all times. Listen to your children and be alert for unusual behaviors from them and others in your household.

Secondary Prevention

Assess for and intervene with risk factors:

Parent abused as a child

Multiple caretakers for the child

Caretaker or parent who has multiple sexual partners

Drug and/or alcohol abuse

Stress associated with poverty

Social isolation and family secrecy

Child with poor self-esteem or other vulnerable state

Other family members abused

Gang member associations

Tertiary Prevention

Counseling is recommended to prevent or minimize the complications of sexual abuse. Sexually abused children and adolescents can suffer a range of short- and long-term problems that include depression, anxiety, guilt, fear, sexual dysfunction, withdrawal, eating disorders, substance abuse, promiscuity, and acting out. Many of these problems can continue into adulthood. Revictimization is also a common phenomenon among adults abused as children, and studies have shown that they are more likely to be the victims of rape or to be involved in physically abusive relationships than adults with no abuse history.

RESOURCES

Child Sexual Abuse—MedLine Plus: www.nlm.nih.gov/medlineplus/childsexualabuse.html

National Center for Victims of Crime: www.ncvc.org/ncvc/main.aspx?dbName=DocumentViewer&DocumentID=32315

National Children's Advocacy Center: www.nationalcac.org

A National Protocol for Sexual Assault Medical Forensic Exams Adult/Adolescents: www.ncjrs.gov/pdffiles1/ovw/206554.pdf

Rape, Abuse & Incest National Network: www.rainn.org

Sexual Assault Nurse Examiner (SANE) Development & Operation Guide: www.ovc.gov/publications/infores/sane/saneguide.pdf

REFERENCES

Botash, A. (2008). *Pediatrics, child sexual abuse.* Retrieved from http://emedicine.medscape.com/article/800770-overview

Ernoehazy, W., & Murphy-Lavoie, H. (2008). *Sexual assault.* eMedicine. Retrieved from http://emedicine.medscape.com/article/806120-overview

Groth, A. N., & Birnbaum, H. J. (1978). Adult sexual orientation and attraction to underage persons. *Archives of Sexual Behavior, 7*(3), 175–181.

Kellogg, N., & the Committee on Child Abuse and Neglect. (2005). The evaluation of sexual abuse in children. *Pediatrics, 116,* 506–512.

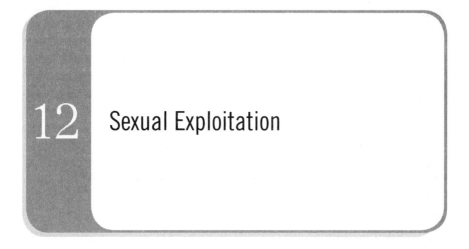

12 Sexual Exploitation

DEFINITIONS

Child sexual exploitation is a complex problem that involves possession, manufacture, and distribution of child pornography; online enticement of children for sexual acts; child prostitution; child sex tourism; and trafficking. *Commercial sexual exploitation of children* (CSEC) exists for economic gain. It involves physical abuse, pornography, prostitution, and the smuggling of children for unlawful purposes. Children throughout the world are kidnapped and sold into the illegal sex industry; some are sold by impoverished families who sell their children to traffickers in the hope of giving the children a better life. Children may be held captive in slavelike conditions where they are beaten, malnourished, threatened, and sexually exploited. In the United States, children are more likely to be sexually exploited for monetary gain by family and friends. This cycle of exploitation begins when an adult family member or friend sexually abuses a minor child, escalates to systematic sexual behavior involving multiple children, and then photographs and/or videotapes the sexual abuse and distributes it via the Internet.

Child Prostitution

Prostitution is illegal in most places of the United States and minors who take money for sex are usually taking part in that illegal activity; however, they are also victims of crime. Most minors who become involved in prostitution are runaway or throwaway children from abusive or otherwise dysfunctional homes. They are usually lured into prostitution by sophisticated criminals (frequently pimps) who convince them that they will earn money to survive and they will be taken care of in a secure, loving environment that they lacked at home. However, the pimps take the child's money and often engage in severe physical abuse to build a relationship of dependency.

Child Pornography

Federal law defines *child pornography* as any visual depiction, including any photograph, film, video, picture, or computer or computer-generated image or picture, whether made or produced by electronic, mechanical, or other means, of sexually explicit conduct, where:

- The production of the visual depiction involves the use of a minor engaging in sexually explicit conduct
- The visual depiction is a digital image, computer image, or computer-generated image that is, or is indistinguishable from, that of a minor engaging in sexually explicit conduct
- The visual depiction has been created, adapted, or modified to appear that an identifiable minor is engaging in sexually explicit conduct

Federal law also criminalizes knowingly producing, distributing, receiving, or possessing with intent to distribute, a visual depiction of any kind, including a drawing, cartoon, sculpture, or painting, of a child that:

- Depicts a minor engaging in sexually explicit conduct and is obscene.
- Depicts an image that is, or appears to be, of a minor engaging in graphic bestiality, sadistic or masochistic abuse, or sexual intercourse, including genital-genital, oral-genital, anal-genital, or oral-anal, whether between persons of the same or opposite sex and such depiction lacks serious literary, artistic, political, or scientific value.

Sexually explicit conduct is defined under federal law as actual or simulated sexual intercourse (including genital-genital, oral-genital, anal-genital, or oral-anal, whether between persons of the same or opposite sex), bestiality, masturbation, sadistic or masochistic abuse, or lascivious exhibition of the genitals or pubic area of any person.

Human Trafficking

Human trafficking is modern-day slavery. It is the recruitment, harboring, transportation, provision, or obtaining of a person for labor or services through the use of force, fraud, or coercion for the purpose of involuntary servitude, debt bondage (peonage), or slavery. Trafficking is different from smuggling, which is the crime of getting paid to assist another in illegally crossing a border. However, if the smuggler sells or brokers the smuggled individual into a condition of servitude, or if the smuggled individual is forced to work the debt off, the crime turns from smuggling into human trafficking. Contrary to a common assumption, human trafficking is not just a problem in other countries—cases have been reported in all 50 states, Washington, DC, and some U.S. territories.

Victims of human trafficking are young children, teenagers, men, and women who are subjected to force, fraud, or coercion to compel them to engage in commercial sex or involuntary labor. Any child who has engaged in commercial sex is a victim of human trafficking. Approximately 600,000 to 800,000 victims are trafficked across international borders annually, and more than half of these victims worldwide are children. Child victims of trafficking:

- Are exploited for commercial sex, including prostitution, pornography, and sex tourism.
- Are exploited for labor, including domestic servitude, migrant farming, landscaping, and hotel or restaurant work.
- Most frequently come from the Pacific Islands, the former Soviet Union, Latin America, Southeast Asia, and Africa as well as developing countries.
- Can be trafficked by close family members.

The reasons for coming to the United States vary, but most children succumb to exploitation under the guise of opportunity. They may believe they are coming to the United States to be united with family, to work in a legitimate job, or to attend school. Children may also be subject to psychological intimidation or threats of physical harm to self or family members.

Child Sex Tourism

Sex tourism is defined as traveling to a foreign country with the intent to engage in sexual activity with a child. Sex tourism is a lucrative industry that spans the globe. Asian countries, including Thailand, India, and the Philippines, have long been prime destinations for child-sex tourists, but in recent years, tourists have increasingly traveled to Mexico and Central America for their sexual exploits as well. Child sex tourists are individuals that travel to foreign countries to engage in sexual activity with children. End Child Prostitution, Child Pornography, and the Trafficking of Children (ECPAT) estimates that more than 1 million children worldwide are drawn into the sex trade each year (United Nations Children's Fund, 2007). Child sex tourists are usually males who come from all income brackets. Most perpetrators hail from Western European nations and North America, including the United States—it is a crime for a U.S. citizen or permanent resident to travel abroad to have sex with a minor, and it is a crime for a U.S. citizen or permanent resident to actually have sex with a minor while abroad.

The child sex tourism trade profits from the exploitation of child prostitutes in developing countries. The lives of child prostitutes, many of whom are younger than 10, are appalling. Studies indicate that these children serve between 2 and 30 clients per week, leading to a shocking estimated base of anywhere between 100 to 1,500 clients per year, per child (U.S. Department of Justice Child Exploitation and Obscenity Section, n.d.-a). Child prostitutes live in constant fear: fear of sadistic acts by clients, fear of being beaten by pimps, and fear of being apprehended by the police. Not surprisingly, victims often suffer from depression, low self-esteem, substance abuse, and feelings of hopelessness, leading many to suicide.

Many also suffer from physical ailments, including tuberculosis, exhaustion, infections, and physical injuries resulting from violence inflicted upon them. Sexually transmitted infections run rampant among these children, and they rarely receive medical treatment until they are seriously or terminally ill. Living conditions are poor, and meals are inadequate and irregular. Children who fail to earn enough money are punished severely, often through beatings and starvation. While child sex tourism involves children who are living outside the United States, health care providers can still help minimize this problem by participating in campaigns to stop this horrible crime.

PREVALENCE

The U.S. Department of Justice estimates the number of children involved in prostitution, child pornography, and trafficking to be between 100,000 and 3 million. About 293,000 American youth are currently at risk of becoming victims of commercial sexual exploitation (U.S. Department of Justice Child Exploitation and Obscenity Section, n.d.-b). However, these children are often difficult to locate, reluctant to acknowledge their age and exploitation, and potentially engaged by multiple institutions that do not routinely share information; thus, it is extremely difficult to assess accurately the true nature and extent of the problem.

Approximately 55% of street girls engage in formal prostitution, and 75% work for a pimp. Pimp-controlled CSEC is linked to escort and massage services, private dancing, drinking and photographic clubs, major sporting and recreational events, major cultural events, conventions, and tourist destinations. Approximately one-fifth of these children become entangled in nationally organized crime networks and are trafficked throughout the United States by a variety of means—cars, buses, vans, trucks, or planes—and are often provided counterfeit identification to use in the event of arrest. The average age at which girls first become victims of prostitution is 12–14. For boys and transgender youth, the average age of entry into prostitution is 11–13.

ETIOLOGY

Unfortunately, much of the etiology boils down to greed, since predators exploit children for monetary purposes. There are also correlates with each type of sexual exploitation.

Child Pornography

There is limited research about the motivations of people who possess child pornography, but Wolak, Mitchell, and Finkelhor (2003) suggest that child pornography possessors are a diverse group, including people who are:

- Sexually interested in prepubescent children or young adolescents and who use child pornography for sexual fantasy and gratification,
- Sexually "indiscriminate," and are thus constantly looking for new and different sexual stimuli,
- Sexually curious, downloading a few images to satisfy their curiosity,
- Interested in child pornography to profit financially by selling images or setting up Web sites requiring payment for access.

In a study by Wolak et al. (2005) of 1,713 people arrested for the possession of child pornography over a 1-year period, the possessors ran the gamut in terms of income, education level, marital status, and age. Virtually all of those who were arrested were men, 91% were White, and most were unmarried at the time of their crime, either because they had never married (41%) or because they were separated, divorced, or widowed (21%). Forty percent of those arrested were "dual offenders," who sexually victimized children and possessed child pornography, with both crimes discovered in the same investigation. An additional 15% were dual offenders who attempted to sexually victimize children by soliciting undercover investigators who posed online as minors (Wolak et al., 2005).

The producers of pornography create the pornography for economic reasons. Based on information provided by law enforcement to the National Center for Missing and Exploited Children's (NCMEC) Child Victim Identification Program, more than half of the child victims of pornography were abused by someone who had legitimate access to them such as parents, other relatives, neighborhood/family friends, babysitters, and coaches.

Prostitution

Prostitution is a very classic example of a crossover of victim blended with offender. Selling sex for money is illegal in most areas of the United States. The person selling sex, male or female, is an offender in the eyes of the law regardless of age. However, many young people who sell sex have a history of sexual violence in their past. Child sexual abuse is often a precursor to adolescent prostitution. This is true related to a chronic nature of the abuse.

Children who are sexually abused over and over by a family member or member of the community learn that their bodies do not belong to them, and they also learn to dissociate during sex. They learn that others can take their bodies sexually as they wish to do so, and they learn to dissociate or remove themselves psychologically from an unwanted and not desired sexual encounter. These two "skills" set the victim up for prostitution because these skills are what are required to sell oneself for sex or be sold for sex by an adult.

Most American victims of commercial sexual exploitation are runaway or throwaway youth who live on the streets and become victims of prostitution. These children usually come from homes where they have been abused or from families that have abandoned them. These children become involved in prostitution as a way to support themselves financially or to get the things they want or need. Other young people are recruited into prostitution through forced abduction, pressure from parents, or through deceptive agreements between parents and traffickers. Once involved in prostitution, the children are often forced to travel far from their homes and as a result are isolated from their friends and family. Few children in this situation are able to develop new relationships with peers or adults other than the person who is victimizing them. The lifestyle of such children revolves around violence, forced drug use, and constant threats.

Human Trafficking

The victim and offender line is also crossed via human trafficking. Human trafficking, whether it occurs from another country into the United States or whether it occurs from one part of America into another part of America, is often for sexual exploitation. Human beings can be trafficked for various types of services, but sexual service is most common.

In other words, a victim can be recruited into prostitution. Most are victims forced into prostitution from other countries.

These people, often young adolescents, are brought to America under false pretenses. Their passports are taken from them, and they are forced to serve as prostitutes while the money goes to their captors. A lesser-known, but more common, form of human trafficking is enticement of victims into prostitution from somewhere in the United States. These victims are usually young adolescents who are troubled or running away from home. They are found in drug rehabs, living on the streets, or in bus stations and are recruited by someone who offers shelter, food, clothing, and often a relationship. When victims arrive at their new "home," they are forced into prostitution by the recruiter as payment for shelter, food, clothing, and often drugs. These youths have no job skills and relatively few life skills. As a result, they become prostitutes as a way of life.

ASSESSMENT

General Principles

The case histories of child sexual exploitation victims often reveal a continuum of abuse, frequently starting with abuse by a family member. However, some children are at higher risk for exploitation than others:

- Children who run away from home—many of these children are running away from abusive situations.
- Children who run away from juvenile and other institutions—including group homes, foster homes, and psychiatric facilities.
- Throwaway youth—children who are abandoned or forced to leave their homes and not permitted to return.
- Homeless children—those not counted in the throwaway and runaway groups.
- Children ages 10–17 living in public housing.
- Female gang members—some become victims of sexual exploitation as a result of their gang membership.
- Transgender street youth—these youth identify themselves as members of the opposite sex to which they were born; includes male to female, female to male, and youth born with the sex organs of both genders.

Health issues seen in trafficking victims include:

- Sexually transmitted diseases, HIV/AIDS, pelvic pain, rectal trauma, and urinary difficulties from working in the sex industry.
- Pregnancy, resulting from rape or prostitution.
- Infertility from chronic untreated sexually transmitted infections or botched or unsafe abortions.
- Infections or mutilations caused by unsanitary and dangerous medical procedures performed by the trafficker's so-called doctor.

- Malnourishment and serious dental problems.
- Infectious diseases like tuberculosis.
- Undetected or untreated diseases, such as diabetes.
- Bruises, scars, and other signs of physical abuse and torture. Sex-industry victims are often beaten in areas that won't damage their outward appearance, like their lower back.
- Substance abuse problems or addictions either from being coerced into drug use by their traffickers or by turning to substance abuse to help cope with or mentally escape their desperate situations.

The majority of children who appear in child pornography have not been abducted or physically forced to participate. In most cases, they know the producer—who may even be their father—and are manipulated into taking part by subtle means. Nonetheless, being the subject of child pornography can have devastating physical, social, and psychological effects on children. These children are first victimized when their abuse is perpetrated and recorded, and they are continuously victimized each time that record is accessed. Victims of child pornography have described the physical pain (e.g., around the genitals), accompanying somatic symptoms (such as headaches, loss of appetite, and sleeplessness), and feelings of psychological distress (emotional isolation, anxiety, and fear). However, most also feel pressured to cooperate with the offender and not to disclose the offense, both out of loyalty to the offender and a sense of shame about their own behavior. In later years, victims report that initial feelings of shame and anxiety did not fade but intensified to feelings of deep despair, worthlessness, and hopelessness. Their experience provided them with a distorted model of sexuality, and many had particular difficulties in establishing and maintaining healthy emotional and sexual relationships.

History and Physical Assessment

Other than what is noted above, little is known about child victims of pornography. However, health care providers should assess them for sexually transmitted infections and psychiatric sequelae. Most health care information is on victims of trafficking; however, much of this applies to children who are victimized by prostitution as well since many are victims of CSEC. Health care providers, especially those in emergency departments, are a frontline of defense for these children, and thus need to learn how to recognize them. Signs of human trafficking victimization include:

- Sleeping and eating disorders
- Sexually transmitted infections, HIV/AIDS, pelvic pain, rectal trauma, and urinary difficulties
- Fear and anxiety
- Depression, mood changes
- Guilt and shame
- Cultural shock from finding themselves in a strange country
- Posttraumatic stress disorder
- Suffers from traumatic bonding (Stockholm syndrome)—perpetrator instills in the victim fear as well as gratitude for being allowed to live or for any other perceived favors
- Refers to trafficker/pimp by familial titles, such as uncle, aunt, or cousin because perpetrator may indeed be a relative or because the perpetrator conditions them to use title
- Unexplained absences from school for a period of time, and is therefore a truant
- An inability to attend school on a regular basis
- Chronically runs away from home
- Makes references to frequent travel to other cities
- Exhibits bruises or other physical trauma, withdrawn behavior, depression, or fear
- Lacks control over her or his schedule or identification documents
- Hungry, malnourished
- Inappropriately dressed for weather conditions
- Signs of drug addiction
- Sudden change in attire, behavior, or material possessions (e.g., has expensive items)
- Makes references to sexual situations that are beyond age-specific norms ("boyfriend" who is noticeably older (10+ years)
- Makes references to terminology of the commercial sex industry that are beyond age-specific norms
- Engages in promiscuous behavior
- Labeled "fast" by peers

Health care providers can use the following screening questions to identify children who are victims of CSEC. Choose questions according to child's developmental status, but realize that even very young children are "working." Examples of appropriate interview questions include:

- Can you leave your job or situation if you want?
- Can you come and go as you please?
- Have you been threatened if you try to leave?
- Have you been physically harmed in any way?
- What are your working or living conditions like?
- Where do you sleep and eat?
- Do you sleep in a bed, on a cot, or on the floor?
- Have you ever been deprived of food, water, sleep, or medical care?
- Do you have to ask permission to eat, sleep, or go to the bathroom?
- Are there locks on your doors and windows so you cannot get out?
- Has anyone threatened your family?
- Has your identification or documentation been taken from you?
- Is anyone forcing you to do anything that you do not want to do?

Interview questions should be developmentally and culturally appropriate, and health care providers should have an understanding of the child's community and background if they have been trafficked from another country or are part of an immigrant community here in the United States. Children may have serious concerns about immigration and the safety of their siblings or other family members, which may hinder their providing information. Trained interpreters should be part of the investigative team. Child protection needs to be involved at the outset of any investigation, and multidisciplinary responses are most appropriate for these trafficking cases as they are for all cases involving minor victims. Health care providers should be aware of issues these children may have as survivors of abuse, neglect, and trauma. Do not make promises you cannot keep; faulty assurances will not help to heal these victims who have already been abused and betrayed.

Diagnostic Testing

Victims of CSEC require screening for sexually transmitted infections, as well as other infections related to lifestyle difficulties, such as tuberculosis.

INTERVENTION

Many of these children will have suffered from medical neglect and thus may need general pediatric services, such as immunizations and dental care. All will need psychiatric referral for at least an evaluation, and most will need referral to social services to arrange for placement. Law enforcement should be notified, as well as immigration services, when appropriate. Contact the National Human Trafficking Resource Center (1-888-373-7888). They will help determine if you have encountered victims of human trafficking, will identify local resources available in your community to help victims, and will help you coordinate with local social service organizations to help protect and serve victims so they can begin the process of restoring their lives.

PREVENTION/PATIENT TEACHING

Primary Prevention

Given that most child victims of CSEC have a history of physical and sexual abuse, preventing child abuse is the main goal of primary prevention. This can include encouraging positive parenting (see the American Academy of Pediatrics' Connected Kids Program at www.aap.org/con nectedkids); parent education programs and support groups that focus on child development, age-appropriate expectations, and the roles and responsibilities of parenting; family support and family strengthening programs that enhance the ability of families to access existing services, and resources to support positive interactions among family members; and public awareness campaigns that provide information on how and where to report suspected child abuse and neglect.

Parents need to know that good communication with their children is one of the best ways to prevent sexual abuse. Children should know they *can* and *should* talk with their parents about anything that makes them sad, scared, or confused. They should also be encouraged to talk to their health care provider.

Secondary Prevention

Adolescents who are "troubled" and running away or planning to run away from home are targets for the industry of prostitution. Working with families of troubled adolescents would help prevent prostitution. Referring adolescents with mental health issues to mental health professionals for evaluation and treatment may help reduce prostitution.

Tertiary Prevention

There are programs in the United States that work to get prostitutes off the street by offering them shelter and treatment for drug abuse. Giving the young prostitute a place to live, drug treatment, and social work assistance, while also assisting them in getting an education and developing life skills, can help victims of CSEC from repeated victimization.

Assistance with appropriate legal documents is necessary if the victim is from another country and/or is lacking appropriate identification. This assistance is provided via the Federal Bureau of Investigation (FBI) for victims from another country or via the prosecutor's office for American citizens. From the health care perspective, finding appropriate health care is difficult for prostitutes who do not have legal identification, do not have a Social Security number, and do not have health insurance. Thus, assistance from social services is imperative in these matters.

Child pornography is a federal crime and is almost always distributed across state lines. Therefore, federal prosecution is the most common remedy for the distribution of child pornography.

RESOURCES

ECPAT International (End Child Prostitution, Child Pornography and Trafficking of Children for Sexual Purposes): www.ecpat.net
National Center for Missing and Exploited Children: www.missingkids.com
National Human Trafficking Resource Center: www.acf.hhs.gov/trafficking/hotline/index.html
U.S. Immigration and Customs Enforcement: Child Exploitation Crimes: www.ice.gov/pi/childexploitation/index.htm

REFERENCES

Crane, P. (2007). More information from IAFN on human trafficking. *On the Edge,* *13*(2), 3–4.
Estes, R., & Weiner, N. (2001). *The commercial sexual exploitation of children in the U.S., Canada and Mexico: Executive summary of the U.S. national study.* Retrieved from www.sp2.upenn.edu/~restes/CSEC_Files/Exec_Sum_020220.pdf
Klain, E., Davies, H., & Hicks, M. (2001). *Child pornography: The criminal-justice-system response.* Washington, DC: National Center for Missing & Exploited Children. Retrieved from www.missingkids.com/en_US/publications/NC81.pdf

Prevent Child Abuse America. (1999). *Fact sheet: Child sexual abuse.* Retrieved from www.preventchildabuse.org/learn_more/research_docs/sexual_abuse.pdf

United Nations Children's Fund (UNICEF). (2007). UNICEF calls for increased efforts to prevent trafficking of children. Retrieved from www.unicef.org/media/media_40002.html

U.S. Department of Justice Child Exploitation and Obscenity Section. (n.d.-a). Child sex tourism. Retrieved from www.justice.gov/criminal/ceos/sextour.html

U.S. Department of Justice Child Exploitation and Obscenity Section. (n.d.-b). Child prostitution. Retrieved from www.justice.gov/criminal/ceos/prostitution.html

U.S. Health and Human Services. (n.d.). *Looking beneath the surface.* Retrieved from www.acf.hhs.gov/trafficking

Wolak, J., Mitchell, K., & Finkelhor, D. (2003). *Internet sex crimes against children: The response of law enforcement.* National Center for Missing and Exploited Children. Retrieved from http://www.missingkids.com/en_US/publications/NC132.pdf

Wolak, J., Mitchell, K., & Finkelhor, D. (2005). *Child pornography possessors arrested in internet related crimes.* National Center for Missing and Exploited Children. Retrieved from www.missingkids.com/en_US/publications/NC144.pdf

Wortley, R., & Smallbone, S. (2006). *Child pornography on the internet.* U.S. Department of Justice Community Oriented Policing Services (COPS) Problem-Oriented Guides for Police, Problem-Specific Guides Series No. 41. Retrieved from www.cops.usdoj.gov/files/ric/Publications/e04062000.pdf

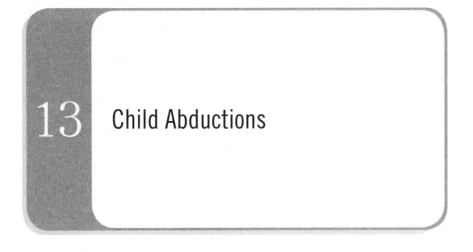

13 Child Abductions

DEFINITIONS

Few things frighten parents as much as a missing child. Most abducted children are taken by someone they know, including a parent. Others are taken by strangers, as is the case in the majority of infant (hospital) abductions.

Family abductions. Parental kidnapping describes the wrongful removal or retention of a child by a parent; however, since child kidnappings are frequently committed by other family members, the term *family abduction* is more accurate. Victims of family abduction are ripped from their homes and deprived of their other parent, often told that parent does not love them or is dead. They often live lives of deception, moving frequently and lacking the stability needed for healthy development. Parental kidnappings may be criminal, civil, or both.

Nonfamily abductions. The National Incidence Studies of Missing, Abducted, Runaway, and Throwaway Children (NISMART) describes a nonfamily abduction as an episode in which a nonfamily member takes a child by the use of physical force or threat of bodily harm or detains the child for at least an hour without parental authority or lawful permission, or an episode in which a child younger than 15 or mentally incompetent is detained or voluntarily accompanies a nonfamily perpetrator who takes the child unlawfully or without parental permission and who conceals the child's whereabouts, demands ransom, or expresses the intent to keep the child permanently. A *stereotypical nonfamily abduction* occurs when a child is detained overnight, transported at least 50 miles, held for ransom, abducted with intent to keep the child permanently, or killed by a stranger or slight acquaintance. A *stranger* is a perpetrator who is unknown to the family or who has an unknown identity, and a *slight acquaintance* is a perpetrator whose name is unknown to the child or family prior to the abduction and whom the child or family didn't know well enough to speak to, or a recent acquaintance who the child or family knows for less than 6 months or known for longer than 6 months but seen less than once a month. In one study, the child was killed in 40% of stereotypical kidnappings, and the child was not recovered in 4% of stereotypical kidnappings (Finkelhor, Hammer, & Sedlak, 2002).

Infant (hospital) abductions. Infant abductions refer to the unsanctioned taking of an infant less than 6 months of age by a nonfamily member. The term "infant abduction" has replaced hospital abduction due to the decrease in the latter and the increase in taking of infants outside hospital facilities, including the taking of fetuses from pregnant women.

PREVALENCE

Family abductions. A child is reported missing about every 40 seconds, and research shows that family abductions are the most prevalent child abduction type. More than 350,000 family abductions occur each year, accounting for about 1,000 per day. Approximately, 163,000 of these cases involve the concealment of a child, transporting out of state, or intent to keep the child permanently (Hammer, Finkelhor, & Sedlak, 2002).

Nonfamily abductions. About 3,000 to 5,000 nonfamily abductions are reported to police each year, most of which are short-term sexually motivated cases. Six percent of these cases make up the most serious cases where the child was murdered, ransomed, or taken with the intent to keep. Most high-profile cases are stereotypical abductions—children abducted, frequently sexually assaulted, and killed. However, not all nonfamily abductions are stereotypical. Most children are abducted by people they know: babysitters, boyfriends/ex-boyfriends (teen's or parent's), classmates, and neighbors. Some are detained for short periods of time, as when one child confines another in the school bathroom to sexually assault her or when a babysitter refuses to let the children go home to their parents because she wasn't paid for prior babysitting duties. The majority of stranger abductions take place in streets, parks, wooded areas, highways, and other public, generally accessible places. Acquaintance abductions typically occur in the home, but 25% of these kidnappings take place in public places. Both strangers and acquaintances rarely abduct from schools or school grounds.

Infant (hospital) abductions. There were approximately 0 to 12 infant abductions per year from 1983 to 2002. Prior to 1983, only 7 cases were reported in the media; from 1983 to 2002, 217 cases were reported. The increase may be due to improved identification of the problem and/or a greater willingness by health care facility administrators to report abductions. Since 1993, more abductions have taken place in homes and in public places such as shopping malls, parking lots, and social services offices.

ETIOLOGY

Family abductions. Studies have revealed several reasons for parental abductions. Some are motivated by an effort to force reconciliation or to continue interaction with the left-behind parent. Others have a desire to blame, spite, or punish the other parent. Some abducting parents fear losing legal custody or visitation rights, while others want to protect the child from a parent who is perceived to molest, abuse, or neglect the child. Finally, some parents abduct because of delusional thinking or a total disregard for the law.

Nonfamily abductions. Nonfamily motivations vary. Some abduct children for sexual gratification or for use in the sex trade (pornography or prostitution), while others abduct children for ransom. Some may abduct for revenge or out of anger, and others to create their own "family."

Infant abductions. Perpetrators may abduct an infant to save a relationship with their significant other. They may want to replace a baby that died or may be incapable of conception. Some may be involved in a fertility program at or near the facility from which they attempt to abduct an infant.

ASSESSMENT

While no one can guarantee that perpetrators will fit into specific sets of criteria, health care providers can still increase their awareness of these specific characteristics.

Family abductors. A high percentage of parental abductions take place between separation and divorce, especially in cases where the separation is quite bitter. The presence of one or more of these profiles in a parent does not mean that abduction is inevitable, not does the absence mean that abduction is not possible.

Profile 1: The parent who has committed a prior credible threat or abduction. This profile is usually combined with one or more of the others, as it is important to understand why the parent abducted the child. Other risk factors of flight include the parent is homeless, unemployed, and without ties to the area; the parent has divulged plans to abduct and has the resources to do so; and the parent has liquidated assets and maxed out credit cards or borrowed from other sources.

Profile 2: The parent who suspects or believes that abuse has occurred. Many parents abduct their children because they truly believe that the other parent is abusing, molesting, or neglecting their child. They feel the authorities have not taken their allegations seriously and have not properly investigated their concerns. These parents "rescue" the child with help from supporters who concur with their beliefs, including underground networks that help them obtain new identities and safe locations. Risk increases if the parent has a fixed belief that the abuse is occurring, has support of family or friends, or makes repetitive and increasingly hostile accusations.

Profile 3: The parent who is paranoid delusional. These parents demonstrate paranoid, irrational, and sometimes psychotic beliefs and behaviors toward the other parent. They may claim that the other parent exercises mind control over the child or that the other parent harmed the child. This disorder is rare, but these parents are often dangerous, especially if they have a history of domestic violence, substance abuse, or hospitalization for mental illness. The psychotic parent doesn't see the child as a separate person. Instead they perceive the child as fused with themselves as a victim or as part of the hated parent, which may cause them to abandon or kill the child. Marital dissolution and custody investigation can result in the psychotic parent committing murder-suicide.

Profile 4: The parent who is severely sociopathic (antisocial). These parents have contempt for authority, including the legal system, and often have flagrantly violated it. They're self-serving, manipulative, and exploitive. They hold exaggerated beliefs about their own superiority and entitlement and are highly gratified by their ability to exert power and control over others. They typically have a history of domestic violence, and, like paranoid abductors, they do not see the child as having separate rights and needs. Thus, they use their children as instruments of revenge and punishment or as trophies in their fight with their ex-partner. This profile is also rare.

Profile 5: The parent who is a citizen of another country. These parents have strong ties with their country of origin and have long been recognized as potential abductors. The risk is very high at the time of separation when these parents feel cast adrift in a foreign land and desire to reconnect with their ethnic or religious roots. Parents at greatest risk are those who idealize their own family, homeland, and culture and deprecate the American culture.

Profile 6: The parent who feels alienated from the legal system and who has support in another community. Several subgroups feel alienated and rely on their own networks of kin, who may live in another geographical community, to resolve family problems. These subgroups are:

- Parents who are indigent and poorly educated about custody laws and who cannot afford legal representation or counseling that would help them solve their dispute appropriately.
- Parents who have prior negative experience with criminal or civil courts and who thus do not expect the family courts to be responsive to their plight. Many of these parents have a police record.
- Parents who belong to certain ethnic, religious, or cultural groups that hold childrearing beliefs contrary to prevailing custody laws.
- The mother who has a transient, unmarried relationship with her child's father and who often views her child as her exclusive property.
- Parents who are victims of domestic violence, especially when the courts have failed to take the steps necessary to protect them and hold the abuser accountable.

In general, look for these risk factors as suggested by the Polly Klass Foundation at www.stopfamilyadbductionsnow:

- Volatile parental relationship with frequent arguments over visitation
- A parent who has abducted or threatened to abduct in the past
- A parent who accuses the other parent of abuse and who has the support of family or friends about these allegations
- A parent who is paranoid delusional or severely sociopathic

- A parent from another country who is ending a mixed-culture marriage
- A parent who feels alienated from the legal system and who has support in another community
- A parent who has no job, financial ties, or connections to the child's home state
- A parent who is engaged in quitting a job, selling a home, terminating a lease, closing a bank account, or applying for passports, birth certificates, or school and medical records, or other activities that may indicate preparation for flight

Nonfamily abductors. The health care provider would do best to focus on teaching families and children how to prevent nonfamily abductions. Extra attention should be spent on "vulnerable" children, as they are at higher risk for nonfamily abductions.

Infant abductors. Hospital infant abductors tend to have the following characteristics:

Female, aged 12 to 50, and usually overweight

Compulsive

Manipulative and deceitful to gain access

Claims to have lost a baby or be unable to conceive

Lives in or is familiar with the community where the abduction occurs

Will be able to provide good care for the baby after the abduction

Usually married or living with a man

Visits various nursery and obstetrical units before the abduction and asks detailed questions about procedures and unit layout

Plans the abduction, but does not necessarily target a specific infant; usually takes a victim of opportunity

Frequently impersonates a nurse or other health care provider

Frequently becomes familiar with facility staff and routines, as well as with parents of intended victims

Infant abductors who kidnap from nonhealth care settings differ. They have the first five characteristics, as well as four others:

Usually single while claiming to have a partner

Targets a mother and tries to meet the target family

Plans the abduction and brings a weapon, although the weapon might not be used

Impersonates a health care or social services professional when visiting the home

INTERVENTION

Family and nonfamily abductions. Assure that all medical records are up-to-date and easily accessible for the family and law enforcement should the need arise. Assist the family in obtaining emotional support during the crisis, and ensure that family members maintain their own health. In cases of potential parental abductions, assist the custodial parent in obtaining legal help.

Infant abductions. Utilize *For Healthcare Professionals: Guidelines on Prevention of and Response to Infant Abductions* (Raburn, 2009) to assure that your facility safeguards infants from abductions, requiring:

A comprehensive program of policies, procedures, and processes

Education and a teamwork approach by nursing personnel, parents, physicians, security, and risk-management personnel

Coordination of physical and electronic security. (Electronic security measures are simply modern tools used to "back up" policies, procedures, and the actions of personnel.)

PREVENTION/PATIENT TEACHING

Primary Prevention

Enable families to be prepared for the unthinkable. Teach parents to:

1. Keep a complete description of their children, including date of birth, height, weight, hair and eye color, and other identifying characteristics (birthmarks, braces, glasses, body piercings, tattoos).

2. Take ID photo of their children every 6 months—every 3 months for children under 2. ID-type head and shoulder photos, taken from different angles, are preferable to school and family pictures.
3. Know where the children's medical records are located and know how to access them. Make sure they contain information that can help identify the children.
4. Make sure their children have up-to-date dental records and that parents know how to access them.
5. Have their children fingerprinted by their local police department and keep the fingerprint card in a safe place. The police will not keep records themselves.
6. Consider having their children's DNA tested. Fingerprints provide accurate identification, but DNA is far more accurate.
7. Make sure custody documents are in order.
8. Never leave young children unattended, not even for a few seconds.

Family abductions. If you recently separated from your spouse/partner, and if he or she fits into any of the risk categories or profiles, you need to take appropriate steps to prevent your child from being abducted by the noncustodial parent.

General Strategies

Most custodial parents benefit from these steps:

■ Keep a friendly, at least civil, relationship with your ex. This helps reduce the anger and frustration that often leads to abduction.

■ Communicate openly with your child, reinforcing that you love her and always want her, no matter what anyone else says. Let her know she has the right to reach you and make sure she knows how to make a long-distance phone call to you.

■ Have certified copies of your custody agreement readily available and make sure the agreement gives the police the right to recover your child.

■ Speak to your attorney immediately so that he or she can take the legal steps necessary to thwart abduction.

- Keep a discrete list of your ex's information: Social Security number, driver's license number, car registration number, and checking and savings account numbers. Use caution when obtaining them so as not to set off an abduction.

- Don't ignore abduction threats. Get advice from the police, a counselor, and your attorney.

- Notify your child's school or day care that your child is not to be released to anyone, including your ex, without your permission.

- If you're not married, get a custody agreement anyway because state laws vary as to whether the mother automatically gets custody in these cases.

- Find out if your state has an agreement with the Office of Child Support Enforcement of the U.S. Department of Health and Human Services, allowing state officials to use the Federal Parent Locator Service (FPLS, www.acf.hhs.gov/programs/cse/newhire). The FPLS is a national network that can help find an abducting parent in child custody, visitation, or criminal custodial interference cases. It is most effective when the abductor is receiving federal benefits or when the child has been missing for 6 months or more.

Strategies for Specific Profiles

The strategies for the specific profiles were released by the Office of Juvenile Justice and Delinquency Prevention (Johnston, Sagatun-Edwards, Blomquist, & Girdner, 2001) and resulted from a series of research studies.

Profile 1: Previous threat or abduction—A court order should be obtained that specifies which parent has custody, defines arrangements for the child's contact with the noncustodial parent, designates which court has jurisdiction, and requires written consent of the custodial parent or the court before the noncustodial parent can take the child out of the area. If visitation is unsupervised, the plan should include dates, times, places of exchange, and so forth. The courts should also specify consequences for failure to observe the custody provisions.

The child's passport can be marked with the requirement that she not travel without authorization. School and day care officials, as well as medical personnel, should be presented with a copy of the custody agreement and can be told not to release any information on the child to the noncustodial parent.

Supervised visitation is a stringent way of preventing abductions and is typically used to prevent recidivism in serious cases. It is usually difficult to convince a judge to curtail a parent's visitation unless there is substantial proof that the parent has committed a crime.

Profile 2: The parent who suspects abuse—The priority strategy is to ensure that a careful and thorough investigation takes place. Accusing parents tend to calm down when they feel investigators are taking their concerns seriously. During the investigation, authorities must ensure that there is no ongoing abuse or protect the accused parent, who may be innocent, from further allegations. Precautions include supervised visitation or even suspended visitation if the child demonstrates emotional or behavioral disturbances to the parent's visits. Counseling is beneficial for both parents and the child, and a legal representative may be appointed for the child in the event of further legal action.

Profile 3: The paranoid delusional parent—Courts need to have procedures in place to protect children from severely delusional parents. If the noncustodial parent is psychotic, visitation may be supervised in a high-security facility and the parent assisted with maintaining the child's safety at other times. However, the psychotic parent's visitation may be suspended if he repeatedly violates the visitation order; highly distresses the child with his visits; or uses his time with the child to malign the custodial parent, obtain information on the custodial parent's whereabouts, or transmit threats of harm or abduction.

If the custodial parent is psychotic, extreme care must be taken during litigation and evaluation to prevent abduction or violence. The family court may need to obtain emergency psychiatric screening and use ex parte (without notice to the psychotic parent) hearings to effect temporary placement of the child with the other parent or third party while investigators undertake a more comprehensive evaluation.

Profile 4: The sociopathic parent—When a parent is diagnosed as having a sociopathic personality, counseling and therapeutic mediation are inappropriate and potentially dangerous. These parents lack the capacity to develop a working relationship with a counselor and may even hide behind professional confidentiality to manipulate and control the other parties to achieve his or her own ends. If the sociopathic parent blatantly violates visitation orders, supervised or suspended visitation is appropriate. Courts also need to respond quickly and decisively with fines and/or jail time to any overt disregard of the explicit custody and access orders. Counseling may then be appropriate once control mechanisms are in place.

Profile 5: The parent who is a citizen of another country—The range of actions suggested for Profile 1 are appropriate, especially those regarding passport and travel. Problems occur when the child has dual citizenship since foreign embassies are not under obligation to honor restrictions when the request is made by the U.S. citizen parent. The court may require the foreign national parent to request and obtain these assurances of passport control from his or her embassy before allowing unsupervised visitation. The foreign national parent can also post bond that would be released to the other parent in the event of abduction. During times of acute risk, authorities can monitor the airline schedules so that an abducting parent and child can be intercepted at the airport before leaving the country.

Profile 6: The parent who feels alienated from the legal system— Alienated parents, particularly mothers, have the best prognosis for effective interventions to prevent abductions. These strategies include access to affordable counseling and legal services; family advocates to bridge cultural, religious, and economic gaps; and the inclusion of important members of their informal social network into brief intervention services.

Nonfamily abductions. Being prepared is not enough. Both you and your child need strategies to prevent abductions.

General Safety Strategies

- Make sure your child knows her full name, address, and phone number. Older children should also know parent's names, work addresses, and work phone numbers.
- Keep communication lines open. Don't belittle your child's fears or concerns.
- Talk to your child. Kids who talk regularly with their parents have higher levels of self-esteem and assuredness, making them less vulnerable to predators.
- Be sensitive to changes in her behavior.
- Don't let her wear clothing with her name on it. The perpetrator will use her name to gain her confidence.
- Set boundaries as to where your child can go. Young children should not leave the yard unsupervised, older children should ask permission. Teens should phone home to tell you where they are.

- Establish a parental back-up system so your child has somewhere to go in an emergency.
- Instruct her to tell you if an adult asks her to "keep a secret" or if someone offers her money, gifts, or drugs or asks to take her picture.
- Tell her that adults don't usually ask children for directions or help finding their puppy or kitten.
- Instruct her to not go near the car of a person who tries to talk to her. Your child should learn which cars she may ride in. Share a code word with your child known only to family members.
- Tell her to go for help—police station, neighbor's house, store—if someone is following her on foot or in a car.
- Carefully choose babysitters, nannies, day care providers, preschools, and after-school programs. Check their references, and, if possible, see if you can have access to their background information. Several states will allow you to access criminal and sex abuse registries.
- Know your child's friends and their parents.
- Know your neighbors.
- If someone demonstrates a great deal of interest in your child, find out why.
- Beware of gadgets that promise to keep your child safe.
- Don't rely on martial arts or self-defense training to keep your child safe. It may, however, build up her confidence.
- Teach online safety.
- If home alone, your child should not answer the door or tell anyone that she is home alone.
- Tell her to say "NO" to anyone who tries to take her somewhere, touches her, or makes her feel uncomfortable in any way.
- Inform her to not go into anyone's home without your permission.
- Have a plan should you and your child become separated while away from home.
- Tell her to not look for you if you become separated while in a public place or shopping area. She should go to the nearest checkout counter, security office, or lost and found, and tell them she's lost. She should never go to the parking lot without you.
- Instruct her to scream, "You're not my parent!" if someone tries to take her away.

Age-specific safety guidelines follow.

Preschool-Aged Children

- Never leave your child unattended and never leave her alone in a car, carriage, stroller, or yard.

- Make sure she knows how to dial 911 or another emergency number.

- Teach her to go to safe people—police officers, firefighters, and teachers—to ask for help when needed.

- Play the license number and state reading game so that she will be able to recognize license plates.

- Talk to her about "strangers." Preschoolers possess magical thinking, so they picture strangers as unusual-looking men with trench coats, sunglasses, and a moustache. And have you ever tried to get a 4-year-old to NOT talk! Yikes. How can you get them to not talk to strangers? Teach them:

  - To be on the lookout for unusual situations and actions, rather than unusual people.

  - To be polite, but also let them know it is okay to be suspicious of any adult asking for help or directions.

  - It's okay to say "no" to adults if they feel uncomfortable, scared, or confused in any way.

  - To not let anyone touch them in areas where their bathing suit touches their body and to not touch anyone one else on those areas if that person asks them to do so.

School-Aged Children

- Have your child use the buddy system whenever away from you, including walking to school.

- Make sure she checks in with you when going from one site to another.

- Tell her to follow her gut—if she feels uncomfortable, get out of there.

- Teach her how to find a pay phone and call from it. Make sure she knows how to call long-distance.

- Instruct her to never hitchhike.

- Tell her to avoid dark or abandoned places and to come home before dark.

- Tell her to avoid adults who hang around playgrounds.

Teenagers

- Continue to use the buddy system.

- Tell her that nothing she owns is worth risking her life for. If someone threatens her for an item, the safest thing to do is to give it up. And encourage her to tell you if such an incident occurs.

- As tough as she thinks she is, it's not tough enough when it comes to perpetrators. Make sure she practices safety.

Infant abductions. Encourage parents to be concerned and watchful with the following guidelines:

- Never leave your baby alone. If you need to go to the bathroom, call the nurse to take the baby back to the nursery.

- Don't give your baby to anyone who lacks proper hospital identification. Know the staff and the unit.

- If strangers enter your room or ask about your baby, call the nurse immediately.

- Know when and where your baby will be taken for tests or procedures and know who authorized them.

According to Burgess, Carr, Nahirny, and Rabun (2008), the site of infant abductions seems to be showing a trend away from health care facilities and toward homes. This may reflect a rise in parental injury and a greater use of weapons during abduction (abductors might anticipate stronger opposition from parents than from health care facility staff). Abductors also tend to "case" homes more frequently than health care settings. These prior visits to non–health care abduction sites may show that is it more important for abductors to familiarize themselves with homes than health care settings. Burgess et al (2008) suggest that parents be cautioned to be watchful of anyone they do not know well, especially anyone whom they met during the pregnancy, anyone who shows excessive interest in their infant, and anyone who arrives at their home unannounced or who can't provide checkable identification.

Secondary Prevention

In the event that your child is missing or abducted, take the following steps:

- Act immediately. Search your house inside and out, especially places where children can get trapped like old refrigerators and trunks.

- Check with your neighbors and your child's friends to see if she is with them.

- If you still have not found her, call the police immediately. Describe your child, including the clothes she was wearing when last seen. If the case meets criteria, an AMBER (America's Missing: Broadcast Emergency Response Alerting System) alert is issued.

- The AMBER Alert System was created in 1996 as a legacy to 9-year-old Amber Hagerman, who was kidnapped and murdered while riding her bike in Arlington, Texas. Once initiated, the child's descriptive information is transmitted to radio stations designated under the Emergency Alert System who in turn send it to area radio and TV stations for broadcasting. TV stations run a "crawl" on the screen along with the photo of the child. Some states, including Pennsylvania, incorporate the information into their electronic highway billboards to alert the public of an AMBER alert. These signs display pertinent descriptive information on the child, as well as the suspected abductor's vehicle information if available.

- Contact the National Center for Missing and Exploited Children at 1-800-THE-LOST (1-800-843-5678) (TDD Hotline 800-826-7653) to report your child missing.

- Check for clues that will help find your child: notes, letters, items you don't recognize.

- Examine your phone bill for unfamiliar calls that may indicate where she has gone.

- Check the neighborhood for clues, and don't forget to ask children if they've seen your child.

- Look for clues in all areas of your child's life: school, activities, friends, and clubs.

- Tell everyone you meet your child is missing and ask for help and communicate a sense of love for your child.

- In urban areas, check generally inaccessible areas like basements and roofs.

- In rural areas, check barns, mines, boats, and caves.

- Contact the media and provide interviews.

- Post "missing child" flyers with a recent photo and description as well as contact information. Post these anywhere and everywhere you can.

- If you can afford it, hire a reliable private investigator (check references).

- Ask that your child's name and identifying information be immediately entered into the National Crime Information Center (NCIC) Missing Person File.

- Use the National Center for Missing and Exploited Children Web site for further information: www.missingkids.com.

- Take care of yourself. You can't help your child if you're falling apart. Counseling can help ease both your pain and any guilt you may feel.

If your child vanishes in a store, notify the security office or store manager. Then immediately call police. Many stores have a *Code Adam* plan of action. If a child goes missing in a store, employees immediately mobilize to look for the missing child.

Tertiary Prevention

The emotional consequences of abduction can be significant for the child and family. The child may experience depression, loss of trust and stability, excessive fearfulness, anger, disruption in identity formation, and abandonment fears, as well as disorders such as posttraumatic stress disorder and separation anxiety. Some may experience Stockholm syndrome (sense of loyalty to the abductor). The parents can face a number of devastating emotional, and possibly financial, problems, especially if the child is never returned. Siblings feel frightened and confused. The victim and family members should be referred for counseling, preferably to a professional versed in the effects of abductions. If the family cannot afford transportation and lodging to pick up their child once found, they should contact the National Center for Missing and Exploited Children, since it has a program to provide assistance.

RESOURCES

Family Abduction: Prevention and Response: www.missingkids.com/en_US/publica tions/NC75.pdf

For health care professionals: Guidelines on Prevention of and Response to Infant Ab ductions: www.missingkids.com/en_US/publications/NC05.pdf

National Center for Missing and Exploited Children: www.missingkids.com

What About Me? Coping with the Abduction of a Brother or Sister: www.ncjrs.gov/pdf files1/ojjdp/217714.pdf

You're Not Alone: The Journey from Abduction to Empowerment: www.ncjrs.gov/pdf files1/ojjdp/221965.pdf

REFERENCES

Amber Alert Registry. (n.d.). Retrieved from www.amberalertregistry.org

Burgess, A., Carr, K., Nahirny, C., & Rabun, J. (2008). Nonfamily infant abductions, 1983–2006. *American Journal of Nursing, 108*(9), 32–38.

Burgess, A., & Lanning, K. (2003). *An analysis of infant abductions.* National Center for Missing and Exploited Children. Retrieved from http://www.missingkids.com/ en_US/publications/NC66.pdf

Chiancione, J. (n.d.). *Parental abductions: A review of the literature.* Office of Juvenile Justice and Delinquency Prevention. Retrieved from www.ncjrs.gov/pdffiles1/ ojjdp/190074.pdf

Finkelhor, D., Hammer, H., & Sedlak, A. (2002). *Nonfamily abducted children: National estimates and characteristics.* The National Incidence Studies of Missing, Abducted, Runaway, and Throwaway Children (NISMART). Retrieved from www.ncjrs.gov/pdf files1/ojjdp/196467.pdf

Hammer, H., Finkelhor, D., & Sedlak, A. (2002). Children abducted by family members: National estimates and characteristics. The National Incidence Studies of Missing, Abducted, Runaway, and Throwaway Children (NISMART). Retrieved from http:// www.ncjrs.gov/pdffiles1/ojjdp/196466.pdf

Hoff, R. (2008). *Family abduction: Prevention and response* (6th ed.). National Center for Missing and Exploited Children. Retrieved from http://www.missingkids.com/ en_US/publications/NC75.pdf

Johnston, J., Sagatun-Edwards, I., Blomquist, M., & Girdner, L. (2001). Early identification of risk factors for parental abduction. Office of Juvenile Justice and Delinquency Prevention. *Juvenile Justice Bulletin*. NCJ 185026. Retrieved from http://www.ncjrs.gov/pdffiles1/ojjdp/185026.pdf

Miller, J., Kurlycheck, M., Hansen, J., & Wilson, K. (2008). Examining child abduction by offender type patterns. *Justice Quarterly, 25*(3), 523–543.

Muscari, M. (2004). *Not My Kid 2: Protecting Your Children from the 21 Threats of the 21st Century*. Scranton, PA: University of Scranton Press.

Raburn, J. (2009). *For healthcare professionals: Guidelines on prevention of and response to infant abductions*. National Center for Missing and Exploited Children. Retrieved from http://www.missingkids.com/en_US/publications/NC05.pdf

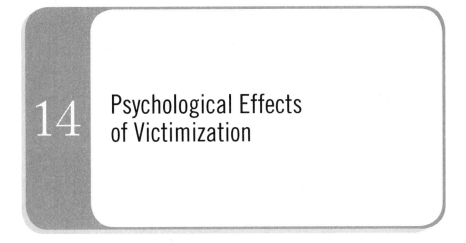

14 Psychological Effects of Victimization

A violent crime may only last seconds, but its effects can last a lifetime. Child maltreatment (abuse and/or neglect) substantially contributes to child mortality and morbidity and has long-lasting effects on mental health, substance abuse, risky sexual behavior, obesity, and criminal behavior, which persist into adulthood. Numerous studies have examined the long-term consequences of relationship violence during childhood. These studies have suggested that physical and sexual abuse in early life can lead to problems in adulthood, including poor mental and physical health, as well as higher rates of substance abuse. In one study, 1,458 (6.7%) and 1,429 (6.5%) out of 21,000 participants reported childhood physical and sexual abuse, respectively (Draper et al., 2007). Multivariate models indicated that participants who had experienced either childhood sexual or physical abuse had a greater risk of poor physical and mental health. Older adults who reported both childhood sexual and physical abuse also had a higher risk of poor physical and mental health.

Child abuse and neglect, or more specifically child maltreatment, victims may suffer physical, psychological, social, and/or financial trauma. The impact on each child depends upon a number of factors, including age of the child when abuse began, severity of the abuse, frequency of the abuse, the child's relationship to the abuser, availability of support persons, and the child's ability to cope. The effects can also be compounded when children are exposed to more than one type of maltreatment, including exposure to intimate partner and community violence. Children who are exposed to one type of maltreatment are frequently exposed to other types on several occasions or continuously.

PHYSICAL CONSEQUENCES

The physical effects of abuse vary according to the type of abuse perpetrated and may stem from physical or sexual abuse or from neglect. Some effects may be short-term, such as bruising or a minor fracture, while others may be permanent. Victims may suffer from brain damage from head injury or functional disabilities from spinal cord injuries. Newborns may suffer the effects of intimate partner violence committed during pregnancy. Shaken baby syndrome (acute head trauma, AHT) may cause problems that are not immediately noticeable and that may include bleeding in the eyes or brain, damage to the spinal cord and neck, and rib or bone fractures (please refer to Chapter 9 for further information on this maltreatment).

A literature review by Turnera, Finkelhor, and Ormrod (2006) revealed multiple effects of child maltreatment. These include strong associations between child maltreatment and obesity, which persist after accounting for family characteristics and individual risk factors, such as childhood obesity; an association between child sexual abuse and eating disorders, such as bulimia and anorexia nervosa; and relationships between multiple child adversities, including child maltreatment, and a range of health outcomes in adulthood, including ischemic heart disease, cancer, chronic lung disease, skeletal fractures, and liver disease.

Physical effects of sexual assault. The physical consequences of sexual assault can be quite severe. Forced sexual contact can result in genital injuries and gynecological complications, such as bleeding, infection, chronic pelvic pain, pelvic inflammatory disease, and urinary tract infections, depending on the victim's age. Sexual violence can put all girls at risk of sexually transmitted infections, including HIV/AIDS and postpubertal girls at risk for unwanted pregnancies. The unwanted pregnancies may lead to unsafe abortions or to injuries sustained during an abortion. Women can also suffer injuries resulting from physical abuse that may accompany the sexual assault.

Physical effects of intimate partner violence on fetal development. A study of 2,562 women showed that those exposed to spousal violence (n = 1,307) were 50% more likely to experience a single or repeated stillbirth or spontaneous abortion (Alio, Nana, & Salihu, 2009). In this group, physical violence was most common (39%), followed by emotional abuse, defined as verbal or physical public humiliation or verbal threatening of the woman or her family (31%), and sexual abuse (15%). Physical assault during pregnancy can result in placental separation; antepartum hemorrhage; fetal fractures; rupture of the uterus, liver, or spleen; preterm labor; low birth-weight babies; and risk for urinary tract infections, sexually transmitted diseases, and poor prenatal care. Research also suggests an association between intimate partner violence and preterm labor, premature delivery, and miscarriage. Abusive partners may also pressure their wives or girlfriends not to gain weight, or abuse could cause stress, which has in turn been associated with smoking, low weight gain, and consequent low birth-weight.

PSYCHOLOGICAL EFFECTS

Children can experience both immediate and long-term psychological effects from violence. Depression remains the most common response, and depression and withdrawal symptoms have been seen in abused children as young as 3. Children may also experience acute or posttraumatic stress disorder (PTSD).

Data on *acute stress disorder (ASD)* are limited since it was only formally recognized in 1994. However, the main cause of acute stress disorder is exposure to severe trauma. The impact of trauma is influenced by several factors, including the severity of the event, the duration of the event, the proximity to the event (whether the event was directly experienced or witnessed), the type of the event, and the intent (whether the event was planned or accidental). Human acts of violence, especially those that are particularly cruel, create a greater risk for this disorder than natural events. Individuals with ASD develop dissociative responses and may experience decreased emotional responsiveness, often finding it difficult to experience pleasure and frequently feeling guilty. Symptoms appear during or immediately after the trauma, last for at least 2 days, and resolve within 4 weeks after the conclusion of the traumatic event or when the diagnosis is changed. Symptoms lasting more than 4 weeks may warrant a diagnosis of PTSD, provided the full criteria for that disorder are met.

The criteria for ASD per the *Diagnostic and Statistical Manual of Mental Disorders* (American Psychiatric Association [APA], 2000) are:

1. The person was exposed to a traumatic event in which the person experienced, witnessed, or was confronted with an event(s) that involved actual or threatened death or serious injury to themselves or others and the person's response involved intense fear, helplessness, or horror;

2. While experiencing or after experiencing the distressing event, the individual has three (or more) of the following dissociative symptoms: a subjective sense of numbing, detachment, or absence of emotional responsiveness, a reduction in awareness of his or her surroundings, derealization, depersonalization, or dissociative amnesia;

3. The traumatic event is persistently reexperienced in at least one of the following ways: recurrent images, thoughts, dreams, illusions, flashbacks, a sense of reliving the experience, or distress on exposure to reminders of the traumatic event;

4. Marked avoidance of stimuli that cause recollections of the trauma;

5. Marked symptoms of anxiety or increased arousal, such as difficulty sleeping, poor concentration, hypervigilance, or exaggerated startle response;

6. The disturbance causes clinically significant distress or impairment in social, occupational, or other important areas of functioning;

7. The disturbance lasts for a minimum of 2 days, a maximum of 4 weeks, and occurs within 4 weeks of the traumatic event; and

8. The disturbance is not due to substance abuse or a general medical condition, is not better accounted for by Brief Psychotic Disorder, and is not merely an exacerbation of a preexisting psychiatric disorder.

Data on ASD in children is minimal; however, the Child Stress Reaction Checklist (CSRC), a 30-item questionnaire, was developed to identify symptoms of ASD in children as rated by a parent or nurse. The score range is from 0 to 60, and higher scores indicate more symptoms of ASD.

Posttraumatic stress disorder (PTSD) often presents in primary and community care, but goes unrecognized. Failure to identify and treat PTSD has adverse effects on client health since PTSD is associated with increased health complaints, health services utilization, morbidity, and mortality. Persons with PTSD have persistent frightening thoughts and memories of the incident and feel emotionally numb, especially with people they were once close to. They may experience sleep disturbances, feel numb or detached, or be easily startled.

The American Psychiatric Association (2000) revised the diagnostic criteria for PTSD in the *DSM-IV-TR*. The criteria now include a history of exposure to a traumatic event that meets two criteria and symptoms form three clusters: intrusive recollections, avoidant or numbing symptoms, and hyperarousal symptoms. Additional criteria address symptom duration and functioning. To be diagnosed with PTSD, the person must have experienced, witnessed or faced an event that involved actual or perceived threatened death or serious harm to them or others that evoked intense fear, horror, or helplessness. The person must meet at least one intrusive recollection criterion, such as recurrent and intrusive images, thoughts or perceptions of the event, flashbacks or the sensation of reliving the event. The person must meet at least three avoidant or numbing criteria, such as efforts to avoid conversations associated with the trauma, inability to remember critical aspects about the trauma, significantly decreased participation in important activities, feeling detached from others, or a sense of a shortened future. The person must also manifest at least two hyperarousal criteria, such as hypervigilance, difficulty sleeping, outbursts of anger or irritability, difficulty concentrating, or an exaggerated startle response. Symptoms need to last more than one month and must cause significant distress or impairment in social, occupational, or other important areas of functioning. PTSD often presents with comorbid disorders, including depression, substance abuse, and other anxiety disorders. Thus health care providers need to consider other symptoms not specific to PTSD as they may indicate an additional psychiatric disorder.

PTSD may not present itself in children the same way it does in adults, and thus, criteria for PTSD now include age-specific features for some symptoms. According to the National Center for PTSD, the following age-specific features are noted:

Very young children may present with few symptoms, possibly because eight of the PTSD symptoms require a verbal description of one's feelings and experiences. They may instead report more generalized fears such as stranger or separation anxiety, avoidance of situations that may or may not be related to the trauma, sleep disturbances, and a preoccupation with words or symbols that may or may not be related to the trauma. Young children may also display posttraumatic play in which they repeat themes of the trauma and/or they may lose an acquired developmental skill (such as toilet training) as a result of experiencing a traumatic event.

Elementary school-aged children may not experience visual flashbacks or amnesia for aspects of the trauma, but they do experience "time skew" (mis-sequencing trauma-related events when recalling the memory) and "omen formation" (belief that there were warning signs that predicted the trauma) that are not typically seen in adults. Thus, children often believe that they can recognize warning signs and avoid future traumas. School-aged children may also exhibit posttraumatic play or reenactment of the trauma in play, drawings, or verbalizations.

Adolescent symptoms of PTSD may begin to more closely resemble those in adults. However, there some differences. Adolescents may engage in traumatic reenactment, in which they incorporate aspects of the trauma into their daily lives. They are also more likely than younger children or adults to exhibit impulsive and aggressive behaviors.

Stockholm syndrome is a psychological state in which victims identify with their offenders. It was originally used in cases of kidnapping and hostage situations, but has been extended to other forms of violence, including intimate partner violence and child abuse.

There is no universally accepted definition of Stockholm syndrome, but it has been suggested that it is present if one or more of the following is observed: positive feelings by the captive toward his or her captor, negative feelings by the captive toward the police or authorities trying to win his or her release, and positive feelings by the captor toward his or her captive.

These conditions must be met for Stockholm syndrome to occur:

- A perceived threat to survival and a belief that the captor is willing to carry out that threat
- A perception by the captive of some small kindness from the captor within the context of terror
- Isolation from perspectives other than those of the captor
- Perceived inability to escape

BEHAVIORAL EFFECTS

Not all abused children develop behavioral consequences, but those who do may have behavior problems that include:

Risky sexual behaviors. Most studies that have examined the relation between child maltreatment and sexual behavior in adolescence and adulthood have focused on outcomes for sexual abuse. In one prospective study, Wilson and Widom (2008) reported a significant association between physical or sexual abuse or neglect and arrest for prostitution or being paid for sex (13% of cases vs. 4% of controls for girls, $p = 0.001$; 15% vs. 8% for boys, $p = 0.17$), but no significant associations with promiscuity or teenage pregnancy.

Substance abuse. Abused children are more likely to smoke cigarettes, abuse alcohol, or take illicit drugs during their lifetime than nonabused children. A report from the National Institute on Drug Abuse (Swan, 1998) notes that as many as two-thirds of people in drug treatment programs reported being abused as children.

Juvenile delinquency and adult criminality. Abused children are more likely to be arrested for criminal behavior as a juvenile, more likely to be arrested for violent and criminal behavior as an adult, and more likely to be arrested for one of many forms of violent crime as a juvenile or adult.

Abusive behavior. Abusive parents often have experienced abuse during their own childhoods, and it is estimated approximately one-third of abused and neglected children will eventually victimize their own children.

COGNITIVE EFFECTS

Child abuse and neglect may cause important regions of the brain to fail to form or fail to grow properly, resulting in impaired development. These changes in brain maturation have long-term consequences for cognitive, language, and academic abilities. Child maltreatment is associated with long-term deficits in educational achievement. Studies, such as one by Boden and colleagues (2007), have shown that abused children have lower educational achievement than their peers, and are more likely to receive special education. Abuse can have long-term economic consequences as abused children are more likely to end up in menial and semiskilled jobs than their nonabused peers.

INTERVENTIONS

Physical interventions are found throughout this text in specific crime-related chapters. This section provides basic interventions for all victims, as well as those with psychological, safety, and financial problems. Health care providers must be aware of victim rights and needs, as well as victim safety, including how to direct them to obtain orders of protection.

Victim Rights

The American Bar Association's Criminal Justice Section (2009) developed a Child Victim's "List of Rights" for courts to provide to child victims and their guardians:

- You have the right to know what is happening in the court case that came about from the report you made.

- You have the right to be in court whenever the judge and the prosecutor are there to discuss the case, before a trial starts.

- You have the right to request to speak to the judge anytime the judge makes a major decision in the case.

- If you lost money or something valuable was stolen from you or damaged as a result of the crime, you have the right to ask the court to make the defendant pay you back for what you have lost.

- If your property was stolen and has been recovered, you have a right to get your property back as soon as possible.

- If you are scared or feel threatened, you have the right to ask the judge to provide reasonable protection before, during, and after the trial.

- There are services and people you can talk to outside of the courtroom about what you are feeling.

- If you would like to talk to someone privately without your parents or legal guardian knowing, you may ask the judge to appoint a guardian or an attorney to represent you.

■ You have the right to ask the judge to allow your parents, your guardian, or another adult whom you trust to be present with you during your testimony.

■ Whether or not there is a trial, you have a right to know if the defendant is sent to jail or prison, and, if so, when the defendant is expected to be released.

Victim Needs

The Office for Victims of Crime (OVC) states that there are three critical needs for all victims:

1. *Victims need to feel safe.* People usually feel helpless, vulnerable, and frightened by victimization. When working with victims, be sure to follow these guidelines:

■ Introduce yourself by name and title and briefly explain your role.
■ Ensure privacy during your interview. Assure confidentiality when possible (extent of confidentiality depends on your role).
■ Reassure victims of their safety. Pay attention to your own words, posture, mannerisms, and tone of voice. Use body language to show concern, such as nodding your head, using natural eye contact, placing yourself at the victim's level, keeping an open stance, and speaking in a calm, sympathetic voice. Tell victims that they are safe and that you are there for them.
■ Ask victims to tell you in just a sentence or two what happened, and ask if they have any physical injuries. Tend to medical needs first.
■ Offer to contact a family member, friend, victim advocate, or crisis counselor.
■ Ask simple questions to allow victims to make decisions, assert themselves, and regain control over their lives, such as "How would you like me to address you?"
■ Ask victims if they have any special concerns or needs.
■ Develop a safety plan before leaving them. Pull together personal or professional support for the victims. Give victims a pamphlet listing resources available for help or information, including contact information for local crisis intervention centers and support groups, the prosecutor's office and the victim-witness

assistance office, the state victim compensation/assistance office, and other nationwide services, including toll-free hotlines and Web addresses.

■ Give them your name and information on how to reach you in writing. Encourage them to contact you if they have any questions or if you can be of further help.

2. *Victims need to express their emotions.* Victims need to express their emotions and tell their story after the trauma. They need to have their feelings accepted and have their story heard by a nonjudgmental listener. They may feel fear, self-blame, anger, shame, sadness, or denial, and most will say, "I don't believe this happened to me." Some may have a reaction formation and act opposite to how they feel, such as laughter instead of crying. Some feel rage at the sudden, unpredictable, and uncontrollable threat to their safety or lives, and this rage can even be directed at the professionals who are trying to help them. When working with victims, be sure to follow these guidelines:

■ Listen. Show that you are actively listening to victims through your facial expressions, body language, and comments such as "Take your time; I'm listening" and "We can take a break if you like. I'm in no hurry."

■ Notice victims' body language, to help you understand and respond to what they are feeling as well as to what they are saying.

■ Assure victims that their emotional reactions are not uncommon. Sympathize with the victims by saying things such as, "You've been through something very frightening. I'm sorry."

■ Counter self-blame by victims by saying things such as, "You didn't do anything wrong. This was not your fault."

■ Ask open-ended questions.

■ Avoid interrupting victims while they are telling their story.

■ Repeat or rephrase what you think you heard the victims say for validation.

3. *Victims need to know "what comes next" after their victimization.* Victims usually have concerns about their role in the criminal investigation and legal proceedings. They may also be concerned about payment for health care or property damage. You can help relieve some of their anxiety by telling victims what to expect in the aftermath of the crime and by preparing them for upcoming

stressful events and changes in their lives. When working with victims, be sure to follow these guidelines:

- Refer the victim to a victim's advocate who will assist the victim through the investigative and legal proceedings.
- Tell victims about subsequent law enforcement interviews or other kinds of interviews they can expect.
- Discuss the general nature of medical forensic examinations the victim will be asked to undergo and the importance of these examinations for the legal proceedings.
- Counsel victims that lapses of concentration, memory losses, depression, and physical ailments are normal reactions for crime victims. Encourage them to reestablish their normal routines as quickly as possible to help speed their recovery.
- Give victims a listing of resources that are available for help and information, as noted above.
- Ask victims whether they have any questions. Encourage victims to contact you if you can be of further assistance.

Treatment of Acute and Posttraumatic Stress Disorders

Treatment should be individualized and may include:

Cognitive-behavioral therapy (CBT) has been shown to be the most effective treatment of PTSD in adults. CBT for children generally includes the child discussing the traumatic event (exposure), anxiety management techniques such as relaxation and assertiveness training, and correction of inaccurate or distorted trauma-related thoughts. There is some controversy regarding exposing children to the events that scare them, but exposure-based treatments seem to be most relevant when memories or reminders of the trauma distress the child. Children can be exposed gradually and taught relaxation techniques so they can relax while recalling the painful experiences and learn that they do not have to be afraid of their memories. CBT also involves challenging children's distorted beliefs.

Psychoeducation and *parental involvement* are used in conjunction with CBT. Children and parents are educated about PTSD symptoms and their effects. The better parents cope with the trauma, and the more they support their children, the better their children will function. Thus, parents need to seek treatment for themselves in order to develop the necessary coping skills that will help their children. This includes the abusive parent who will be reunited with his children.

Play therapy uses games, drawings, and other techniques to help the children process their traumatic memories. It can be used to treat young children who are not able to deal with the trauma more directly.

Eye movement desensitization and reprocessing (EMDR) combines cognitive therapy with directed eye movements. EMDR has been shown to be effective in treating both children and adults with PTSD, but studies indicate that it is the cognitive intervention rather than the eye movements that accounts for the change.

Psychopharmacology may be indicated. However, due to the minimal research in this area, it is too early to evaluate the effectiveness of medication therapy.

RESOURCES

National Association of Crime Victim Compensation Boards (NACVCB): www.nac vcb.org
National Center for PTSD: www.ptsd.va.gov
Office for Victims of Crime: http://ovc.gov/

REFERENCES

Alio, A., Nana, P., & Salihu, H. (2009). Spousal violence and potentially preventable single and recurrent spontaneous fetal loss in an African setting: Cross-sectional study. *The Lancet, 373*(9660), 318–324.
American Bar Association. (2009). Child victim rights. *Criminal Justice Section Newsletter,* Winter, *17*(2). Retrieved from www.abanet.org/crimjust/committees/childvictim rights.pdf
American Psychiatric Association. (2000). *Diagnostic and statistical manual of mental disorders* (4th ed., text rev.). Washington, DC: Author.
Boden, J., Horwood, L., & Fergusson, D. (2007). Exposure to childhood sexual and physical abuse and subsequent educational achievement outcomes. *Child Abuse & Neglect, 31*(10), 1101–1114.
Child Welfare Information Gateway. Retrieved from www.childwelfare.gov/pubs/fact sheets/long_term_consequences.cfm
Draper, B., Pfaff, J., Pirkis, J., Snowdon, J., Lautenschlager, N., Wilson, I., et al. (2007). Long-term effects of childhood abuse on the quality of life and health of older people:

Results from the Depression and Early Prevention of Suicide in General Practice Project. *Journal of the American Geriatrics Society, 56*(2), 262–271.

Duffy, F., Craig, T., Moscicki, E., West, J., & Fochtmann, L. (2009). Performance in practice: Clinical tools to improve the care of patients with posttraumatic stress disorder. *Focus: The Journal of Lifelong Learning in Psychiatry, 7*, 186–203.

Gilbert, R., Spatz-Widom, C., Browne, K., Fergusson, D., Webb, E., & Janson, S. (2009). Burden and consequences of child maltreatment in high-income countries. *The Lancet, 373*, 68–81.

Jonker, B., & Hamrin, V. (2007). Acute stress disorder in children related to violence. *Journal of Child and Adolescent Psychiatric Nursing, 16*(2), 41–51.

King, L. (2003). Child stress disorders checklist: A measure of ASD and PTSD in children. *Journal of the American Academy of Child and Adolescent Psychiatry, 42*, 972–978.

Swan, N. (1998). Exploring the role of child abuse on later drug abuse: Researchers face broad gaps in information. *NIDA Notes, 13*(2). Retrieved from www.nida.nih.gov/NIDA_Notes/NNVol13N2/exploring.html

Turnera, H., Finkelhor, D., & Ormrod, R. (2006). The effect of lifetime victimization on the mental health of children and adolescents. *Social Science & Medicine, 62*, 13–27.

Wilson H., & Widom, C. (2008). An examination of risky sexual behavior and HIV in victims of child abuse and neglect: A 30-year follow-up. *Health Psychology, 27*, 149–158.

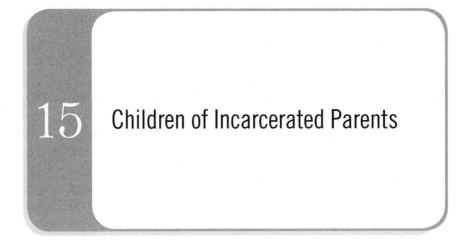

Children of Incarcerated Parents

DEFINITION

More than 1.7 million children in this country have a parent serving a sentence in a state or federal prison. Children of incarcerated parents face unique difficulties. Many experience the trauma of sudden separation from their sole caregiver, and are most are vulnerable to feelings of fear, anxiety, anger, sadness, depression, and guilt. They may be moved from caretaker to caretaker and have significant behavioral consequences, including emotional withdrawal, failure in school, delinquency, and risk of intergenerational incarceration.

Parental incarceration has profound effects on children. When parents are sent to prison, children who live in single-parent households must move, sometimes to foster care and the homes of strangers. In other families, the children's caregivers must carry out family responsibilities often with reduced financial resources and increased expenses. Caregivers must manage childrearing with limited, if any, support and involvement from the children's imprisoned parents. Many of these caregivers are the children's grandparents, who may also be dealing with aging and chronic illness.

Children usually are confused about their parents' absence, have ambivalent feelings, and may wonder if their parents care about them. They may be teased by peers, creating embarrassment and shame. Many children adjust remarkably well, while others experience problems in school, act out in socially undesirable ways, or suffer depression.

Few children see their incarcerated parents on a regular basis, and most do not see their incarcerated parents at all. Prisons are usually difficult to reach using public transportation and may be a distance from the family, and many prisons are not conducive to the presence of children. Visiting policies are restrictive and visiting procedures at many institutions are humiliating and demeaning for adults and children. Telephone calls can be costly, with some institutions charging more than $30 for a 30-minute prison-based collect phone call.

Without contact, children begin to view their parents as strangers, making their adjustment more challenging and reunification with their parents even more difficult. The literature shows that regular contact decreases the risk of parental reoffending and intergenerational incarceration. However, there are little data to guide decisions related to the impact of prison visitation on child physical and emotional health or on the long-term impact of the incarceration of a parent on child outcomes. Health care providers seeking information regarding outcomes for children of incarcerated parents often rely on data related to children's reactions to divorce or death of a parent.

PREVALENCE

Incarcerated parents (52% of state inmates and 63% of federal inmates) reported having an estimated 1,706,600 minor children, accounting for 2.3% of the U.S. resident population under age 18. More than 10 million children live with a parent who has come under some form of criminal justice supervision at some point in the child's life (Glaze, & Maruschak, 2008).

ETIOLOGY

Incarcerated parents typically have a history of being raised by adults who were chemically dependent, abusive, or both. They may have learned to cope and adapt to trauma by striking out at others and/or by self-medicating with drugs or alcohol. Incarcerated parents can lack the ability to attach to others and may not have internalized adequate or healthy models of child rearing. For many, rage, depression, and addiction have been a part of life followed by the criminal activity related to substance abuse. Some perpetrators are incarcerated because of crimes against their family members, including parents imprisoned for domestic or sexual violence, or homicides involving their own children or partner. However, these are relatively rare cases and are not typical of incarcerated parents and their children.

ASSESSMENT

General Principles

Parental incarceration creates challenges for families that often result in financial instability and material hardship, with financial problems the most severe for already vulnerable families and caregivers who support contact between the incarcerated parent and his or her child; instability in family structure and relationships, as well as residential mobility; school behavior and performance problems; loss of pre-incarceration support systems; and shame and stigma.

History and Physical Assessment

Children may experience multiple psychological problems including sadness, low self-esteem, anxiety, guilt, shame, and fear, and negative behavioral manifestations that include withdrawal, decline in school performance, truancy, and use of drugs or alcohol, and aggression. Many children of incarcerated parents exhibit symptoms of posttraumatic stress disorder, attention deficit disorder, and attachment disorders. Dr. Denise Johnston, Director of the Center for Children of Incarcerated Parents at Pacific Oaks College in Pasadena, California, has studied the impact of parental crime, arrest, and incarceration on children's development. She outlined the effects according to developmental stages:

Infancy (0–2 years): Impaired parent-child bonding

Early childhood (2–6 years): Anxiety, developmental regression, acute traumatic stress, survivor guilt

Middle childhood (7–10 years): Acute traumatic stress and reactive behaviors

Early adolescence (11–14 years): Rejection of limits on behavior, trauma-reactive behaviors

Late adolescence (15–18 years): Premature termination of parent-child relationship; intergenerational crime and incarceration

There is a continuum of risk. At one end of the continuum are families that are in serious danger, while at the other, are families with adequate support systems that are coping well. In between are large numbers of families that are barely managing and are under extreme pressure. There are some variables that can influence a child or family's ability to cope with the incarceration of a family member. Screening for the presence of these positive supports could be included in a routine health care visit for families of incarcerated parents by assessing:

- Family's economic stability
- Health status and emotional capacity of caregivers
- Quality of the child's school
- Job satisfaction level (teens and adults)
- Support versus isolation in the community environment: urban, suburban, or rural
- Available community resources
- Child and family spirituality
- Racial and ethnic prejudices

INTERVENTION

The involvement of the criminal justice system in the lives of children is in and of itself an issue for consideration by health care providers. Learn the rules of prison visitation. These rules are very restrictive and can create difficulty for child visitation. For example, only two visitors may be allowed at any time; children must be accompanied by a parent or legal guardian and the legal guardian must submit proof of guardianship; religious garments are not permitted without prior permission of the assistant warden; and visitors may be subjected to searches. Many prisons post their visiting guidelines on their Web sites.

Caregivers may request that the child's health records be sent to the incarcerated parent to facilitate caregiver consultation by phone with the parent in prison. Caregivers may express an urgent need to toilet train or wean a child from bottle or pacifier to make prison visiting easier. Understanding prison rules helps health care providers to respond more effectively to these and other issues. Health care providers may also need details related to prison visitation in order to answer parent's questions and address issues related to exposure to TB, HIV, and Hepatitis C. There are no known cases of these diseases being transmitted to prison visitors, but concerned adults in the lives of children of prisoners will sometimes use the fear of exposure to these diseases as reason to object to prison visits for children. It is important to ask about the rules and realities of prison visiting before giving advice or making recommendations. Each facility is different.

Family members may be hesitant to reveal details about the incarcerated parent to health care providers. When caregivers do reveal information about their involvement in the criminal justice system, health care providers should react in a nonjudgmental manner and fully address the questions and concerns without discomfort or avoidance. It is important to remember that while many families of prisoners share common characteristics, there are also many variations.

When health care providers are aware of the typical stress points, emotional reactions, and behavioral responses of children and families of prisoners, they can use this awareness to formulate checkpoints for anticipatory guidance. Health care professionals can ask about the child's adjustment, the visits at the prison, and how the caregiver is coping. These statements let the family know that they are comfortable talking about incarceration and its impact. Children and family members with "slow to warm" temperament styles may need several such encounters with the provider before they can open up or even respond at all.

Grandparents raising grandchildren of incarcerated parents. An increasing number of children of incarcerated parents are being raised by their grandparents. These grandparents face a number of important challenges, beginning with how to help the children deal with the parent's incarceration. Health care providers can use these suggestions as guidelines when offering support to such grandparents (modified from the AARP, 2008):

■ Children want to know what happened, and it is best to tell them the truth.

■ Grandparents should talk to the children in a developmentally appropriate manner. Give young children a simple explanation of what happened and older children, the complete story. Most children can understand what you mean when you say that the parent did something wrong and is being punished.

- Children feel many conflicting emotions when their parent is incarcerated. They may feel angry and shameful, while still feeling very loyal to the parent. They may fear that they will never see the parent again and that you may leave them too. Let your grandchildren know that you love them and that you are not going anywhere. Listen, and let them know that it's "okay" to feel the way they do, even if their feelings are different from others'. Some children miss their parent and want to see the parent often, while their grandparents may be angry at the parent and want no contact.

- Respect the child's feelings and do not try to change those feelings.

- Except in extreme circumstances, children should stay in touch with their parent. It gives them a chance to make peace and to adjust more easily when the parent comes home. Staying in touch could even help the parent turn his or her life around since offenders with strong family ties usually do better after they leave prison. Children can talk with an incarcerated parent on the telephone or swap letters with the parent.

- Mail cards on special holidays, send report cards and other school papers, and remind the parent to send cards on the children's birthdays. If possible, take the children to visit the parent in prison. The prison may be a distance away, travel may be costly, and the prison may not be child friendly. However, talk to your health care provider to help you get assistance. Children do better at home if they can visit a parent in jail since they tend to think that prison conditions are much worse than they really are. Seeing the parent in prison can set their minds at ease.

- Do not force the child to visit the incarcerated parent. Some children don't want to have any contact with an incarcerated parent. Instead, try to gently convince the child to stay in touch by phone or mail. If this does not work, try to get the parent to contact the child.

- Sometimes children are severely affected by their parent's incarceration. They may cry often, withdraw, or become aggressive. If this happens, talk to your health care provider.

Grandparents can also feel the same stressors as any parent, as well as stress from aging and chronic illnesses. Raising grandchildren can cause financial and social stress, as well as legal problems if the grandparents have not been made legal custodians. Therefore, referral to social and legal services, as well as other agencies, may be helpful.

PREVENTION/PATIENT TEACHING

Primary Prevention

Since many incarcerated parents are imprisoned because of drug offense, health care professionals can minimize this by utilizing measures to prevent substance abuse.

Secondary Prevention

Health care providers can minimize the effects of incarceration on families by supporting policies and programs that:

Actively encourage kinship care placements.

Ensure that child welfare authorities remain in touch with incarcerated parents.

Facilitate visitation between children and incarcerated parents.

Make appropriate reunification services available to incarcerated parents.

Explore alternatives to incarceration that could make child welfare intervention and child removal unnecessary in many cases.

Tertiary Prevention

Tertiary prevention involves recidivism prevention. Regular contact between incarcerated parents and their children can decrease the chances of the parent reoffending, as well as decrease the chances of the children going to prison later in life.

RESOURCES

Children of Incarcerated Parents: A Bill of Rights: www.norcalserviceleague.org/images/billrite.pdf

GrandCare Tool Kit: Resources for Grandparents Raising Children: www.aarp.org/family/grandparenting/articles/grandcare_toolkit.html

Incarcerated Parents Manual: www.prisonerswithchildren.org/pubs/ipm.pdf

National Resource Center on Children and Families of the Incarcerated (NRCCFI) at Family and Corrections Network (FCN): http://fcnetwork.org

REFERENCES

AARP. (2008). Grandparent tool kit. Retrieved from http://www.aarp.org/family/grand parenting/articles/grandcare_toolkit.html

Adalist-Estrin, A. (2003). National Resource Center on Children and Families of the Incarcerated (NRCCFI) Family and Corrections Network (FCN). *Challenges for health care providers* CPL 302. Retrieved from http://fcnetwork.org/wp/wp-content/uploads/cpl302-challenges.pdf

Bouchet, S. (2008). *Children and families with incarcerated parents: Exploring development in the field and opportunities for growth.* A Report Prepared for the Annie E. Casey Foundation. Retrieved from www.aecf.org/~/media/Pubs/Topics/Child%20 Welfare%20Permanence/Permanence/ChildrenandFamilieswithIncarceratedPar entsExp/Children%20and%20families%20with%20incarcerated%20parents.pdf

Community Legal Services, Inc., and the Center for Law and Social Policy. (2002). *Every door closed: Barriers facing parents with criminal records.* Retrieved from www.clasp. org/admin/site/publications_archive/files/0092.pdf

Glaze, L., & Maruschak, L. (2008). *Parents in prison and their minor children.* Bureau of Justice Statistics Special Report NCJ 222984. Retrieved from www.ojp.usdoj.gov/bjs/pub/pdf/pptmc.pdf

LaLiberte, T., & Snyder, E. (2008). *Children of incarcerated parents.* University of Minnesota Center for Advanced Studies in Child Welfare. Retrieved from www.cehd. umn.edu/SSW/cascw/attributes/PDF/publications/CW360.pdf

Simons, C. (2000). *Children of incarcerated parents.* California Research Bureau. Retrieved from www.library.ca.gov/crb/00/notes/V7N2.pdf

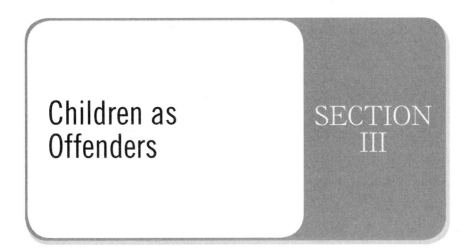

Children as Offenders

SECTION
III

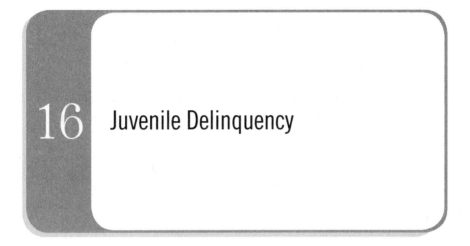

16   Juvenile Delinquency

DEFINITIONS

According to the law, the only difference between a juvenile delinquent and an adult offender is age. However, health care providers should realize that juveniles are not responsible for the bulk of crime, that adult offenders almost always began offending in childhood, and that most childhood offenders grow up to be law-abiding citizens.

The term "juvenile delinquency" is a legal term that refers to single or multiple acts that violate the law by persons who are minors, generally under age 18. In most states, the juvenile court has original jurisdiction over youth who were charged with a law violation and who were younger than 18 years of age at the time of the offense, arrest, or referral to court. However, not all states use age 17 as the oldest age for original juvenile court jurisdiction in delinquency matters. In 2004, the age was 15 in Connecticut, New York, and North Carolina, and 16 in Georgia, Illinois, Louisiana, Massachusetts, Michigan, Missouri, New Hampshire, South Carolina, Texas, and Wisconsin. (See Appendix B, "State Age Parameters in the Juvenile Justice System.")

Many states have higher upper ages of juvenile court jurisdiction in status offense, abuse, neglect, or dependency matters (typically through age 20), and many states grant the juvenile court original jurisdiction over young adults who committed offenses while juveniles. Many states have statutory exceptions to age criteria, such as excluding married or otherwise emancipated juveniles from juvenile court jurisdiction. Other exceptions, such as the nature of the alleged offense and/or prior court history, place certain youth under the original jurisdiction of the criminal court. In some states, a combination of the youth's age, offense, and prior record places the youth under the original jurisdiction of both the juvenile and criminal courts. In the latter cases, the prosecutor has the authority to decide which court will initially handle the case.

Status offenses. Law violations for minors include all violations for which adults are held accountable, as well as status offenses. *Status offenses* are offenses that would not be crimes if committed by an adult. Status offenses include running away, violating curfew, underage drinking, truancy, and incorrigibility. Status offenders are no longer classified as delinquents in most states. Instead, they are considered persons in need of supervision and family assistance. But status offenses are illegal, and the term "delinquency" is often used to refer to both status and other offenses committed by juveniles.

In addition to the above definitions, health care providers should become familiar with the following terminology as it relates to juveniles (from Office of Juvenile Justice and Delinquency Prevention, 1999):

- *Adjudication* is a judicial determination that a youth is responsible for the delinquent or status offense that is charged in a petition.

- *Delinquent act* is an act committed by a juvenile that would be a criminal act if committed by an adult. Delinquent acts include crimes against persons, crimes against property, drug offenses, and crimes against public order.

- *Dependent child* typically refers to a child who has been placed in the legal custody of either the state or the county foster care system by the courts. This usually results from abandonment, abuse, or neglect of the child by its parents or other caregivers.

- *Detention* is the placement of a youth in a secure facility under court authority at some point between the time of referral to court intake and disposition.

- *Disposition* refers to the sanction ordered or treatment plan decided upon in a particular case. Case dispositions are usually coded as follows:

- *Waiver to criminal court.* These are cases that were transferred to a criminal court as the result of a judicial waiver hearing in the juvenile court.

- *Placement.* These are cases in which youth were placed in a residential facility for delinquents or status offenders, or cases in which youth were removed from their homes and placed elsewhere.

- *Probation.* These are cases in which youth were placed on informal/voluntary or formal/court-ordered probation or supervision.

- *Dismissed/released.* These cases are dismissed or otherwise released, including those where the youth were warned and counseled, with no further sanction or consequence anticipated. Among cases handled informally, some may be dismissed by the juvenile court because the matter is being handled in another court or agency.

- *Other sanction.* These may include fines, restitution, community service, referrals outside the court for services with minimal or no further court involvement anticipated, and dispositions coded as "other" in a jurisdiction's original data.

- *Manner of handling* is a general classification of case processing within the court system. Manner of handling can be further classified as "petitioned" or "nonpetitioned."

  - *Petitioned* refers to formally handled cases that appear on the official court calendar in response to the filing of a petition or other legal instrument requesting the court to adjudicate the youth a delinquent, status offender, or dependent child, or to waive jurisdiction and transfer the youth to criminal court for processing as a criminal offender.

  - *Nonpetitioned* refers to informally handled cases in which duly authorized court personnel decide not to file a formal petition after screening the case. Duly authorized personnel include judges, referees, probation officers, other officers of the court, and/or staff of an agency statutorily designated to conduct petition screening for the juvenile court.

- *Petition* refers to a document filed in juvenile court alleging that a juvenile is a delinquent or a status offender and asking that the court assume jurisdiction over the juvenile, or that an alleged delinquent be transferred to criminal court for prosecution as an adult.

Unfortunately, high-profile, highly publicized cases tend to shape professionals' perceptions of juvenile offenders. Juvenile offenders are a heterogeneous group who commit offenses that range from underage drinking to homicide, and all tend to have considerable health care needs. Working in juvenile justice settings can be challenging for health care providers. Secure juvenile correctional settings present a stark contrast to more traditional health treatment settings, and youths dressed in correctional attire, chained, or handcuffed may elicit a wide range of responses in clinicians. In many states, juveniles as young as 9 and as old as 20 are held in the same correctional facility, creating even more challenges, particularly for mental health care.

Juvenile Correctional Facilities and Juvenile Correctional Health

Juvenile correctional facilities can be divided into two main categories: local detention facilities and state-run institutions for longer-term incarceration. Detention facilities administered by local jurisdictions hold preadjudicated youths (those who are awaiting court decisions). These facilities are used for short-term detention or until sentenced youth are transferred to long-term facilities. Some local jurisdictions operate camps and treatment programs, including mental health units. States generally run long-term institutions such as training schools or youth prisons, although some states use private group homes and prisons.

The federal government and court rulings set minimal standards of care, but each state regulates the local facilities and may conduct inspections with variable oversight. The American Academy of Pediatrics (AAP, 2001) and the Society for Adolescent Medicine (SAM, 2000) have published position papers on care of juveniles in correctional facilities, and voluntary accreditation by several national bodies, such as the National Commission on Correctional Health Care (NCCHC) and the American Correctional Association (ACA), assures minimal standards but cannot assess actual day-to-day practices. In 2004 the NCCHC published an updated version of Standards for Health Services in Juvenile Detention and Confinement Facilities. These standards contain seven performance measures meant to determine the actual outcomes of health services. Unfortunately, despite these advances there is no universal accrediting body or universal standardization of care for incarcerated juveniles in the United States.

PREVALENCE

The true extent of delinquent behaviors is unknown, especially since these behaviors often go undetected. Estimates of the extent come from two major sources: data from criminal justice agencies (such as arrest data) and information on offending and victimization based on self-report. Self-report data suggest that delinquent behavior, particularly minor delinquencies like petty theft, underage alcohol use, and truancy, is fairly widespread.

The latter part of the teen years, ages 15 to 19, are the peak period for delinquency; however, there is some evidence of an increase in very young offenders (see Chapter 17, "Child Delinquents"). An estimated 2.18 million juveniles were arrested in 2007. There were 2% fewer juvenile arrests in 2007 than in 2006, and juvenile violent crime arrests declined 3%. These latest data show increases in some offense categories but declines in most (changes being less than 10% in either direction). Other recent findings from the FBI's Uniform Crime Reporting (UCR) Program (n.d.) include the following:

- Juveniles accounted for 26% of all property crime and 16% of all violent crime arrests in 2007.
- In 2007, the juvenile murder arrest rate was 4.1 arrests per 100,000 juveniles ages 10 through 17, which was 24% more than the 2004 low of 3.3, but 72% less than the 1993 peak of 14.4.
- Between 1998 and 2007, juvenile arrests for aggravated assault decreased more for males than for females (22% vs. 17%).
- Although Black youth accounted for just 17% of the youth population ages 10 through 17 in 2007, they were involved in 51% of juvenile Violent Crime Index arrests and 32% of juvenile Property Crime Index arrests.

HEALTH PROBLEMS OF JUVENILES

Many juveniles have conditions that may have resulted from parental neglect; mental health disorders; or physical, drug, or sexual abuse. Others suffer from the consequences of early sexual activity, violence, weapon use, and gang involvement. Detained youths have higher rates of depression and suicide than the general population.

There is substantial evidence that delinquent youths are more likely to display mental health disorders compared to youths in the general population. The most common disorders are substance abuse disorders, and disruptive behavior disorder diagnoses including conduct disorder, oppositional defiant disorder, and attention deficit hyperactivity disorder. Mood and anxiety disorders, although less common, also significantly exceeded rates among nondelinquent youth, and comorbidity is particularly common in offenders displaying conduct problems from early childhood. Many juveniles may also be suffering from traumatic brain injury.

Substance abuse disorders. Persistent juvenile substance abuse is often accompanied by an array of problems, including academic difficulties, health-related consequences, poor peer relationships, family problems, mental health issues, and involvement with the juvenile justice system.

- *Academic difficulties:* declining grades, absenteeism from school and other activities, increased potential for dropping out, cognitive and behavioral problems disrupting learning by their classmates

- *Health-related consequences:* accidental injuries, physical disabilities and diseases, the effects of possible overdoses; danger of contracting HIV or other sexually transmitted diseases; alcohol-related traffic fatalities

- *Poor peer relationships:* alienation from and stigmatization by their peers

- *Mental health issues:* depression, developmental lag, apathy, withdrawal; higher risk for mental health problems, including suicidal thoughts, attempted suicide, completed suicide, depression, conduct problems, and personality disorders; interference with short-term memory, learning, and psychomotor skills from marijuana use; alterations in motivation and psychosexual/emotional development

- *Family life:* disruption resulting in family dysfunction, profound effects on siblings and parents, draining of family financial and emotional resources

■ *Involvement with the juvenile justice system:* high economic and social costs from monetary expenditures and emotional distress related to alcohol- and drug-related crimes, increased burdens for the support of adolescents and young adults who are not able to become self-supporting, and greater demands for medical and other treatment services for these youth.

Conduct disorder. Delinquency can involve a single act, but conduct disorder involves a pattern of behavior over time and behavior domains, and includes some behaviors that are not illegal such as deceitfulness. Conduct disorder is a repetitive and persistent pattern of behavior in which the basic rights of others, or major rules and values of society are violated, as shown by the presence of three (or more) of the following behavior patterns in the past 12 months, with at least one behavior pattern present in the past 6 months: aggression to people and animals (such as often bullies, threatens, or intimidates others; often initiates physical fights; has used a weapon that can cause serious physical harm to others; has been physically cruel to animals; or forced someone into sexual activity); destruction of property (has deliberately engaged in fire-setting with the intention of causing serious damage; has deliberately destroyed others' property, other than by firesetting); deceitfulness or theft (has broken into someone else's house, building, or car; often lies to obtain goods or favors or to avoid obligations [cons]; has stolen items of nontrivial value without confronting a victim [shoplifting, but without breaking and entering; forgery]); serious violations of rules (often stays out at night despite parental prohibitions; has run away from home overnight at least twice while living in parental or parental surrogate home, or once without returning for a lengthy period; is often truant from school). Conduct disorder can have a child, adolescent, or unspecified onset, and can range in severity from mild to severe.

Oppositional defiant disorder. A diagnosis of oppositional defiant disorder refers to age- inappropriate and persistent angry, irritable, defiant, and oppositional behavior. The pattern of negativistic, hostile, and defiant behavior lasts at least 6 months and includes at least four of the following: often loses temper; often argues with adults; often actively defies or refuses to comply with adults' requests or rules; often deliberately annoys people; often blames others for his or her mistakes or misbehavior; is often touchy or easily annoyed by others; is often angry and resentful; and is often spiteful or vindictive.

Attention deficit hyperactivity disorder. The core symptoms of ADHD include inattention, hyperactivity, and impulsivity. Most children experience transient episodes of these symptoms, especially younger ones. These symptoms indicate ADHD when they occur over an extended period of time, typically for at least 6 months; begin before age 7; appear in different settings; and occur at a level that is both performance impairing and developmentally inappropriate. Youth affected by ADHD may appear functionally impaired in many areas and may engage in a broad array of problem behaviors that frustrate and disrupt family, school, and peer relationships. Their inability to pay attention and sit still in class may lead to school failure, truancy, and dropping out. Untreated ADHD can continue into adolescence and adulthood. These individuals may also have comorbid oppositional defiant or conduct disorders, and may abuse substances, and engage in antisocial behavior. Boys with ADHD are at increased risk for engaging in delinquent and antisocial behavior; less is known about girls.

Traumatic brain injury (TBI) results from a blow or jolt to the head or a penetrating head injury that disrupts the normal function of the brain. One study showed that nearly one in five youths (18.3%) reported a lifetime TBI. These juveniles were significantly more likely than youths without TBI to have received a psychiatric diagnosis, report an earlier onset of criminal behavior/substance use, report lifetime suicidality, be impulsive, be fearless, have an external locus of control (feel that others or fate determine events in their lives), and have been criminally victimized in the year preceding incarceration. However, the causal role of TBIs in the pathogenesis of comorbid conditions remains unclear.

TBI can cause supervision and treatment issues in adult prisoners that also may be applicable to juveniles. These issues include the following:

- Attention deficits can make it difficult for the prisoner to focus on a required task or respond to directions given by a correctional officer. These can be misinterpreted, leading to an impression of deliberate defiance.
- Memory deficits can make it difficult to understand or remember rules and directions, which can lead to disciplinary actions.
- Uncontrolled anger can lead to an incident with another prisoner or correctional officer and to further injury for the person and others.
- Slowed verbal and physical responses may be interpreted by correctional officers as uncooperative behavior.

■ Uninhibited or impulsive behavior, including unacceptable sexual behavior, may provoke other prisoners or result in disciplinary action by jail or prison staff.

Home and lifestyle factors put juvenile delinquents at risk for certain problems that may affect their general health, including sexually transmitted infections (STIs) such as human immunodeficiency virus (HIV) infection; other communicable infections; and issues regarding pregnancy and parenting. Conditions occurring at a greater rate in incarcerated youth include tuberculosis (confirmed by positive results of skin testing); dental caries or missing, fractured, or infected teeth; cardiac problems; orthopedic problems; otolaryngologic conditions. They also have conditions that occur in any population of youth, such as obesity, asthma, hypertension, acne, and diabetes.

ASSESSMENT

General Principles

Delinquent youth have the same health care needs as all other youth; however, additional attention should be paid to those issues more prevalent in this population.

History and Physical Assessment

Delinquent youths are often disenfranchised from traditional health care services in the community. Therefore, special attention should be focused on immunization status, dental care, developmental and psychosocial issues, and establishing a plan of continued health care. All children should be evaluated for emergent, acute, and chronic conditions.

Detained juvenile offenders should receive a health screening upon arrival or within 24 hours to rule out emergent needs, contagious conditions, and the need to continue current medications. A complete assessment and health maintenance examination with necessary interventions should be performed within 3 to 7 days.

Diagnostic Testing

Since early sexual activity, sexual abuse, and sexual offending are all associated with delinquency, STD screening should be performed when appropriate. Young postpubertal females should also be screened for the possibility of pregnancy.

INTERVENTION

Juvenile offenders should receive mental health care in a timely manner to meet their acute and chronic emotional conditions. All children should be assessed for suicidal ideation, and precautions must be implemented for those children at risk. Psychological counseling, drug cessation programs, anger management programs, and parenting classes should be available, as should appropriate education. Some children may require psychotropic medication, and provisions need to be made to provide ongoing evaluation as standing orders for their administration may be considered inappropriate.

Detention can present a unique opportunity to address the basic health needs of these children and provide health education. However, factors can impede this process. The provision of health care in these facilities is multifaceted with the potential for conflict of interests regarding custody versus care issues. Juveniles who are released and those who are not ordered detained easily fall through the cracks, their health care neglected.

The American Academy of Pediatrics (AAP) made recommendations in its 2001 policy on health care for children and adolescents in the juvenile correctional care system. The recommendations are presented here with minor modifications for health care providers:

- Youths confined in detention/correctional care facilities should be provided with health care services as recommended by the AAP (Guidelines for Health Supervision III34) and at least equivalent to those accepted as standards of care in the community. Many of these juveniles have not had primary health care, and thus special attention should be focused on immunization status, developmental and psychosocial issues, and establishing primary health care before release.
- Juveniles confined in detention/correctional care facilities should receive recommended comprehensive preventive pediatric and adolescent health services during the period of detention/incarceration. Confinement can be used as an opportunity to provide health maintenance for the youth, including a complete medical history and physical and dental examinations; STI testing for the most common pathogens, including N gonorrhoeae and C trachomatis; and gynecologic examinations for teenage girls. Other appropriate examinations should be conducted as needed, includ-

ing child and adolescent psychiatry; psychopharmacology; other mental health and substance abuse evaluations; neuropsychologic, educational, and projective testing; and pediatric neurology assessments. Immunizations should be provided as recommended by the AAP, the Advisory Committee on Immunization Practices of the Centers for Disease Control and Prevention, and the American Academy of Family Physicians.

- Prenatal services, parenting classes, and substance cessation programs should be available for males and females during their period of incarceration.
- Child and adolescent health care specialists should be consulted about health care policies and procedures governing all detention/correctional care facilities in which juveniles are detained/incarcerated.
- Children and adolescents should be detained or incarcerated only in facilities with developmentally appropriate programs, structure, and staff trained to deal with their unique needs. When youths are housed in adult correctional care facilities, they should be separated from the adult population by sight and sound and provided with a developmentally appropriate environment.
- Health care professionals should work with their professional organizations, the juvenile justice sections of their state judiciary and bar associations, and state legislators to make certain that the medical, educational, and emotional needs of juveniles are appropriately addressed while they are confined and that appropriate state funding (including continued eligibility for Medicaid) is available for provision of these needed services.
- Health care providers should encourage all correctional care facilities to adopt and comply with the National Commission on Correctional Health Care's Standards for Health Services in Juvenile Detention and Confinement Facilities.

In addition, recommendations for the mental health assessment and treatment of all juveniles in detention facilities and correctional institutions have been made by the American Academy of Child and Adolescent Psychiatry (AACAP, 2005) and include the following:

- Clinicians should have an awareness and an understanding of the operations of the juvenile correctional facility and the issues that affect it, including the interface with multiple systems.

- All juveniles should be screened for mental or substance use disorders, suicide risk factors and behaviors, and other emotional or behavioral problems.
- All juveniles should receive continued monitoring for mental and substance abuse disorders, emotional and behavioral problems, and especially suicide risk.
- Any juvenile with recent or current suicidal ideation, attempts or symptoms of a mental or substance abuse disorder during their period of incarceration [or detention] should be referred for an additional evaluation by a mental health clinician.
- Clinicians who work in juvenile justice settings must be vigilant about personal safety and security issues and be aware of actions that may compromise their own safety and/or the safety and containment of the incarcerated [detained] juveniles.
- All qualified mental health care professionals should clearly define and maintain their clinician role with juvenile offenders and their families.
- Adequate time and resources are needed to perform mental health assessment using a biopsychosocial approach with special attention to gender, family, cultural, and other relevant youth issues.
- Clinicians should be alert to symptoms, behaviors, and other clinical presentations of malingering, secondary gain, and manipulative behaviors by incarcerated [detained] juveniles.
- Mental health professionals should be aware of the unique therapeutic and boundary issues that arise in the context of the juvenile correctional setting.
- All referred juveniles should be evaluated for current and future risk of violent behavior.
- Clinicians should be knowledgeable about their facility's policies and procedures regarding seclusion, physical restraints, and psychotropic medication, and, in support of humane care, should advocate for the selective use of restrictive procedures only when needed to maintain safety or when less restrictive measures have failed.
- Clinicians should use psychotropic medications in a safe and clinically appropriate manner and only as a part of a comprehensive treatment plan.
- Clinicians should be involved in the development, implementation, and evaluation of a juvenile's individual treatment plan while in the juvenile setting, as well as with the reentry planning process,

which should include multidisciplinary, culturally competent, and family-based treatment approaches.

■ It is critical that clinicians be aware of relevant financial, fiscal, reimbursement, agency, and role issues that may affect their ability to provide optimal care to incarcerated [detained] juveniles and consultation to the juvenile correctional system.

Further information on these parameters is available at www.aacap.org/galleries/PracticeParameters/JAACAP%20Juvie%20Det%20Corr%20Fac.pdf.

PREVENTION/PATIENT TEACHING

Primary Prevention

Health care and criminal justice professionals should strive to promote protective factors through family education and by assisting schools in developing programs that foster these factors. Schools should also be encouraged to implement policy and curriculum to address issues such as anger management and bullying. The most promising school and community prevention programs integrate:

Classroom and behavior management programs

Social competency promotion curriculums

Conflict resolution and violence prevention curriculums

Bullying prevention

Afterschool recreation programs

Mentoring programs

Comprehensive community interventions

Secondary Prevention

The risk factors for delinquency are usually categorized in four domains: individual, family, peer, and community. Health care providers should assess for these risk factors during routine wellness exams and when juveniles present with suspicious signs, such as bruised knuckles, intoxication, and drug overdose. Health care providers should be aware that multiple risk factors and processes interacting across multiple life domains lead to serious delinquency, rather than single factors or processes (Shader, n.d.).

> *Individual risk factors:* impulsivity, hyperactivity, difficult temperament, ADHD, learning problems, neurological and cognitive impairments, substance abuse, antisocial attitudes
>
> *Family risk factors:* harsh and abusive parenting, lack of or inconsistent discipline, lack of support and attachment, family conflict, antisocial parents
>
> *School/peer risk factors:* early conduct problems in school, lack of commitment to school and lack of school attainment; delinquent friends or whose friends approve of delinquency, gang membership
>
> *Community risk factors:* crime, chronic violence, and disorganization in the neighborhood

At-risk youth require intervention, either from their primary health care provider or referral to an appropriate counseling agency.

Tertiary Prevention

Health care providers should participate in the aftercare of juvenile offenders to assure that they have an adequate plan to return to society. Aftercare is a combination of services, planning, supervision, and support that begins at the disposition, continues through placement, anticipates release, continues when the youth is discharged from the court supervision, and extends thereafter through opportunities, supports, and services.

RESOURCES

Juvenile Offenders and Victims 2006 National Report: http://ojjdp.ncjrs.gov/ojstatbb/nr2006/downloads/NR2006.pdf
National Commission on Correctional Health Care: www.ncchc.org
Office of Juvenile Justice and Delinquency Prevention: http://ojjdp.ncjrs.org/

REFERENCES

American Academy of Child and Adolescent Psychiatry. (2005). Practice parameter for the assessment and treatment of youth in juvenile detention and correctional facilities. *Journal of the American Academy of Child and Adolescent Psychiatry, 44*(10), 1085–1098.

American Academy of Pediatrics, Committee on Adolescence. (2001). Health care for children and adolescents in the juvenile correctional care system. *Pediatrics, 107,* 799–803.

American Psychiatric Association. (2000). *Diagnostic and statistical manual of mental disorders* (4th ed., text rev.). Washington, DC: Author.

Dickenson, T., & Crowe, A. (1997). *Capacity building for juvenile substance abuse treatment.* Office of Juvenile Justice and Delinquency Prevention Juvenile Justice Bulletin NCJ 167251. Retrieved from http://www.ncjrs.gov/html/ojjdp/jjbul9712-1/jjbdec97.html

Federal Bureau of Investigation Uniform Crime Reporting Program. (n.d.). Retrieved from www.fbi.gov/ucr/ucr.htm

Griel, L., & Loeb, S. (2009). Health issues faced by adolescents incarcerated in the juvenile justice system. *Journal of Forensic Nursing, 5,* 162–179.

Morris, R. (2005, March). Health care for incarcerated adolescents: Significant needs with considerable obstacles. *Virtual Mentor, 7*(3). Retrieved from http://virtualmentor.ama-assn.org/2005/03/pfor2-0503.html

Office of Juvenile Justice and Delinquency Prevention. (1999). Offenders in juvenile court, 1996. Juvenile Justice Bulletin July 1999, NCJ 175719. Retrieved from http://www.ncjrs.gov/html/jjbulletin/9907_2/contents.html

Perron, B., & Howard, B. (2008). Prevalence and correlates of traumatic brain injury among delinquent youths. *Criminal Behaviour and Mental Health, 18,* 243–255.

Puzzanchera, C. (2009). *Juvenile arrests 2007.* Office of Juvenile Justice and Delinquency Prevention Bulletin 225344. Retrieved from www.ncjrs.gov/pdffiles1/ojjdp/225344.pdf

Shader, M. (n.d.) Risk factors for delinquency: An overview. Office for Juvenile Justice and Delinquency Prevention. Retrieved from http://www.ncjrs.gov/pdffiles1/ojjdp/frd030127.pdf

Smith, C. (2008). Juvenile delinquency: An introduction. *The Prevention Researcher, 5*(1), 3–9.

Society for Adolescent Medicine. (2000). Health care for incarcerated youth. Position paper of the Society for Adolescent Medicine. *Journal of Adolescent Health, 27,* 73–75.

Stern, K. (2001, May). *A treatment study of children with attention deficit hyperactivity disorder.* Office of Juvenile Justice and Delinquency Prevention Fact Sheet #20. Retrieved from www.ncjrs.gov/pdffiles1/ojjdp/fs200120.pdf

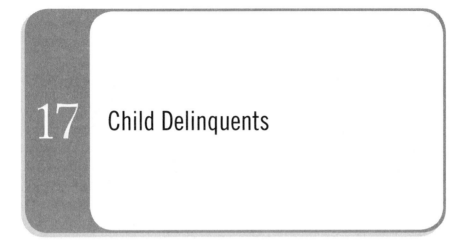

17 Child Delinquents

DEFINITION

Child delinquents are those who become adjudicated before the age of 13. The minimum age for which a child can be adjudicated varies per state. According to the National Juvenile Defender Center (n.d.), 13 states specify a minimum age for delinquency adjudication, while most of the remaining states have no statute that specifies a minimum age under which a child cannot be adjudicated delinquent. In these states, the juvenile court statute typically defines a child as being younger than 18 (or another age). Minnesota's Court of Appeals sets a minimum age of 10 for delinquency adjudications. States that set a minimum age of 10 are Arkansas, Colorado, Kansas, Louisiana, Mississippi, South Dakota, Texas, and Vermont. Arizona has a minimum of 8, while Maryland, Massachusetts, and New York set their minimum at 7. North Carolina's minimum age is 6.

PREVALENCE

Many child delinquents are referred directly to the court by family members, social service agencies, and schools, but most make their first contact with the legal system after arrest by law enforcement. From 1988 to 1997, child offender arrests for property crimes dropped 17%, while arrests for violent crimes increased 45%. In 1997, children under age 13 made up 9%, or approximately 1 in 11, of all juvenile arrests with crimes that varied from arson (35%) to sex offenses (19%) and murder (1%) (McGarrell, 2001).

These children tend to have longer criminal careers than juveniles who become delinquent at a later age, and they constitute a disproportionate threat to public safety and property. Juveniles who enter the court system at a young age run a very high risk of continued offending. Approximately 60% of children aged 10–12 years who are referred to juvenile courts subsequently return to court. For those offending a second time, the chance of return soars to 80%. However, because most of these children do not commit serious or violent offenses and because they have not yet accumulated a long record, child delinquents tend not to get much attention from juvenile justice officials, even though they are more amenable to services and sanctions than teen offenders.

Racial minorities are overrepresented in nearly every aspect of the juvenile justice system. Even though non-White youths constituted about 20% of the U.S. juvenile population in 1997, they were involved in 37% of the court cases of juveniles younger than 13 years. Non-White juveniles are also more likely to be remanded to detention while awaiting court disposition (16% vs. 7%), be placed on the court docket (45% vs. 37%), and be ordered to out-of-home placement when adjudicated delinquent (23% vs. 17%).

Arson. Although legal definitions vary from state to state, under modern statutes arson is the intentional and wrongful burning of someone else's property or one's own property. Juveniles are arrested for a greater share of this crime than any other—juveniles accounted for 49% of persons arrested for arson in 2001 (Federal Bureau of Investigation, 2002). Curiosity and the desire to learn attract children to fire; thus, they need to learn its ability to harm and destroy. This attraction leads some children to fireplay and firesetting (both typically done without malice), which may be the precursors of arson.

Sex offenses. The percent of child delinquents arrested for forcible rape grew from 4% in 1980 to 12% in 1997. The rate of arrests for other sexual offenses rose from 11% to 19% in the same time period. Research in the area of prepubertal sex offenders is still in its infancy, but one literature review (Araji, 1997) revealed that some children are sexually aggressive as early as age 3 or 4, although the most common age of onset appears to be between 6 and 9. Contrary to findings regarding adolescent sex offenders, girls were represented in much greater numbers among preadolescent offenders. Furthermore, these girls often engaged in behaviors that were just as aggressive as the boys' actions. Victims of child sex offenders range in ages from 1 to 9, and many offenders have multiple victims.

Homicide. Homicides by child delinquents remain relatively rare, and only 26% of these murders are committed by children 10 and under. The majority of children murderers are male, with 48% of these being White, 50% Black, and the remaining percent American Indian or Asian. More than one-third of their victims are also younger than 13, and half of their homicides are committed with handguns.

Although not represented in delinquency reports, two other aggressive acts bear mentioning here: bullying and animal cruelty. Both are forms of violence, and both may serve as predictors for other violent and antisocial behaviors.

Bullying. Although not typically a criminal offense, bullying is a form of violence among children. School bullying has come under more scrutiny amid reports that it may have been a factor in many of the school shootings, including those in Littleton, Colorado, Santee, California, and Williamsport, Pennsylvania. Bullying behavior has been linked to other forms of antisocial behavior, such as vandalism, shoplifting, truancy, fighting, and substance use. Bullying behavior can also lead to criminal behavior later in life—60% of males who were bullies in Grades 6 through 9 were convicted of at least one crime as adults.

Animal cruelty. Children under 12 represent only a small number of animal abuse cases. However, children who are cruel to animals are at greater risk of committing acts of violence toward humans. Animal cruelty is one of the criteria for conduct disorder—possibly the earliest sign, and it is typically associated with other antisocial behaviors, such as bullying, truancy, and vandalism.

ETIOLOGY

The Pittsburgh Youth Study (Kelley, Loeber, Keenan, & DeLamatre, 1997) demonstrated three pathways to juvenile offending, all of which are predicted by less serious behaviors in childhood. The *overt pathway* begins with minor aggression (bullying, annoying others), is followed by physical fighting, and then by violence (assaults, rape). The *authority conflict pathway* begins with stubborn behaviors, followed by defiance (disobeying), and then truancy and running away from home. The *covert pathway* begins with minor infractions (shoplifting), escalates to property damage (firesetting), and proceeds to more serious property crimes (burglary).

Behaviors that place a child at risk for child delinquency may be present as young as 2 years of age. Thus the preschool period is a critical time for building a foundation to prevent the development of disruptive behavior and delinquency. Disruptive problem behavior that chronically violates the rights of others is the most common source of referral to mental health services for preschool children, and studies have documented a predictive relationship between problem behaviors in preschool and later conduct disorder and child delinquency. Many important developmental skills begin during this period, and difficulties in these skills may weaken the foundation of learning and contribute to later disruptive behavior. Language is the primary means by which parents and others affect children's behavior. Delayed language development may increase a child's stress level, impede normal socialization, and be associated with later criminality up to age 30. Difficult temperament (and temperament misfit between the child and parent) early in life may be a marker for the early antecedents of antisocial behavior and behavior problems. Low attachment to caregivers, especially the early mother-infant bond, plays an important role in later behavior and delinquency problems, and the closer a child is to the mother, the less likely a child is to be at risk for delinquency.

ASSESSMENT

General Principles

Child delinquents present a challenge to both the judicial and health care systems, particularly since the majority of them will be returning to a society that may have forgotten them. Parents and communities tend to lose interest in these children when their success in school begins to decline. When schools fail to respond to these children, their delinquent behavior escalates.

History and Physical Assessment

When assessing a known child offender, health care providers should perform a comprehensive exam that includes a complete history and physical, with a neuropsychiatric assessment to monitor for the possibilities of underlying neurologic and psychiatric disorders, including cranial lesions, conduct disorder, attention deficit hyperactivity disorder, bipolar disorder, and substance abuse. If the child has had any health problems in the past that have affected activity or shows any variance in expected growth, he or she should also be assessed for chronic illness such as asthma and orthopedic disorders.

Diagnostic Testing

Laboratory evaluation should rule out lead poisoning and hyperthyroidism, which may manifest in behavioral problems. Since many of these children come from violent families, each should be carefully evaluated for signs of abuse with radiographic studies for suspicious injuries and trauma and laboratory studies to rule out sexually transmitted diseases (STDs) when sexual abuse is suspected. Toxicology studies may be warranted to assess for substance abuse.

INTERVENTION

Child offenders have the same health maintenance needs of their nonoffender peers. In addition, these children need substantial psychosocial interventions for themselves and their families.

Research specific to the health needs of child delinquents is lacking; however, some inferences can be made from resources on the needs of the general juvenile delinquent population. Many of these children have conditions that may have resulted from parental neglect; mental health disorders; or physical, drug, or sexual abuse. Others suffer from the consequences of early sexual activity, violence, weapon use, and gang involvement. Detained youths have higher rates of depression and suicide than the general population.

PREVENTION/PATIENT TEACHING

Primary Prevention

Given the potential for recidivism, prevention is critical. Health care providers can promote preventive measures through direct contact with children and families or through indirect contact via consultation with schools and other youth organizations, public presentations, and publications. Health care providers can promote mentoring programs, community volunteering, and school involvement, and they can develop and implement parenting classes for those at risk, hopefully identifying these parents during the prenatal period to minimize the chance of child abuse and neglect.

Prevention should focus on the *reduction of risk factors* and the *promotion of protective factors*. Risk factors include those already noted from the Hennepin County "Delinquents Under 10" Project (Loeber & Farrington, 1999), as well as the following from the New York State Delinquency Prevention Program for 7- to 15-year-olds (New York State Division of Criminal Justice Services, 2002):

Risk Factors

> Drug use in the home and the community
>
> Long-term unemployment in their areas
>
> Lack of school involvement
>
> Lack of positive peer influence
>
> High levels of family and community violence

Protective Factors

> Healthy self-esteem
>
> A sense of responsibility
>
> Tolerance and respect for others
>
> High adequate parental attention and supervision
>
> Involvement in school
>
> Positive peer influence

Nurse-Family Partnership

Another helpful prevention program is the Nurse-Family Partnership® (NFP; www.nursefamilypartnership.org). This evidence-based program helps change the lives of vulnerable first-time moms and their babies through ongoing home visits from registered nurses. Each mother is partnered with a registered nurse early in her pregnancy and receives ongoing nurse home visits that continue through her child's second birthday. This early intervention allows for any critical behavioral changes needed to improve the health of the mother and child.

Secondary Prevention

Screening is especially important because child delinquents are not legally defined the same way in every state, and many states have no defined age of criminal responsibility (minimum age of arrest). This variation, along with the "several bites of the apple" effect, can allow children to go undetected and untreated in the criminal justice system, making detection and intervention all the more critical in health care settings.

Health care providers should screen all children for violent and other antisocial behavior during wellness visits and during episodic visits where manifestations suggest the possibility of these behaviors. Questions regarding vandalism, habitual stealing, fighting, and animal cruelty can be integrated, along with questions regarding inappropriate sexual behavior, into the routine psychosocial history. Health care providers can also use the psychosocial history to screen for the following risk factors based on the Hennepin County "Delinquents Under 10" Project. Risk factors that may emerge from the psychosocial history include:

Abuse, neglect, and/or violence in the home

Delinquent or criminal behavior in parents or siblings

School failure or poor attendance

Multiple problems in daily family functioning

Absence of supportive relationships

Children with multiple risk factors have higher recidivism rates and account for the majority of new offenses committed by young juveniles. Therefore, health care providers should consider early intervention strategies, such as counseling and academic support, for multiple-risk children, regardless of whether they have committed any criminal activities.

Tertiary Prevention

Children with serious disruptive behavior disorders require several different services simultaneously in a continuum of care that involves multiple agencies. A comprehensive model that integrates family mental health care, substance abuse treatment, parenting classes, graduated sanctions, aftercare, and community interventions would best address child delinquency.

RESOURCES

National Council of Juvenile and Family Court Judges: Child Delinquents: http://www. ncjfcj.org/content/view/195/239

REFERENCES

Araji, S. (1997). *Sexually aggressive children: Coming to understand them.* Thousand Oaks, CA: Sage Publications.

Federal Bureau of Investigation. (2002). Crime in the United States, 2001. Washington, DC. Retrieved from http://www.fbi.gov/ucr/01cius.htm

Fox, J. (2002).The violent family. In J. Fox (Ed.). *Primary health care of children* (2nd ed., pp. 335–338). St. Louis, MO: CV Mosby.

Kelley, B., Loeber, R., Keenan, K., & DeLamatre, M. (1997). Developmental pathways in boys' disruptive and delinquent behavior. Office of Juvenile Justice and Delinquency Prevention. *Juvenile Justice Bulletin.* Retrieved from http://www.ncjrs.gov/html/ojjdp/jjbul9712-2/jjb1297.html#contents

Loeber, R., & Farrington D. (1999). Etiology and delinquency prediction. Program and abstracts of the Delinquents Under 10—Targeting the Young Offender Conference, September 30–October 2, Minneapolis, Minnesota.

Loeber, R., & Farrington, D. (Eds.). (2001). *Child development, intervention and service needs.* Thousand Oaks, CA: Sage Publications.

Loeber, R., Farrington, D., & Petechuk, D. (2003). *Child delinquency: Early intervention and prevention.* Office of Juvenile Justice and Delinquency Prevention Bulletin NCJ 186162. Retrieved from www.ncjrs.gov/pdffiles1/ojjdp/186162.pdf

McGarrell, E. (2001). *Restorative justice conferences as an early response to young offenders.* Office of Juvenile Justice and Delinquency Prevention Juvenile Justice Bulletin NCJ 187769. Retrieved from www.ncjrs.org/html/ojjdp/jjbul2001_8_2/contents. html

National Juvenile Defender Center. (n.d.) *Minimum age for delinquency adjudication.* Retrieved from www.njdc.info/state_data_minimum_age.php

New York State Division of Criminal Justice Services. (2002). New York State juvenile delinquency prevention program fact sheet. Retrieved from http://www.criminaljus tice.state.ny.us/ofpa/juvdelprevfactsheet.htm

Snyder, H., Espiritu, R., Huizinga, H., Loeber, R., & Petechuk, D. (2003). *Prevalence and development of child delinquency.* Office of Juvenile Justice and Delinquency

Prevention. Child Delinquency Bulletin Series. NCJ 13411. Retrieved from www.ncjrs.gov/pdffiles1/ojjdp/193411.pdf

Wasserman, G., Keenan, K., Tremblay, R., Coie, J., Herrenkohl, T., Loeber, R., et al. (2003). *Risk and protective factors of child delinquency.* Office of Juvenile Justice and Delinquency Prevention Bulletin NCJ 193409. Retrieved from www.ncjrs.org/pdffiles1/ojjdp/193409.pdf

Wilder Research Center. (2000). *Delinquents under 10: Targeted early intervention.* Retrieved from www.wilder.org/download.0.html?report=1142&summary=1

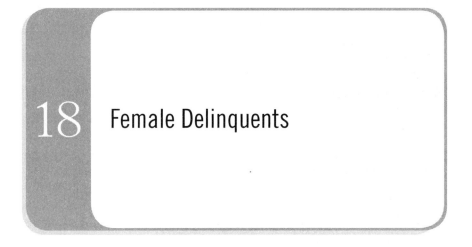

18 Female Delinquents

DEFINITIONS

The majority of juveniles arrested are male; thus, the majority of research on juvenile delinquents has been performed on a mostly male population that does not account for differences between girls and boys. Few studies have examined which girls become delinquent or why, and intervention programs have been traditionally designed with boys in mind, with little known about how well girls respond to these interventions.

Context of girl violence. The Girls Study Group (Zahn et al., 2008) suggests that, while more data are needed, girls' violence occurs in the following context:

- *Peer violence.* While both boy and girl violence is targeted chiefly toward same-sex peers, girls fight with peers to gain status, to defend their sexual reputation, and to defend themselves against sexual harassment.

- *Family violence.* While boys target persons outside the home, girls fight more frequently at home with parents. Girls' violence against parents is multidimensional. For some girls, it represents striking back against their perceived overly controlling structure; for other girls, it is a defense against or an expression of anger originating from being sexually and/or physically abused by members of the household.

- *School violence.* Girl fighting in schools may result from teacher labeling, self-defense, or a general sense of hopelessness.

- *Neighborhood violence.* Girls in disadvantaged neighborhoods are more likely to perpetrate violence because of the increased risk of victimization (self-defense), parental inability to counteract negative community influences, and lack of opportunities for success.

Female juvenile sex offenders (JSO). The average female JSO is 14 years old and exhibits greater variability in her sexual arousal and behavior patterns than adult male/female sex offenders. The most common sexual offenses committed by female adolescents are nonaggressive acts, such as mutual fondling, that occur during a caregiving activity such as babysitting. They rarely commit sex offenses against adults. Their victims are typically young acquaintances or relatives, with male and female children equally at risk for sexual victimization by female adolescents.

Female JSOs are similar to their male JSOs in the level of diversity that exists within their population. They commit a wide range of illegal sexual behaviors, ranging from limited exploratory behaviors committed largely out of curiosity to repeated aggressive acts. Some have histories of multiple nonsexual behavior problems or prior nonsexual juvenile offenses, but many are otherwise well-functioning youth with limited behavioral problems. While some female JSOs experience high levels of individual and family psychopathology, others have limited psychological problems and minimal family dysfunction. Female JSOs differ from male JSOs with regard to physical and sexual abuse history. On average, female JSOs have experienced more extensive and severe physical and sexual maltreatment during their childhood than male JSOs. Female JSOs are also sexually victimized at younger ages and are more likely to have had multiple perpetrators.

Female gang members. Male teens are much more likely to join gangs than female teens. Female gang members are less likely to be involved in criminal behavior than males, but they reported being involved in gang fights, carrying a weapon for protection, and attacking someone with a weapon. Female gangs may be autonomous or allied with male gangs, or female gang members may be part of a fully gender-integrated gang (Moore & Hagedorn, 2001).

However, there is not enough information to determine how each kind of gang structure affects the members' behavior. Existing information does indicate, however, that joining a gang, regardless of its structure, is a significant act for an adolescent female, often with important consequences later in life. According to the Girls Study Group (Zahn et al., 2008), survey research has shown a number of factors associated with girls' involvement in gangs, including attitudes toward school, peers, delinquency, drug use, and early sexual activity. Qualitative research has addressed the role of disadvantaged neighborhoods and families with multiple problems (violence, drug and alcohol abuse, neglect). Girls associated with primarily male gangs exhibit more violence than those in all-female gangs. In general, girls in gangs are more violent than other girls but less violent than boys in gangs.

PREVALENCE

Females accounted for 29% of juvenile arrests in 2007. Law enforcement agencies made 641,000 arrests of females under age 18 in 2007 (Puzzanchera, 2009). From 1998 through 2007, arrests of juvenile females decreased less than male arrests in most offense categories, including aggravated assault, burglary, and larceny-theft, but in some categories, including simple assault, drug abuse violations, and driving under the influence (DUI), female arrests increased, while male arrests decreased. Male juvenile offenders are not only more likely than females to be arrested, but, once arrested, they are more likely to be petitioned, more likely to be adjudicated, and more likely to receive residential placement as a sanction. Females are also less likely to be tried as adults.

ETIOLOGY

The literature on female delinquency is sparse, and data on etiology, extremely limited and more specific for girl violence. Like other types of violence, the etiology of girl violence is viewed as multifactorial. Few juvenile violence studies have included females, and those that included girls often did not conduct gender-based analyses. Thomas (2003) showed that violent girls differed from nonviolent girls with regard to their loneliness, level of connectedness to school, and anger intensity. Some studies show that age of onset for violence is later for girls than boys.

ASSESSMENT

General Principles

Research from the University of Adelaide (2009), Australia, shows that the physical and mental health needs of juvenile offenders should be treated as a priority if offenders held in detention are to have any real hope of rehabilitation.

History and Physical Assessment

When evaluating female adolescents, assess for risk factors, as discussed by the Girls Study Group (Zahn et al., 2008):

Risk Factors Associated With Delinquency That Do Not Differ for Girls and Boys

> Negative family dynamics
>
> Lack of structure and stability
>
> Lack of supervision and control
>
> Family criminality
>
> Family violence
>
> Lack of school involvement

Gender-Sensitive Risk Factors

> Early puberty
>
> Depression and anxiety
>
> Witnessing family violence
>
> Cross-gender peer influence
>
> Responsivity to religion
>
> Attachment and bonding to school
>
> Neighborhood disadvantage

Other Potential Risk Factors

Psychological dysfunction as a response to traumatic events

Maltreatment and sexual assault

Family involvement in prostitution or drug use

Girls are more influenced by the delinquency of romantic partners

Female delinquents have the same issues as males (Chapter 16), as well as issues related to pregnancy, pelvic inflammatory disease, and eating disorders, all of which appear to be more prevalent in this population when compared to nondelinquent females.

INTERVENTION

Female delinquents have a high frequency of mental health problems, suggesting that effective prevention efforts should target the mental health needs. Diverting girls with mental health problems who come into the juvenile justice system to community-based treatment programs would not only improve their individual outcomes, but allow the juvenile justice system to focus on cases that present the greatest risk to public safety.

Evidence is emerging that gender-specific treatment methods can be effective for female offenders, especially when treatment targets multiple aspects of offenders' lives, including family and peer environments. But it is also becoming clear that female offenders are not a homogeneous group and that treatment ultimately should be tailored to suit individual needs defined more specifically than by gender alone (Cauffman, 2008).

PREVENTION/PATIENT TEACHING

Please also refer to Chapter 16, "Juvenile Delinquency," for further information.

Primary Prevention

Targeting girls at risk may prevent delinquent behaviors in some. Some girls manage to achieve success despite the difficulties they encounter in their lives. Positive experiences in life can strengthen a child's ability to become resilient to the difficult situations—abuse, neglect, poverty, witnessing violence—that can lead to delinquency. Protective factors vary. For some girls, caring adults, school connectedness, school success, and religiosity helped to prevent specific forms of delinquency during early adolescence. In other cases, these protective factors were not strong enough to mitigate the impact of the risks. Thus one delinquency prevention program cannot be tailored to the needs of all girls who are at risk for delinquency. However, health care providers can reinforce these resilient factors to prevent delinquency in the hopes to at least reach some girls:

Support from a caring adult. Girls who had a caring adult in their lives during adolescence were less likely to commit status or property offenses, sell drugs, join gangs, or commit simple or aggravated assault during adolescence. They also were less likely to commit simple assault as young adults.

Success in school as measured by grade point average. Girls who experienced success in school during adolescence committed fewer status and property offenses and were less likely to join gangs in adolescence. School success helped protect them from involvement in simple and aggravated assault in adolescence and young adulthood.

Religiosity. Girls who placed a high importance on religion during adolescence were less likely to sell drugs in early adolescence.

Secondary Prevention

Health care providers can assess girls for risk factors and refer those with positive results to appropriate counseling agencies. The factors that equally increase the risk of delinquency for both sexes include:

- Negative family dynamics (i.e., how parents supervise and monitor a child, family history of criminal behavior, child maltreatment)
- The youth's lack of involvement in school
- Negative community (e.g., poverty level, crime rate, employment rate)
- Lack of community-based programs

A number of factors influence girls' behavior more strongly than boys' behavior. Some factors increase a girl's risk of delinquency more than a boy's, including:

- Antisocial females tend to exhibit a pattern of greater right frontal activation (more like that of normative males), while antisocial males exhibit no asymmetry at all.
- Early puberty increases girls' risk for delinquency, especially if they come from disadvantaged neighborhoods and have dysfunctional families. The disparity between biological and social maturity can lead to increased conflict with parents or negative associations with older boys or men.
- Sexual abuse or maltreatment increases girls' risk for delinquency. Girls experience more sexual victimization overall, including sexual assaults, rapes, and sexual harassment; however, all types of maltreatment (sexual, physical, and neglect) can increase the risk of delinquency for both sexes.
- Depression and anxiety disorders have been associated with delinquency and girls receive these diagnoses more frequently than boys.
- When a youth's boyfriend or girlfriend commits a crime, he or she may also engage in delinquent behavior. For less serious crimes, girls are influenced more by their boyfriends than boys are by their girlfriends, but for serious crimes, they are equally affected.

Tertiary Prevention

Health care providers should participate in the aftercare of female juvenile offenders to assure that they have an adequate plan to return to society. Aftercare is a combination of services, planning, supervision, and support that begins at the disposition, continues through placement, anticipates release, continues when the youth is discharged from the court supervision, and extends thereafter through opportunities, supports, and services.

RESOURCES

Girls Study Group: http://girlsstudygroup.rti.org/index.cfm?fuseaction=dsp_home
Juvenile Offenders and Victims 2006 National Report: http://ojjdp.ncjrs.gov/ojstatbb/nr 2006/downloads/NR2006.pdf
Office of Juvenile Justice and Delinquency Prevention: http://ojjdp.ncjrs.org/

REFERENCES

Cauffman, E. (2008). Understanding the female offender. *The Future of Children: Juvenile Offenders, 18*(2), 119–142.
Moore, J., & Hagedorn, J. (2001). *Female gangs: A focus on research.* Office of Juvenile Justice and Delinquency Prevention Juvenile Justice Bulletin 186159. Retrieved from www.ncjrs.gov/pdffiles1/ojjdp/186159.pdf

Office of Applied Studies, Substance Abuse and Mental Health Services Administration. (2004). Female youths and delinquent behaviors. *The NSDUH Report.* Retrieved from www.oas.samhsa.gov/2k4/girlDelinquents/girlDelinquents.htm

Puzzanchera, C. (2009, April). Juvenile arrests 2007. Office of Juvenile Justice and Delinquency Prevention. *Juvenile Justice Bulletin,* NCJ 225344.

Schmidt, S., & Pierce, K. (2004). *What research shows about female adolescent sex offenders.* National Center on Sexual Behavior of Youth. NCSBY Fact Sheet #5. Retrieved from www.ncsby.org/pages/publications/Female%20ASO.pdf

Thomas, S. (2003). Identifying and intervening with girls at risk for violence. *Journal of School Nursing, 19*(3), 130–139.

University of Adelaide. (2009). Young offenders' health critical to rehabilitation. *Science-Daily.* Retrieved from www.sciencedaily.com/releases/2009/06/090619112333.htm

Zahn, M., Brumbaugh, S., Steffensmeier, D., Feld, B., Morash, M., Chesney-Lind, M., et al. (Girls Study Group). (2008). *Violence by teenage girls: Trends and context. Understanding and responding to girls' delinquency.* Office of Juvenile Justice and Delinquency Prevention. Retrieved from www.ncjrs.gov/pdffiles1/ojjdp/218905.pdf

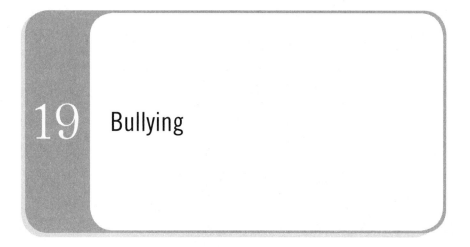

19 Bullying

DEFINITION

Bullying is a form of violent behavior, and bullies can cause serious problems for their victims, as well as for themselves. The American Academy of Pediatrics (2009) defines bullying as a form of aggression in which one or more children repeatedly and intentionally intimidate, harass, or physically harm a victim who is perceived as unable to defend herself or himself. Others note that bullying invokes an imbalance of physical and psychological power between the persons involved. Attacks are unprovoked, systematic, and purposely harmful toward the same individual child. Regardless of the definition, the key factors in bullying are the imbalance of power and the repeated pattern of abuse, as well as the critical point that bullying is not a developmental norm.

Bullying behavior is purposeful and aimed at gaining control over another child. Bullying usually encompasses *direct behaviors,* such as taunting, threatening, hitting, kicking, stealing, and sexual harassment. However, bullying behaviors can also be *indirect (also called relational aggression),* such as gossiping or spreading cruel rumors that cause the victim to be socially isolated by intentional exclusion. Boys tend to prefer direct methods and girls, indirect methods.

Bullying behaviors differ in form and severity. Forms include verbal, physical, and emotional intimidation, as well as racist and sexual bullying. Verbal bullying typically accompanies physical behavior, and includes name calling, spreading rumors, and persistent teasing. Physical bullying, the most obvious form, embodies punching, kicking, biting, hair pulling, pinching, and threatening. Emotional intimidation entails deliberate attacks on the victim's self-esteem, such as deliberate exclusion from a group activity or belittling. Racist bullying takes many forms, including mocking the victim's traditions, voicing racial slurs, and painting graffiti on a victim's locker. Sexual bullying encompasses unwanted physical contacts, such as "wedgies" or bra snapping, as well as derogatory comments. Bullying behaviors range in severity from mild (pushing, spitting, and spreading rumors) to moderate (stealing lunch money, making intimidating phone calls, and using racial slurs) to severe (inflicting bodily harm, threatening with a weapon, and spreading malicious rumors).

Electronic Aggression (Cyberbullying)

Electronic aggression, which encompasses cyberbullying, refers to any kind of aggression perpetrated through technology. Acts include harassment or bullying (teasing, telling lies, making fun of someone, making rude or mean comments, spreading rumors, or making threatening or aggressive comments) that occur through e-mail, a chat room, instant messaging, a Web site (including blogs), or text messaging. Little information exists about whether electronic aggression decreases or increases as young people age. However, as with other forms of aggression, there is some evidence that electronic aggression is less common in 5th grade than in 8th grade, but is higher in 8th grade than 11th grade. Thus electronic aggression may peak around the end of middle school/beginning of high school.

Cyberbullying may be more harmful than traditional bullying because the victim feels that there is no escape. The bullying can take place any time of day or night and anywhere the child has a communication device, including the child's bedroom, which should be a place of safety. Hurtful material may be posted globally and become irretrievable. Unlike victims of schoolyard bullying, victims of cyberbullying may not know the identity of the bully, creating frustration, fear, and feelings of helplessness.

Victims of cyberbullying suffer the same effects as those who are victimized by traditional bullying. Victims may exhibit signs of depression (such as lack of interest in school or pleasurable activities, changes in sleep and eating patterns, depressed mood, and withdrawal), develop school phobias, complain about somatic symptoms such as headaches and abdominal pain, or demonstrate aggressive behaviors. Victims of cyberbullying may not tell their parents about the problem due to their fear of losing their technical devices; they may simply suffer in silence.

Stop Cyberbullying (www.stopcyberbullying.org) describes five types of cyberbullies:

> *Vengeful Angels* believe they are righting wrongs, or protecting themselves or others from the "villain" they are victimizing. They may have been the victims of bullying or may be acting out to protect a friend who has been bullied. This may also be the jilted boyfriend or girlfriend who uses cyberbullying methods to retaliate for the break-up.

> *Power-Hungry Cyberbullies* want to control others and get them to obey their commands. They brag and crave attention to the point that they may escalate their actions to get it.

> *Revenge of the Nerds Cyberbullies* usually target single victims and keep their actions secretive. They rarely appreciate the impact of their actions, and, because of their level of technical skills, can be the most dangerous of cyberbullies.

> *Mean Girls* are typically egotistical, immature, and bored. They use cyberbullying as entertainment and tend to act as a group because they require an audience. This form of cyberbullying is typically fed by admiration, cliques, and the silence of others who let it happen. Mean Girls quit when the entertainment value dissipates.

> *Inadvertent Cyberbullies* may be pretending to be tough or role playing. They don't lash out intentionally and instead behave without thinking.

The National Crime Prevention Council (www.ncpc.org) and Cyberbullying.org (www.cyberbullying.org) note that cyberbullying techniques are as inventive as they are cruel. Techniques used by cyberbullies include the following:

- Pretending they are other people online to trick victims
- Sending cruel, vicious, and sometimes threatening messages via texting, instant messaging, or e-mails
- Creating Web sites that have stories, cartoons, pictures, and jokes ridiculing others

- Posting pictures of classmates online and asking students to rate them, with questions such as, "Who is the biggest ____ (add a derogatory term)?"
- Posting unflattering photos of peers on the Web
- Taking a picture of a person in the locker room using a digital phone camera and sending that picture to others
- Altering pornographic photos by adding a peer's face to the image and sending it to porn sites or posting it in a blog
- Breaking into an e-mail account and sending vicious or embarrassing material to others
- Engaging someone in instant messaging, then tricking that person into revealing sensitive personal information and forwarding that information to others
- Criticizing or defaming teachers and administrators on the Web

Cyberbullies also use *bash boards.* Bash boards are online bulletin boards or chat rooms where youths can anonymously write whatever they want, true or false, creating or adding mean-spirited postings for the world to see. The nature of today's technology makes it possible for cyberbullying to occur more secretly, to spread more rapidly, and to be preserved more easily.

Cyberbully mechanisms have been classified by the Center for Safe and Responsible Internet Use (http://cyberbully.org) as:

Flaming: sending angry, rude, or offensive messages

Harassment: repeatedly sending a person offensive messages

Denigration: sending or posting harmful, false, or cruel statements about a person to other people

Cyberstalking: harassment that includes threats of harm or that is intimidating

Masquerading: pretending to be someone else and sending material that makes that person look bad or places that person in potential danger

Outing and *trickery:* engaging in tricks to solicit embarrassing information about a person and then making that information public

Exclusion: actions that specifically and intentionally exclude a person from an online group, such as blocking a student from an instant messenger buddy list

PREVALENCE

Bullying is prevalent, affecting up to half of children and adolescents worldwide. A 2009 report by the Community Oriented Policy Services (COPS) noted that studies from other counties generally found that between 8% and 38% of students are bullied with some regularity, and that studies conducted in the United States found higher levels of bullying in America than in some other countries (Sampson, 2009).

Estimates vary according to data collection methods, but the problem is probably more prevalent than noted. Bullying frequently goes undetected. Bullies tend to act out at times and places when authority figures are not likely to witness their actions, and victims rarely report the events. Bullies warn victims not to tell, and many adults and other students blame victims for being weak and unable to defend themselves. Children may not report because they fear retaliation, fear not being believed, or fear that things may get even worse if they tell. Young children believe that bullying is acceptable if teachers do not intervene, whereas older students believe that victims are at least partially responsible for bringing the bullying upon themselves. These students believe that bullying "toughens up" a weak person and that bullying teaches victims appropriate behaviors. Other students considered victims to be "weak," "nerds," or afraid to fight back. Parents tend to be unaware of the bullying problem and talk about it only to a limited extent. Teachers seldom or never talk about bullying in their classes, and school personnel may even view bullying as a harmless rite of passage that is best ignored until it crosses the line into theft or assault.

ETIOLOGY

Bullies

Overt bullies act like Scut Farkus in the movie *A Christmas Story*. They behave in an active, outgoing, aggressive manner, using brute force or open harassment, rejecting rules, and rebelling to feel superior and secure. Covert bullies behave in a more reserved manner, not wanting to be recognized as tormentors. They, like Eddie Haskell in *Leave It to Beaver*, control with soft talk and lies, saying the "right thing at the right time," and they draw their sense of power carefully through deception. Both types have the same underlying characteristics—interest in their own pleasure, desire for power over others, willingness to manipulate others to get what they want, and the inability to see things from another's perspective.

Bullies appear to derive gratification from inflicting injury and suffering on others. They have little to no empathy and often defend their actions by claiming their victims provoked them. Bullies have qualities similar to other perpetrators, as they tend to be drawn disproportionately from lower socioeconomic families with poor childrearing techniques, tend to be impulsive, and tend to be unsuccessful in school. Regardless of their degree of intelligence, bullies usually do poorly in school and lack good connections with their teachers. They find it difficult to solve problems without violence. Bullies seem to have little anxiety and strong self-esteem. Contrary to popular belief, little evidence exists to support the idea that bullies victimize because of poor self-esteem. Olweus (1991) noted that bullies tend to be characterized by either unusually low or about average levels of anxiety and insecurity, and their self-image is also about average or even relatively positive.

Children bully for a variety of reasons. Some bully to deal with difficult situations at home; some have been victims of abuse themselves. Bullies may have previously been rejected by their peers because they showed high rates of conflict, aggression, and immature play and because they have trouble taking in the perspective of another child. Many bullies come from families characterized by little warmth and affection. These families have trouble sharing their feelings and tend to be less close to one another. The parents use inconsistent discipline and may be bullies themselves.

Bullying frequently persists because it is rapidly and substantially rewarded. Bullies often get what they want from victims—status, material possessions, and domination. Aggression can then become a problem-solving mechanism early in life, becoming fully incorporated into the child's personality or response repertoire by middle childhood.

Victims

Bullies may target children whose characteristics deviate from the norm in size, appearance, and way of thinking. However, they most often prey upon children who are shy, anxious, or insecure, and who lack social graces and friends. These victims tend to be close to their parents, who may be overprotective. Usually physically weaker and emotionally vulnerable, victims become easy targets who do not fight back.

Passive victims tend to be insecure, reacting passively and anxiously to situations. Many are physically smaller, cautious, sensitive, socially isolated, and quiet. They tend to have a negative view of themselves, seeing themselves as failures and feeling lonely, stupid, ashamed, and unattractive. It is not known the extent to which physical, mental, or speech difficulties, glasses, skin color, weight, hygiene, posture, and dress play a role in victim selection. However, children who have been abused are more likely to be targeted by peers. Other vulnerable populations are children with learning disorders, children with physical disabilities, and children who are experiencing a family crisis or who are actually neglected. In general, it appears that the children who already have much to cope with in terms of physical, emotional, or social disadvantage become victims of bullies.

Provocative victims tend to be quick-tempered and try to fight back if they feel insulted or attacked. They may be hyperactive and have difficulty concentrating. Children who tend to be restless and irritable and who tease and provoke others can become victims. Some experts suspect that some children with attention deficit hyperactivity disorder (ADHD) fit into this category. Provocative victims frequently display the social-emotional problems of victimized children, as well as the behavioral problems of bullies, which may create challenges for treatment.

Other Players

While some refer to the other players as bystanders, these players can be divided into specific groups. Bully buddies are the sidekicks of the bullies. They assist the bully, sometimes luring victims or holding them down. Bully bolsters do not actively attack the victim; however, they give positive feedback to the bully, usually by acting as an audience by laughing and making other encouraging gestures. Victim victors take sides with the victim. They show antibullying behavior by comforting the victim and trying to stop the bully. Bully bystanders do not get involved. They stay in the background and allow the bullying to continue because of their silence.

ASSESSMENT

General Principles

Screen all school-aged and adolescent children during health maintenance examinations, and screen children who present with school phobia, mood and/or behavioral problems, or somatic complaints (trouble sleeping, headaches, enuresis, and stomachaches).

History and Physical Assessment

Victims. When asking children about school, monitor their demeanor to notice whether they behave in a shy or withdrawn manner, especially when discussing peer relationships and activities. Ask children about their route to and from school, because victims may be fearful of walking to and from school or riding the bus. Subtle signs, as well as obvious ones, may be present; however, realize that these signs can indicate other disorders, such as depression and substance abuse, which should be ruled out. Possible signs of victimization include the following:

- Depression and/or suicidal ideation

- Anxiety

- Moodiness or sullenness, as well as withdrawal from family interaction

- Loss of interest in school work

- Aggression; bullying siblings or other children

- Unexplained bruises or injuries

- Arrival at home with torn clothes or unexplained bruises

- Disappearance of personal belongings, asking for extra money or allowance for school lunch or supplies, or stealing money

- Waiting to use the bathroom at home or enuresis

- Crying during sleep or nightmares

- Stomachaches or mysterious illnesses invented to avoid going to school or outright refusal to go to school

- Drastic changes in sleep or eating patterns

- Desire to carry a weapon, such as a knife or gun, for protection

- Unwillingness to discuss the situation at school or improbable excuses for the aforementioned signs

Bullies. Detecting bullies is more difficult than detecting victims because bullies are adept at hiding their mistreatment of others. Parents may have no idea that their child is bullying until a teacher or another parent confronts them about it. Other parents may report that their child has little concern for others, is aggressive or manipulative, abuses animals, or possesses unexplained items or money. Bullies may act cocky, arrogant, and self-assured, and they may have difficulty accepting authority. When asked about bullying, they are apt to be condescending about responding to questions. Because most bullies lack empathy, they also tend to appear pleased or amused when providers ask them how they feel about other children getting hurt. Bullies may also exhibit many of the same signs as victims, especially depression, anxiety, and psychosomatic symptoms; and they may have substance abuse problems.

Repeated bullying may be a sign of conduct disorder. The primary diagnostic features of conduct disorder include aggression, theft, vandalism, violations of rules, and/or lying that have occurred for at least a 6-month period. Bullying has also been linked to other antisocial behaviors, including vandalism, fighting, theft, smoking, substance abuse, truancy, and dropping out of school.

Diagnostic Testing

No diagnostic testing is required.

INTERVENTION

Management of bullying should be multidisciplinary, involving the parents, primary health care provider, teachers, school administrators, school counselors, and other mental health professionals as needed. The health care professional can play a key role by acting as liaison between the affected family (bully or victim) and the school.

Victims. Encourage children and their parents to verbalize their feelings about the bullying. Victims and their parents need reassurance that the health care provider can help them find effective ways to respond to bullying and to change the children's behavior to prevent them from being bullied in the future.

Children are less likely to be bullied in a peer group. Because many victims have poor social skills and few friends, they need to practice socially acceptable behaviors. Structured groups and activities, such as scouting, boys and girls clubs, sports, martial arts, and after-school activities help children develop these skills under the adult supervision. Drama clubs teach children how to act in a manner that does not show what they feel, a skill that can be used when bullied. In addition, health care providers can foster healthy self-esteem and teach problem-solving skills, and they can teach children to be assertive rather than submissive. Parents can make an appointment with their child's teacher, principal, and/or counselor to discuss the problem and to ask about the school's antibullying policy. School personnel should take the problem seriously and investigate incidents of bullying.

Bullies. Intervening with bullies can be a difficult undertaking because both the parent and child may be reluctant to admit to bullying. Health care providers should avoid arguments and advise parents that this behavior will have negative consequences for their child's future. Like victims, bullies benefit from learning appropriate social skills. Thus, they, too, should be encouraged to participate in small group activities, preferably with older children, so that they can engage in cooperative tasks. Adult supervision is warranted during these groups, and bullies should receive positive reinforcement each time they engage in prosocial or caring behaviors, which enables them to learn more positive ways of gaining attention and affection.

Health care providers can work with the parents to help them learn ways to demonstrate caring and affection toward their children, as well as ways to develop more consistent and appropriate disciplinary measures. Parents should be encouraged to become more involved with community activities and other parents. If the child demonstrates significant bullying behavior or signs of a conduct disorder, referral to a mental health professional is appropriate.

PREVENTION/PATIENT TEACHING

Primary Prevention

Violence prevention is a key role for child care providers, and raising resilient children is a key aspect of violence prevention. Providers should institute a plan that encourages resiliency at each wellness visit, such as the American Academy of Pediatrics' *Connected Kids: Safe, Strong, Secure* (www.aap.org/ConnectedKids). Health care providers also can assist parents in raising nonviolent children, as suggested by Muscari (2002a) in *Not My Kid: 21 Steps to Raising a Nonviolent Child.* Some helpful strategies to support nonviolent parenting include:

- Explain the difference between normal and abnormal. For example, it is normal for toddlers to occasionally tantrum, but frequent, difficult-to-control tantrums require investigation.
- Encourage parents to provide plenty of love and attention.
- Foster positive self-esteem. Give praise when praise is due, but do not give false praise. Children see right through that.
- Encourage parents to talk *with* their children, not at them.
- Enforce the importance of parental supervision. Parents should know where their children are and what they are doing, in both the real and virtual worlds.
- Aid parents in setting limits. While occasional toddler tantrums are normal, they are not socially acceptable. Teach parents how to both ignore tantrums and divert the child's attention to minimize tantruming behavior.
- Teach responsibility. Encourage children to take responsibility for their mistakes.
- Assist parents in teaching problem-solving and decision-making skills. Both skills can be developed by having children plan age-appropriate activities, such as having older school-aged children plan a family dinner that everyone will enjoy.
- Help parents help their children minimize and manage stress.
- Foster anger and conflict management. Have children make a self-control chart to learn when they lose it and use self-control.
- Teach tolerance.
- Enforce family values.
- Minimize the effects of peer pressure. Help children help their friends find alternatives to negative behaviors.
- Instruct parents to monitor their children's media usage.
- Help parents keep their children away from drugs. Start talking about drugs and alcohol during the early years, and set a positive example.
- Keep children away from guns. Use the National Rifle Association's Eddie Eagle program (http://www.nrahq.org/safety/eddie/) to teach young children to stay away from guns, and teach older children how to respect them.
- Empower parents to be responsible role models.
- Urge parents to get involved.

Secondary Prevention

Secondary prevention involves early identification and management. All children should be screened at health maintenance visits and when exhibiting signs that may indicate bullying. However, special attention should be paid to those children who demonstrate risk factors, as delineated by the Center for the Study and Prevention of Violence (2006; www.colorado.edu/cspv):

Risk Factors for Victimization

- Cautious, sensitive, or insecure personality
- Difficulty asserting themselves among peers
- Physical weakness (particularly in boys)
- Overprotection by parents (possible risk factor)
- Lack of close friends
- Presence of aggressive students in same or slightly higher grade
- Lack of supervision during breaks
- Indifferent or accepting student and/or teacher attitudes toward bullying
- Inconsistent enforcement of the rules

Risk Factors for Bullying

- Impulsive, hot-headed, or dominant personality
- Difficulty conforming to rules and low frustration tolerance
- Positive attitudes toward violence
- Physically aggressive
- Gradually decreasing interest in school
- Lack of parental warmth and involvement
- Overly permissive or excessively harsh discipline/physical punishment by parents
- Lack of parental supervision
- Friends/peers with positive attitudes toward violence
- Exposure to models of bullying

- Lack of supervision during school-time breaks
- Unsupervised interactions between different grade levels during breaks
- Indifferent or accepting student and/or teacher attitudes toward bullying
- Inconsistent enforcement of the rules

Note that most of these risk factors can place children at risk for victimization and offending for other types of violence as well as bullying.

Health care providers can also teach parents how to deal with their children, be they bully, victim, or both.

For Parents Whose Child Is a Victim

- Do not overreact and do not let your child see that you are upset. Your child may interpret that reaction to mean that you are disappointed with her.
- Talk to your child and listen carefully to her concerns.
- Reinforce the idea that the incident was not your child's fault: "The bully has a problem, not you. She picked on you for no reason. You didn't do anything to cause it."
- Minimize bullying opportunities. Do not allow your child to take valuable possessions to school. Instruct your child to try to avoid places where the bully hangs out. Staying out of harm's way is sensible, not "chicken."
- Teach your child possible strategies to help handle the problem:
  - Instruct your child not to react by crying or becoming upset, because this is what the bully wants. Bullies get bored when they do not get the expected response.
  - Foster friendship and tell your child to walk with a buddy.
  - Encourage your child not to do everything the bully says or wants and not to give any belongings to the bully. Your child needs to repair her self-esteem and recapture her dignity, which will not be accomplished by giving in to the bully.
  - Persuade your child to stand tall, look the bully in the eye, and say something like, "Stop it right now." Tell your child to then walk away and ignore any further comments from the bully.

- Tell your child not to get angry or fight back. These reactions will not solve the problem; they actually make matters worse. It gives bullies what they want and encourages them to come back to taunt again. Fighting can also put your child at greater risk for physical injury.

- Discourage your child from retaliating, because it only reinforces violence as a solution to problems.

- Tell your child to find a teacher or other adult and report the incident.

- Seek professional help if the bullying seems to have affected your child's self-esteem.

For Parents Whose Child Is a Bully

- Stay calm. Try to be objective, even though this may be difficult. Do not become angry or defensive. These reactions tend to make a bad situation even worse.

- Because your child most likely will not confess to the behavior, ask him to tell you exactly what he has been doing. Talk to other parents and teachers to find out what has been happening.

- Explain how your child's behavior constitutes bullying and ask why he thinks he bullies and what might help him to stop this behavior. But do not tolerate any excuses for the behavior.

- Because bullying often stems from unhappiness, try to find out what is bothering your child and help him develop ways to cope with it.

Strategies to help modify your child's bullying behavior include:

- Take the problem very seriously. If your child is a bully, he is at risk for more severe problems later in life.
- Supervise your child more closely, and stay nearby when he plays with other children. If you cannot stay nearby, arrange for other adults to supervise the children, or ask that your child only participate in supervised activities.
- Set limits. Tell your child that bullying will not be tolerated, and make sure your child understands you. Create consequences and follow through on them when needed. For example, limit or remove all media devices if the child engaged in cyberbullying.

- Help your child to understand the rights and feelings of others. Ask how your child would feel if someone bullied him. Use examples from books, television, and movies.
- Encourage your child to apologize to the victims.
- Stop displays of aggression immediately, and help your child find nonviolent outlets to handle frustrations and problems.
- Foster your child's participation in physical activities such as sports so that your child will have healthy ways to feel powerful and strong.
- Praise your child for appropriate behaviors.
- Teach your child to be assertive rather than aggressive.
- Talk to your child's school counselor and teacher and explain that he is trying to improve his behavior, and ask them for their assistance. Support the school if it institutes consequences for the child's bullying behavior.
- If older siblings tease your bullying child, instruct them to stop and administer consequences as needed.
- Be a positive role model. Control your own aggression, including road rage.

Seek professional help. Bullying behavior frequently requires outside assistance. Take advantage of the counseling services offered at your child's school or in your community.

Tertiary Prevention

Referral is warranted once children demonstrate the consequences of bullying. If resources are scarce, be creative and consider alternatives, such as developing an alliance with a university psychiatric nursing, psychology, social work, or counseling program or investigate telepsychiatric services.

Health care providers should also get involved in the community. Work with local schools to develop antibullying policies and procedures, and assist school personnel in differentiating normal peer conflict from bullying. Encourage teachers to use discussions and role play to teach conflict resolution skills, encourage caring behaviors, and develop effective strategies to handle bullies. Other suggestions for schools include:

- Conduct a parental awareness campaign during parent-teacher conference days, through newsletters, and at parent teacher association/organization (PTA/O) meetings to stress the importance of parental involvement.

- Develop an antibullying policy.
- Engage students in formal role-playing exercises and related assignments to show alternatives to bullying methods of interaction and to show students how they can assist victims.
- Implement cooperative learning activities to reduce social isolation.
- Increase adult supervision.
- Conduct in-service programs for teachers and other school personnel.
- Hold serious discussions with bullies. Make them realize that the school is aware of the problem and that such behavior will not be tolerated.
- Create ways to help bullies develop more positive social skills.
- Institute programs, such as the Olweus Bullying Prevention Program (www.clemson.edu/olweus).

RESOURCES

Bullying: American Academy of Child and Adolescent Psychiatrists: www.aacap.org/cs/root/facts_for_families/bullying

Bullying: Medline Plus: www.nlm.nih.gov/medlineplus/bullying.html

Center for Safe and Responsible Internet Use: www.cyberbully.org

Connected Kids Clinical Guide: www.aap.org/connectedkids/ClinicalGuide.pdf

Connected Kids Program: www.aap.org/ConnectedKids/default.htm

Electronic Media and Youth Violence: A CDC Issue Brief for Educators and Caregivers: www.cdc.gov/ViolencePrevention/pdf/EA-brief-a.pdf

Helping Kids Deal With Bullies: http://kidshealth.org/parent/emotions/behavior/bullies.html

National Crime Prevention Council Cyberbullying: www.ncpc.org/cyberbullying

Stop Bullying Now: http://stopbullyingnow.hrs a.gov

Stop Cyberbullying Now: www.stopcyberbullying.org

REFERENCES

American Academy of Pediatrics Committee on Injury, Violence, and Poison Prevention. (2009). Role of the pediatrician in youth violence prevention. *Pediatrics, 124*(1), 393–402.

American Medical Association. (2002). *Proceedings from the educational forum on adolescent health youth bullying.* Retrieved from www.ama-assn.org/ama1/pub/upload/mm/39/youthbullying.pdf

Arseneault, L., Walsh, E., Trzesniewski, K., Newcombe, R., Caspi, A., & Moffitt, T. E. (2006). Bullying victimization uniquely contributes to adjustment problems in young children: A nationally representative cohort study. *Pediatrics, 118,* 130–138.

Center for the Study and Prevention of Violence. (2006). *Fact sheet: An overview of bullying.* www.colorado.edu/cspv/publications/factsheets/safeschools/FS-SC07.pdf

David-Ferdon, C., & Hertz, M. F. (2007). Electronic media, violence, and adolescents: An emerging public health problem. *Journal of Adolescent Health, 41*(Suppl. 1): S1–S5.

Garrity, C., & Baris, M. (1996). Bullies and victims: A guide for pediatricians. *Contemporary Pediatrics, 13,* 90–115.

Lamb, J., Pepler, D., & Craig, W. (2009). Approach to bullying and victimization. *Canadian Family Physician, 55,* 356–360.

Muscari, M. (2002a). *Not my kid: 21 steps to raising a nonviolent child.* Scranton, PA: University of Scranton Press.

Muscari, M. (2002b). Sticks and stones: The NP's role with bullies and victims. *Journal of Pediatric Health Care, 16,* 22–28.

Olweus, D. (1991). Bully/victim problems among school children. In K. Rubin & D. Pepler (Eds.), *The development and treatment of childhood aggression* (pp. 411–448). Hillsdale, NJ: Erlbaum.

Olweus, D. (1993). Victimization by peers: Antecedents and long-term outcomes. In K. Rubin, S. Jens, & B. Asendorpf (Eds.), *Social withdrawal, inhibition, and shyness in childhood* (pp. 315–341). Hillsdale, NJ: Erlbaum.

Sampson, R. (2009). *Bullying in school.* U.S. Department of Justice Office of Community Oriented Policing Services. Problem-Oriented Guides for Police, Problem-Specific Guides Series No. 12. Retrieved from www.cops.usdoj.gov/files/RIC/Publications/e07063414-guide.pdf

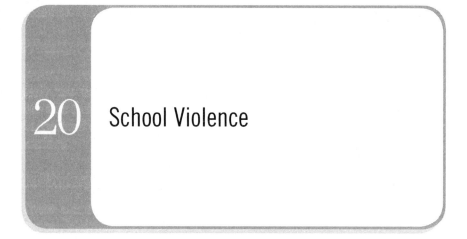

20 School Violence

DEFINITION

Schools should be safe havens for teaching and learning. They should be free from crime and violence because any instance of crime or violence not only affects the individuals involved but also disrupts the educational process and may affect bystanders, the school itself, and the surrounding community. U.S. schools are relatively safe; however, any amount of violence is unacceptable.

The term "school violence" has almost become synonymous with the word "Columbine." However, it is a broader concept. According to the Centers for Disease Control and Prevention (CDC, 2008a), school violence is a subset of youth violence, a broader public health problem. Youth violence includes bullying, fighting, weapon use, and rape. Victims can suffer serious injury, significant social and emotional damage, or even death, and young people may be victims, perpetrators, witnesses, or any combination of these.

PREVALENCE

Collective findings from Indicators of School Crime and Safety: 2008 (Dinkes, Kemp, Baum, & Snyder, 2009), and the CDC show the following:

- Preliminary data show that among youth ages 5–18, there were 35 school-associated violent deaths from July 1, 2006, through June 30, 2007. Of these deaths, 27 were homicides and 8 were suicides.
- In 2006, there were about 1.7 million victims of nonfatal crimes at school among students ages 12–18. These included 909,500 thefts and 767,000 violent crimes (simple assault and serious violent crime).
- During the 2005–2006 school year, 86% of public schools reported that at least one crime occurred at their school.
- In 2007, 8% of students in Grades 9–12 reported being threatened or injured with a weapon in the previous 12 months, and 22% reported that illegal drugs were made available to them on school property.
- In 2005, 24% of students reported gangs at their schools.
- In 2003–2004, 10% of teachers in city schools reported being threatened with injury by students, compared with 6% of teachers in suburban schools, and 5% in rural schools.
- Violent deaths at schools accounted for less than 1% of the homicides and suicides among children 5–18 years of age.
- Most school-associated violent deaths occur during transition times, before and after the school day and during lunch.
- Violent deaths are more likely to occur at the start of each semester.
- Nearly half of all school homicide perpetrators gave some type of warning signal, including making a threat or leaving a note, prior to the event.

ETIOLOGY

A public health model views youth violence as a social problem that can be prevented, using the same approach that has effect on other public health challenges such as drunken driving, use of seat belts, and smoking. Violence is the result of the interaction of multiple individual, situational, contextual, and societal influences. Risk factors for violence and aggression are additive and follow a developmental sequence, and they are also interdependent and are affected by a range of life experiences and influences involving family, peers, community, and culture, as well as an individual's personal physical and mental health status.

Risk factors for school violence and aggression include:

Individual risk factors: history of violent victimization; attention deficits, hyperactivity, or learning disorders; history of early aggressive behavior; involvement with drugs, alcohol, or tobacco; low IQ; poor behavioral control; deficits in social cognitive or information-processing abilities; high emotional distress; history of treatment for emotional problems; antisocial beliefs and attitudes; and exposure to violence and conflict in the family

Family risk factors: authoritarian childrearing attitudes; harsh, lax, or inconsistent disciplinary practices; low parental involvement; low emotional attachment to parents or caregivers; low parental education and income; parental substance abuse or criminality; poor family functioning; and poor monitoring and supervision of children

Peer/school risk factors: association with delinquent peers; involvement in gangs; social rejection by peers; lack of involvement in conventional activities; poor academic performance; and low commitment to school and school failure

Community risk factors: diminished economic opportunities; high concentrations of poor residents; high level of transiency; high level of family disruption; low levels of community participation; and socially disorganized neighborhoods.

ASSESSMENT

Health care providers should assess for violence risk during routine wellness exams and when suspicious circumstances arise in primary care and other settings. When appropriate, they can use specific tools. Even when not using these tools themselves, health care providers should have an understanding of them when working with violent youth.

Pediatric Symptom Checklist (PSC-17). The Pediatric Symptom Checklist (PSC-17) is a brief, validated, psychosocial screening instrument developed to facilitate recognition and referral of child psychosocial problems by primary care pediatricians. The checklist consists of subscales for internalizing (I), externalizing (E), and attentional symptoms (A). Positive scores are PSC17-I ≥ 5; PSC17-A ≥ 7; PSC17-E ≥ 7; Total Score ≥ 15. The checklist can be printed from the WISAAP Web site at www.wisaap.org/WIsper%20Newsletters/Supplements/PSC-17%20Checklist.pdf.

Structured Assessment of Violence Risk in Youth (SAVRY). The SAVRY is composed of 24 items in three risk domains (Historical Risk Factors, Social/Contextual Risk Factors, and Individual/Clinical Factors), drawn from existing research and the professional literature on adolescent development, and violence and aggression in youth. Each risk item has a three-level rating structure with specific rating guidelines (*Low, Moderate,* or *High*). The tool also contains six Protective Factor items that are rated as either *Present* or *Absent.* The SAVRY is useful in the assessment of adolescents between the ages of 12 and 18, and may be used by professionals in a variety of disciplines who conduct assessments and/or make intervention or supervision plans concerning violence risk in youth. The SAVRY is not a formal test or scale; there are no assigned numerical values nor are there any specified cutoff scores. Instead, it helps assist in structuring an assessment so that the important factors will not be missed, and, thus, will be emphasized when formulating a final professional judgment about a youth's level of risk. Further information on the SAVRY can be found at www.fmhi.usf.edu/mhlp/savry/statement.htm.

Psychopathy Checklist: Youth Version (PCL:YV). The PCL:YV is a 20-item rating scale used for the assessment of psychopathic traits in male and female offenders aged 12 to 18. It was adapted from the Hare Psychopathy Checklist-Revised (PCL-R), the most widely used measure of psychopathy in adults, and uses an expert-rater format that emphasizes the need for multidomain and multisource information. The PCL:YV measures interpersonal, affective, and behavioral features related to a widely understood, traditional concept of psychopathy.

Monitor for Early Warning Signs. It is not possible to predict who will be violent. However, health care providers can recognize early warning signs. In some situations and for some youth, different combinations of events, behaviors, and emotions may lead to violent behavior toward self or others. Health care providers can assume that these warning signs, especially when they are presented in combination, indicate a need for further analysis to determine an appropriate intervention. But there is a real danger that early warning signs will be misinterpreted, and therefore, health care providers need to understand basic principles:

Do no harm. The intent should be to get early intervention for the child. Early warning signs should not be used to exclude, isolate, or punish a child, nor should they be used as a checklist for formally identifying, mislabeling, or stereotyping children. Formal disability identification under federal law requires individualized evaluation by qualified professionals, and all referrals to outside agencies based on the early warning signs must be kept confidential and must be done with parental consent (except referrals for suspected child abuse or neglect).

View warning signs within a developmental context. Children at different levels of development have varying social and emotional capabilities. They may express their needs differently at each stage. Know developmentally typical behavior, so that behaviors are not misinterpreted.

Understand that violence and aggression occur within context. Violent and aggressive behavior is an expression of emotion with antecedent factors that exist within the school, the home, and the larger social environment. Certain environments or situations can even trigger violence in at-risk children. Some children may act out if stress becomes too great, if they lack positive coping skills, and/or if they have learned to react with aggression.

Avoid stereotyping. Stereotypes interfere with and can even harm the ability to identify and help children. It is important to be aware of false cues, including race, socioeconomic status, cognitive or academic ability, or physical appearance. Stereotypes can unfairly harm children, especially when the school community acts upon them.

Understand that children typically exhibit multiple warning signs. It is common for troubled children to exhibit multiple signs. Research confirms that most children who are at risk for aggression exhibit more than one warning sign, repeatedly, and with increasing intensity over time. Do not overreact to single signs, words, or actions.

None of the warning signs is sufficient on its own for predicting aggression and violence, and as noted earlier, it is inappropriate and potentially harmful to use these signs as a checklist against which to match individual children. Rather, the signs are offered only as an aid in identifying and referring children who may need intervention. The early warning signs include:

Social withdrawal. The withdrawal frequently stems from feelings of depression, rejection, persecution, unworthiness, and lack of confidence.

Excessive feelings of isolation and being alone. Research has shown that the majority of these children are not violent; however, in some cases, feelings of isolation and not having friends are associated with children who behave aggressively and violently.

Excessive feelings of rejection. All children face rejection at some time or another. But troubled children are often isolated from their mentally healthy peers, and their responses to rejection will depend on many background factors. Without support, they may be at risk of expressing their emotional distress in negative ways, including violence. Some of these children seek out aggressive friends who, in turn, reinforce their violent tendencies.

Being a victim of violence. Children who are victims of violence, including physical or sexual abuse, are sometimes at risk themselves of becoming violent toward themselves or others.

Feelings of being picked on and persecuted. Youth who feel constantly picked on, teased, bullied, and humiliated may initially withdraw socially. If not given adequate support in addressing these feelings, some children may vent them in violent ways.

Low school interest and poor academic performance. It is important to ascertain whether there is a drastic change in performance and/or poor performance becomes a chronic condition that limits the child's capacity to learn. Aggressive behavior may occur in some situations, such as when the low achiever feels frustrated, unworthy, chastised, and denigrated. It is also crucial to assess the emotional and cognitive reasons for the academic performance change to determine the true nature of the problem.

Expression of violence in writings and drawings. Many children produce work about violent themes that is harmless when taken in context. However, an overrepresentation of violence in writings and drawings that is directed at specific individuals (family members, peers, other adults) and used consistently over time may signal emotional problems and the potential for violence. Because there is a real danger in misdiagnosing such a sign, it is important to seek the guidance of a mental health specialist to determine its meaning.

Uncontrolled anger. Anger is a natural emotion; however, anger that is expressed frequently and intensely in response to minor irritants may signal potential violent behavior toward self or others.

Patterns of impulsive and chronic hitting, intimidating, and bullying behaviors. Even mildly aggressive behaviors, such as constant hitting and bullying of others, that occur early in children's lives can later escalate into more serious behaviors if left untreated.

History of discipline problems. Chronic behavior and disciplinary problems may suggest that underlying emotional needs are not being met. These problems can set the stage for the child to violate norms and rules, defy authority, disengage from school, and engage in aggressive behaviors with other children and adults.

Past history of violent and aggressive behavior. Youth who show an early pattern of antisocial behavior frequently and across multiple settings are particularly at risk for future aggressive and antisocial behavior. Similarly, youth who engage in overt behaviors such as bullying, generalized aggression and defiance, and covert behaviors such as stealing, vandalism, lying, cheating, and firesetting also are at risk for more serious aggressive behavior. Problems at an early age may be more significant for later violence than those that first appear at a later age.

Intolerance for differences and prejudicial attitudes. Intense prejudice toward others based on racial, ethnic, religious, language, gender, sexual orientation, ability, and physical appearance, when coupled with other factors, may lead to violent assaults against those who are perceived to be different. Membership in hate groups or the willingness to victimize individuals with disabilities or health problems should also be treated as early warning signs.

Substance abuse. Drug use and alcohol use reduces self-control and exposes children and youth to violence, as perpetrators, as victims, or both.

Affiliation with gangs. Youth who are influenced by antisocial gangs, who emulate and copy their behavior, and/or who become affiliated with them may adopt these values and act in violent or aggressive ways in certain situations. Gang-related violence and turf battles often result in injury and/or death.

Inappropriate access to, possession of, and use of firearms. Youth who inappropriately possess or have access to firearms can have an increased risk for violence. Children who have a history of aggression, impulsiveness, or other emotional problems should not have access to firearms and other weapons.

Serious threats of violence. Idle threats are a common response to frustration. However, *one of the most reliable indicators that a youth is likely to commit a dangerous act is a detailed and specific threat to use violence.* Threats to commit violence against oneself or others should be taken very seriously, and steps must be taken to understand the nature of these threats and to prevent them from being carried out.

Assess for Imminent Warning Signs

Unlike early warning signs, imminent signs indicate that a child is dangerously close to behaving in a violent manner. The following signs require immediate action.

Serious physical fighting with peers or family member

Severe property destruction

Severe rage for apparently minor reasons

Possession or use of firearms or other weapons

Detailed plan to commit a violent act

Immediate intervention by law enforcement officers is needed when a child:

Has presented a detailed plan (time, place, method) to harm or kill others, particularly if the child has a history of aggression or has attempted to carry out threats in the past.

Is carrying a weapon, particularly a firearm, and has threatened to use it.

INTERVENTION

Health care providers should refer at-risk and violent children to appropriate mental health professionals. However, they can also intervene by providing parent and child education including parenting, stress management, coping skills, and problem solving.

PREVENTION/PATIENT TEACHING

Primary Prevention

The American Academy of Pediatrics (AAP) developed its Connected Kids (www.aap.org/ConnectedKids) program to address violence prevention. Designed with input from clinicians, parents, and adolescents from across the country, Connected Kids is a systematic method for enhancing the violence prevention anticipatory guidance that is made up of four elements:

1. Clinical Guide: The Clinical Guide provides an overview to the entire program. It also describes some details of its development and its rationale.
2. Counseling Schedule: The color-coded Counseling Schedule is designed for three separate age groups: GREEN for infancy to early childhood; BLUE for middle childhood; and RED for adolescence. The schedule recommends topics to be introduced, topics to be reinforced, and brochures to be distributed for each health supervision visit. Examples of introductory anticipatory guidance topics include parental frustration for the 2-day to 4-week visit; bullying for 6 years; and conflict resolution for early adolescence.

3. Educational Brochures: Twenty-one educational brochures have been designed for parents and children to reinforce each of the 44 topics covered in Connected Kids. The color codes from the Counseling Schedule are also incorporated into the brochures to facilitate distribution. Topics include Pulling the Plug on TV Violence, and Dating Violence: Tips for Parents.
4. PowerPoint Presentation: The PowerPoint presentation offers an alternative presentation of the material in the Clinical Guide. This presentation may be helpful for personnel in-service training before implementing Connected Kids.

Secondary Prevention

While violence is only one aspect of delinquency, it is probably the most troublesome. Therefore, health care providers also can participate in prevention strategies such as the Centers for Disease Control and Prevention's (CDC) *Best Practices for Violence Prevention* and the Office of Juvenile Justice and Delinquency Prevention's (OJJDP) *The National Juvenile Justice Action Plan.*

The CDC's *Best Practices for Violence Prevention* identifies four strategies for combating the problem of youth violence and offers specific suggestions for implementation. These strategies include:

1. *Family-based strategies* that combine training in parenting skills, education about child development, and exercises to help parents develop skills for communicating with their children and resolving conflict nonviolently.
2. A *home visiting strategy* that brings community resources to at-risk families in their homes, especially for pregnant and first-time parents.
3. A *social-cognitive strategy* that helps children develop the skills they need to deal effectively with difficult situations by teaching nonviolent methods for resolving conflict and establishing (and strengthening) nonviolent beliefs in young people.
4. A *mentoring strategy* that emphasizes the importance of a positive adult role model in reducing risk for violence and delinquent behavior.

The Office of Juvenile Justice and Delinquency Prevention (OJJDP) has developed *The National Juvenile Justice Action Plan,* which is a comprehensive approach to reducing youth violence that combines violence prevention with graduated sanctions for youth offenders. The Action Plan emphasizes five key areas of best practice for communities developing a response to violence. The five key best practices recommend:

1. Mobilizing communities
2. Strengthening the juvenile justice system
3. Decreasing gangs, guns, and drugs
4. Creating opportunities for youth
5. Breaking the cycle of violence through family strengthening and parent education

Tertiary Prevention

Tertiary prevention serves those individuals who have already become violent or chronic offenders and emphasizes punishment and rehabilitation through the justice system. The objective is to help prevent future violent activity. An example of tertiary prevention is a plan coordinated by the health care provider for a student who is in the juvenile justice system. This plan could involve services across school, home, and community. Families may receive such support as training on behavior management skills as well as how to meet their own continuing needs.

RESOURCES

American Medical Association. *Connecting the Dots to Prevent Youth Violence: A Training and Outreach Guide for Physicians and Other Health Professionals:* www.ama-assn.org/ama/pub/physician-resources/public-health/promoting-healthy-lifestyles/violence-prevention/youth-violence-prevention-training-outreach-guide.shtml

Best Practices of Youth Violence Prevention: A Sourcebook for Community Action: www.cdc.gov/ncipc/dvp/bestpractices.htm

Centers for Disease Control and Prevention Youth Violence: www.cdc.gov/violencepre vention/youthviolence/schoolviolence/index.html

Early Warning, Timely Response: A Guide to Safe Schools: www.ncjrs.gov/pdffiles1/172854.pdf

School Health Guidelines to Prevent Unintentional Injuries and Violence (CDC): www.cdc.gov/mmwr/PDF/rr/rr5022.pdf

REFERENCES

Centers for Disease Control and Prevention. (2008a). *Understanding school violence fact sheet.* Retrieved from www.cdc.gov/violenceprevention/pdf/SchoolViolence_FactSheet-a.pdf

Centers for Disease Control and Prevention. (2008b). *Youth violence prevention scientific information: Risk and protective factors.* Retrieved from www.cdc.gov/NCIPC/dvp/YVP/YVP-risk-p-factors.htm

Commission for the Prevention of Youth Violence. (2000). *Youth and violence: Medicine, nursing, and public health: Connecting the dots to prevent violence.* Retrieved from www.ama-assn.org/ama/upload/mm/386/fullreport.pdf

Dinkes, R., Kemp, J., Baum, K., & Snyder, T. (2009). *Indicators of school crime and safety: 2008.* U.S. Department of Education; U.S. Department of Justice Office of Justice Programs, NCES 2009–022; NCJ 226343. Retrieved from www.ojp.usdoj.gov/bjs/pub/pdf/iscs08.pdf

Lipsey, M.W., & Derzon, J.H. (1998). Predictors of violent and serious delinquency in adolescence and early adulthood: A synthesis of longitudinal research. In R. Loeber & D.P. Farrington (Eds.), *Serious and violent juvenile offenders: Risk factors and successful interventions* (pp. 86–105). Thousand Oaks, CA: Sage Publications.

Mercy, J., Butchart, A., Farrington, D., & Cerdá, M. (2002). Youth violence. In E. Krug, L.L. Dahlberg, J.A. Mercy, A.B. Zwi, & R. Lozano (Eds.), *World report on violence and health* (pp. 25–56). Geneva: World Health Organization. Retrieved from www.who.int/violence_injury_prevention/violence/global_campaign/en/chap2.pdf

Resnick, M.D., Ireland, M., & Borowsky, I. (2004). Youth violence perpetration: What protects? What predicts? Findings from the National Longitudinal Study of Adolescent Health. *Journal of Adolescent Health, 35,* 424 e1–e10.

U.S. Department of Health and Human Services. (2001). *Youth violence: A report of the Surgeon General.* Retrieved from www.surgeongeneral.gov/library/youthviolence/toc.html

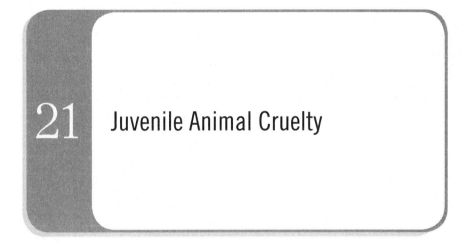

21 Juvenile Animal Cruelty

DEFINITION

Children who abuse animals tend to exhibit more severe conduct disorder problems than other children. *Animal abuse or cruelty* is socially unacceptable behavior that intentionally causes unnecessary distress, suffering or pain, and/or death of an animal. Children who are exposed to violence may in turn abuse animals, and children who abuse animals may become violent toward other humans. *Animal cruelty is associated with other forms of violence including child abuse, domestic violence, elder abuse, and sexual violence.*

All 50 states and the District of Columbia have *anticruelty laws* (www.animal-law.org/statutes), and more than 40 states currently have felony statutes for certain types of animal cruelty. Some felony statutes require psychiatric counseling for convicted abusers.

Animal cruelty is typically classified as follows:

1. *Neglect* occurs when a person deprives an animal of food, water, shelter, and/or veterinary care. Neglect cases are acts of omission rather than commission and do not give satisfaction to the person whose animals are neglected, thus neglect is not a typical form of juvenile animal cruelty. However, household animal

neglect may indicate human neglect or inappropriate parental expectations if the animal was neglected by a child charged with the animal's care.

2. *Physical abuse* results from malicious torturing, maiming, mutilation, or killing. These acts of intentional cruelty are often shocking and usually indicative of a serious human behavioral problem. Juveniles who commit these intentional acts of cruelty may derive satisfaction in causing harm.

3. Animal sexual abuse, or *bestiality,* is the sexual molestation of animals by humans and includes a wide range of behaviors, including fondling; vaginal, anal, or oral penetration; oral-genital contact; penetration with an object; and injuring or killing an animal for sexual gratification. Like rape, this is an eroticization of violence, control, and exploitation. One study found that 96% of their juvenile subjects who had engaged in sex with nonhuman animals also admitted to sex offenses against humans and reported more offenses against humans than other sex offenders their same age and race. They also had histories of more emotional abuse, neglect, and victimization events than other offenders. Thus, sex with animals may be an important indicator of potential or co-occurring sex offenses against humans and may be a sign of severe family dysfunction (Fleming, Jory, & Burton, 2002).

4. *Hoarding,* which is similar to neglect, occurs when a person accumulates a large number of animals; provides minimal standards of nutrition, sanitation, and veterinary care; and fails to act on the deteriorating condition of the animals and/or the environment. Unlike most other perpetrators of animal cruelty, the majority of hoarders are female and adult.

5. *Cock fighting* is the term used when two or more specialty birds, or gamecocks, are placed in an enclosure to fight to the death, sometimes of both birds.

6. Organized *dog fighting* is illegal in the United States and is a felony in all 50 states. Dog fighting is a contest between two specifically bred, conditioned, and trained-to-fight dogs that are placed in a pit to fight. Usually the loser dies, is left to die, or is killed by the owner. Both cock fighting and dog fighting are for the purposes of gambling or entertainment, and both, particularly dog fighting, may be associated with other criminal activity. The American Society for the Prevention of Cruelty to Animals (ASPCA, 2010) notes that police often categorize dog fighting into three groups: (a) *Street fighters* engage in informal dog fights, usually on a street

corner, alley, or playground. They have no fight rules and pit fights are usually triggered by taunts, insults, or turf invasions. Street fights are associated with gang activity, and the fights may be associated with money, drugs, or bragging rights as the pay off. The dogs are bred to be threats to other dogs, and usually also to people. (b) *Hobbyist fighters* are more organized and use fights for entertainment and/or supplemental income. They pay more attention to the care and breeding of their dogs. (c) *Professional dog fighters* have large numbers of animals and earn money from fighting, breeding, and dog sales. They dispose of dogs that do not perform through a variety of methods, including blunt force trauma and shooting. Recently, a group of wealthy fighters have emerged who may make up a fourth category because they have the financial resources of professional fighters but the philosophy of street fighters.

7. During a *hog-dog fight* ("hog-dog rodeo"), a trained dog attacks a trapped feral hog inside an enclosed pit from which there is no escape. Fight organizers give the advantage to the dog by either cutting off the hog's tusks or outfitting the dog in a Kevlar vest. The dog is timed to see how quickly it can pin down the hog by tearing into the hog's snout, ears, and eyes. Hog-dog fight promoters often bill these fights as "family entertainment"; however, they are closely connected to other crimes and forms of violence in addition to cruelty to animals. In some cases, the operator encourages children into a game of "catch the pig." The handler tapes the hog's snout closed and encourages children to chase the terrified animal around the pen.

PREVALENCE

In a 2007 survey of 1,869 perpetrators of animal cruelty, the Humane Society of the United States (2009) noted the following statistics:

- Intentional animal cruelty by children (0–14 years): 5.6% males, 0.2% females
- Intentional animal cruelty by youths (15–20): 19% males, 2.3% females
- Animal fighting by children (0–14): 1% males, 0% females
- Animal fighting by youths (15–20): 12% males, 0.2% females

Diagnostic categories associated with children who commit animal cruelty include attention deficit hyperactivity disorder, oppositional defiant disorder, conduct disorder, and attachment disorders. Other possible diagnostic categories include posttraumatic stress disorder, mood disorder, certain personality disorders (borderline, antisocial), mental retardation, pervasive developmental disorders, and traumatic brain injuries.

ETIOLOGY

Juvenile animal cruelty often represents displaced hostility and aggression that comes from neglect or abuse of the child or of another family member. Animal abuse committed by any family member often means child abuse occurs in that family.

Peers may influence teenage boys to engage in cruelty to gain approval or prove their masculinity—at least half of juvenile cruelty perpetrators act as part of a group. Negative role modeling, particularly behaviors that create chaotic and abusive households, can lead to cruelty. Children mimic these abusive behaviors on others they have some power over, typically animals and/or other children, and some later perpetuate the cycle by continuing to be violent into adulthood. Thus, juvenile animal cruelty can reveal information about the family as well as the child, and therefore may be a marker for family violence—corporal punishment, child abuse, and domestic violence. Pets often do not survive past the age of 2 in violent households because they are either killed, die from neglect, or run away to escape the abuse. Even when overt human violence does not take place, this constant turnover of animals causes the children to suffer repeated cycles of attachment and loss.

ASSESSMENT

General Principles

Assessing for animal cruelty should be part of all routine child health visits and episodic visits for children who present with behavioral problems or signs of child abuse. Children as young as 4 may harm animals, but such behavior is most common during adolescence. Cruelty is often associated with poor academic performance, low self-esteem, few friendships, bullying, truancy, vandalism, and other antisocial behaviors.

Ascione (2001) provides a typology of juvenile animal abusers:

Exploratory/curious animal abusers are likely to be preschoolers or very early school-aged children who are poorly supervised and lack training on the physical care and humane treatment of animals. These children abuse animals out of innocent exploration and do not intend to cause harm. Developmentally delayed children may also fit into this category.

Pathological animal abusers are more likely to be older (but not necessarily). These children may be symptomatic of psychological disturbances of varying severity, and/or may have a history of physical abuse, sexual abuse, or exposure to domestic violence. These children intend to cause harm.

Delinquent animal abusers are typically adolescents with other antisocial behaviors, sometimes gang- or cult-related. Substance abuse may be involved with the cruelty. These children intend to cause harm and may derive pleasure from the animal's suffering.

History and Physical Assessment

The Society & Animal Forum's *AniCare Child: An Approach for the Assessment and Treatment of Childhood Animal Abuse* (n.d.) recommends four steps in assessing juvenile animal cruelty:

1. Ask about the child's relationship with animals.
2. Obtain data from multiple sources (parents and other family members, teachers, guidance counselors, medical and court records, psychological evaluations, principal, previously attended schools, social worker, neighborhood friends, veterinarian).
3. If the child has committed animal cruelty, assess the extent, nature, and motivation.
4. If the child has witnessed cruelty, assess the effects.

To assess extent, nature, and motivation of child animal abuse, assess for the following factors:

1. *Severity:* degree of injury, frequency, and duration; prolonged or immediate injury; number and kind of species, including level

of sentience (degree to which the animal is capable of feeling or sensation); intimacy of injury infliction (shot at a distance or stabbed).

2. *Culpability:* developmental level (were consequences understood); degree of planning; obstacles that were overcome to commit act; solitary or group activity (if group, leader or follower); coerced or dominant individual; videoed or photographed incident.

3. *Psychodynamics/motivation:* curiosity; reaction to fear of the animal; retaliation against human; peer pressure; other antisocial behavior; rehearsing other delinquent behavior; rage; mood enhancement; pleasure from suffering (sadism); sexual arousal; ritualistic features.

4. *Attitudes/beliefs:* level of awareness of physical or psychological needs of the animal: has given little thought to role of animals in society; prejudice against specific species; cruelty as a way to control or discipline an animal; cultural practice/acceptance.

5. *Emotional intelligence:* capacity for empathy; capable of reciprocal relationships; understanding of relationships; capable of forming attachments.

6. *Family history:* domestic violence; child abuse; neglect; animal cruelty; harsh and inconsistent discipline; spanking and other physical punishment.

7. *Mitigating circumstances:* accepts responsibility; expresses remorse, shame, or guilt; seeks to make restitution; assists law enforcement; capable of forming bond with an animal.

Assess the parents. Research demonstrates that parent/family characteristics are essentially related to the development of antisocial behavior in children. Parental stress, psychopathology, social isolation, poor parental relations, child-rearing practices, depression, and substance abuse contribute to aggressive behavior in children.

Observe the child's skin for bites, lacerations, cuts, and scratches that may indicate injuries from an animal that may have fought back.

Diagnostic Tests

The *Children and Animals Inventory (CAI)* is a brief self- and parent-report measure of Ascione's nine parameters of cruelty: severity (based on degree of intentional pain and injury caused to an animal), frequency (the number of separate acts of cruelty), duration (period of time over which the cruel acts occurred), recency (the most recent acts), diversity across and within categories (number of animals abused from different categories and the number of animals harmed from any one category), sentience (level of concern for the abused animal), covertness (child's attempts to conceal the behavior), isolation (whether the cruelty occurred alone or with other children/adults), and empathy (the degree of the child's remorse for the cruel acts).

INTERVENTION

Animal cruelty is not part of normal development. All episodes of abuse, even those done out of curiosity, warrant intervention. Interventions can be based on typology:

1. Exploratory/curious animal abusers: Humane education is likely to be sufficient intervention; however, age should not be the only determining factor as animal cruelty is one of the earliest signs of conduct disorder.
2. Pathological animal abusers: Professional counseling is warranted.
3. Delinquent animal abusers: Both psychiatric and judicial interventions may be required.

Twenty-seven states now recommend or require psychological counseling for persons convicted of animal cruelty. The Doris Day Animal Foundation notes that: (a) a thorough evaluation of the convicted abuser must be conducted *before* a treatment is recommended; (b) prescribing the wrong treatment can do harm, as well as be a missed opportunity; (c) psychological counseling for animal abuse should have the same high standards as other types of counseling; (d) practitioners should not rely on a "one-size-fits-all" approach.

Treatment of juvenile animal cruelty resembles other psychological treatments for children, and thus, the basic theoretical and clinical models of diagnosis and interventions will also apply to children who abuse animals. However, there are some distinguishing features that focus on animal abuse, whether it is central to the treatment, or one component of it. Animals—and the child's relationship with them, attitudes toward them, beliefs about them, learned behavior around them—will be a central feature in the treatment.

If animal-assisted therapy (AAT) is utilized, real animals enter the treatment. The child's interaction and relationship with the animal therapist can be an important tool to teach boundaries, empathy, and foster attachment skills. In some situations, the animals are symbolic and puppets or other toys are used. To teach certain skills, such as problem solving and self-management, therapeutic exercises emphasize situations with animals. Finally, treatment directly addresses problematic behavior and seeks to correct it.

AniCare Child suggests the use of three major therapeutic tasks—connection, expression, and correction—as an organizing framework for treatment. Connection refers to establishing a therapeutic relationship; expression focuses on the importance of identifying, expressing, and regulating feelings; and correction is concerned with therapeutic activity aimed at redirecting the child's behavior.

Animal welfare organizations have developed educational and therapeutic efforts that incorporate "animal-assisted" or "animal-facilitated" components. The underlying theme of many of these programs is that teaching young people to train, care for, and interact in a nurturing manner with animals will reduce any propensity they may have for aggression and violence. Providers should contact their local animal welfare agency to locate programs in their area.

Since laws and penalties vary per state, children may be placed on probation, mandated to perform community service, or adjudicated delinquent and possibly placed in a secure juvenile facility.

PREVENTION/PATIENT TEACHING

Primary Prevention

Teach parents and children humane education:

1. Teach by example; use real-life situations to instill a sense of respect for all life. Encourage children to help feed the birds or rescue a bug. With older children, discuss animal-cruelty cases publicized in the news.
2. Encourage children to speak up for animals.
3. Report animal cruelty. Ignoring it communicates the sense that it is acceptable behavior. Do not engage in physical confrontation, but when appropriate, report the incident to the proper authorities.

4. Practice responsible pet guardianship: (a) obtain annual veterinarian examinations and proper immunizations; (b) provide the best pet food you can afford; (c) assure they get proper love, attention, exercise, and rest; (d) spay and neuter them.
5. Show respect for wildlife.
6. Volunteer at a local shelter or rescue group.

Secondary Prevention

Early identification and prevention of child abuse and parental intimate partner violence minimizes family dysfunction and decreases the risk of juvenile animal cruelty.

Tertiary Prevention

The goal of tertiary prevention is to keep juvenile animal abusers from abusing other animals and from escalating to human violence. This level of prevention utilizes the measures noted in the intervention section, as well as ongoing follow-up to assure that the child remains compliant.

RESOURCES

American Humane Society: www.americanhumane.org
American Society for the Prevention of Cruelty to Animals: www.aspca.org
Humane Society of the United States First Strike Program: www.hsus.org/firststrike
Latham Foundation: www.latham.org
National Association for Human and Environmental Education: http://nahee.org/
People for the Ethical Treatment of Animals: www.peta.com
Society and Animal Forum: www.psyeta.org

REFERENCES

American Society for the Prevention of Cruelty to Animals (ASPCA). (2010). Dog fighting FAQ. Retrieved from http://www.aspca.org/fight-animal-cruelty/dog-fighting/dog-fighting-faq.html

AniCare Child: An approach for the assessment and treatment of childhood animal abuse. (n.d.). Retrieved from http://www.psyeta.org/anicarechild.html

Ascione, F. (2001). *Animal abuse and youth violence.* Office of Juvenile Justice and Delinquency Prevention. Juvenile Justice Bulletin NCJ 188677. Retrieved from www.ncjrs.org/html/ojjdp/jjbul2001_9_2/contents.html

Boat, B. (1998). Abuse of children and abuse of animals. In F. Ascione & P. Arkow (Eds.), *Child abuse, domestic violence, and animal abuse* (pp. 83–100). West Lafayette, IN: Purdue University Press.

Dadds, M. R., Whiting, C., Bunn, P., Fraser, J. A., Charlson, J. H., & Pirola-Merlo, A. (2004). Measurement of cruelty in children: The Cruelty to Animals Inventory. *Journal of Abnormal Child Psychology, 32*(3), 321–334. (Contains instrument on pp. 331–333).

Fleming, W., Jory, B., & Burton, D. (2002). Characteristics of juvenile offenders admitting to sexual activity with nonhuman animals. *Society and Animals: Journal of Human-Animal Studies, 10*(1), 31–45.

Flynn, C. (2000). Why family professionals can no longer ignore violence toward animals. *Family Relations, 49*(1), 87–95.

Humane Society of the United States. (2009). Animal cruelty demographics. Retrieved from http://www.hsus.org/acf/cruelty/publiced/cruelty_demographics.html

Muscari, M. (2004). Juvenile animal abuse: Health policy implications for PNPs. *Journal of Pediatric Health Care, 18*(1), 15–21.

Quinn, K. (2000). Animal abuse at early age linked to interpersonal violence. *The Brown University Child and Adolescent Behavior Letter, 16*(3), 1–3.

Randour, M. (n.d.). *Factors to consider in the assessment of juvenile animal cruelty.* Retrieved from www.jwi.org/atf/cf/%7B3B767476-EF52-4EE7-A902-F97E1597FB88%7D/011008%20Factors%20to%20Consider.pdf

Ross, S. (1998). Green chimneys. In F. Ascione & P. Arkow (Eds.), *Child abuse, domestic violence, and animal abuse* (pp. 367–379). West Lafayette, IN: Purdue University Press.

University of Chicago Survey Lab and the Humane Society of the United States. (2008). *Causes of dog fighting.* Retrieved from www.hsus.org/acf/news/pressrel/university_of_chicago_and_hsus_release_dogfighting_study_042008.html

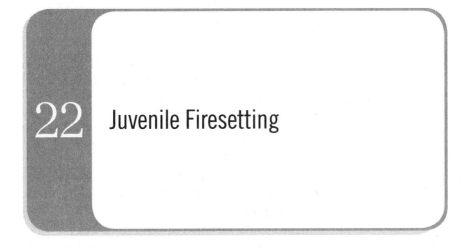

22 Juvenile Firesetting

DEFINITION

Firesetting can serve as a gateway to future delinquent and violent acts, indicating a poor prognosis for these troubled youth. Juvenile firesetting behavior is a frightening yet reliable predictor of adult criminality, and its consequences can be tragic and costly. Fires set by youths destroy more than $300 million worth of property annually and claim the lives of approximately 300 people, with children being the predominant victims of these fires, accounting for 85 of every 100 lives lost.

The Uniform Crime Reporting (UCR) Program of the Federal Bureau of Investigation (FBI) defines *arson* as any willful or malicious burning or attempting to burn a dwelling house, public building, motor vehicle or aircraft, personal property of another, and so forth, with or without intent to defraud. *Fire behavior* follows a development sequence in children and presents in at least three different levels: fire interest, firestarting, and firesetting. These categories represent increasing levels of involvement with fire. Preventive measures allow most children to learn age-appropriate, fire-safe behaviors. However, some children become involved in fire risk behaviors due to a number of factors that include emotional disorders, family dysfunction, and chronic stress. These factors can lead to such behaviors as unsupervised firestarting, and repeated, intentional, and malicious firesetting.

Fire interest. Most children demonstrate fire interest between 3 to 5 years of age. This interest may be expressed through questioning and dramatic play such as dressing up as firemen.

Firestarting. Firestarting begins when children experiment with ignition sources such as matches and lighters. Most boys between ages 3 and 9 experiment with firestarting materials at least once. This best occurs in an adult-supervised, controlled environment, such as lighting candles on a birthday cake. Unfortunately, many firestarts take place in unsupervised settings. Most unsupervised firestarts are single episodes primarily motivated by curiosity, and fires resulting from these incidents are accidental or unintentional, and the children will make an attempt either to put the fire out or get help. Single-episode, unsupervised firestarts usually do not result in a significant fire. However, if children continue to participate in unsupervised firestarts, the probability of starting a significant fire increases dramatically. (The term "fireplay" is often used to convey a low level of intent to inflict harm and an absence of malice.)

Firesetting. Most children have learned many of the rules of fire safety by age 10 and are capable of engaging in age-appropriate firestarting behaviors such as helping to light the family barbecue or building a campfire. With proper guidance, most children achieve a sense of competency and mastery over this powerful yet controllable aspect of their physical environment. However, for some children, fire interest leads to unsupervised firestarts and repeated firesetting. Children ages 7 to 10 may be involved in repeated firesetting. While intentional, it may not be motivated by psychological or social problems but can lead to devastating consequences. Other children are motivated by psychological or social problems, and their firesetting consists of a series of planned firestarts that take place over weeks, months, or years; fire severity varies from small burns to fires that require fire department suppression. These children search for ignition sources and conceal them until needed, and they often gather flammable materials and/or accelerants to hasten the pace of their fires. Their targets often hold specific meaning for them, and once the fire burns, they rarely attempt to extinguish it. Instead, many watch it burn, often from a place where they are safe and undetectable. Some children run away and come back later to view the devastation; others call the fire department and act as the first on the scene. Some volunteer to suppress the fire.

PREVALENCE

According to statistics compiled from national reports by the U.S. Fire Administration (2006):

- 54% of all arson arrests in the United States are of children under 18.
- Juvenile arson arrests were higher, proportionally, than for any other crime.
- Juveniles account for more than half of the arson arrests: one-third are children under the age of 15, and nearly 4% under age 10.
- For fires coded as unintentional child play, 84% involved firesetters under the age of 10.
- The average cost of a juvenile-set structure fire exceeded $20,000.

ETIOLOGY

Putnam and Kirkpatrick (2005) note that the literature suggests that juvenile firesetting may indicate that fire can be an instrument of power or a weapon, as opposed to merely being a product of curiosity. Children typically have less power than adults in society, and many rights and privileges are determined by age, such as voting and drinking alcohol. Access to firearms and other weapons is restricted, but matches and lighters are relatively accessible to youth inclined to act in harmful ways, and a pack of matches can be a formidable weapon used to act out negative behaviors.

The most substantial and pervasive problem for these juveniles seems to be difficulty processing emotions. They tend to feel overwhelmed by negative feelings and do not know how to properly deal with them. Consequently, feelings related to problems such as insecurity and perceived rejection progress into frustration and anger, and they are still unable to face or adequately address these disturbing sensations.

This inability to properly express feelings is usually what drives them to set fires, allowing them to ultimately achieve a sense of relief or domination, or to accomplish an indirect form of revenge, cleansing themselves of their persistent and disabling emotions. The underlying reason for setting fires lies among a broad spectrum of emotions that range from basic boredom to intense suicidal ideation, but some general tendencies typically align with the sex of the individual. Boys seem to set fires more for the purposes of destruction or rebellion, while girls typically obtain a sense of excitement from fire or to use it as a means for self-injury. Regardless of the gender or purpose of firesetting, the act is often reinforced instantaneously, increasing the likelihood of the behavior being repeated in the future.

The literature also shows an association between firesetting and abuse. One study showed that, when compared to the nonabused children, children with histories of maltreatment demonstrated more frequent fire involvement, more versatility regarding ignition sources and targets, and a greater likelihood of an immediate family stressor as a motive for firesetting. They were more likely to become involved with fire out of anger and demonstrated a trend toward higher rates of recidivism (Putnam & Kirkpatrick, 2005). Overall, juvenile firesetting most likely has multiple causes, and firesetters may be of many different types.

ASSESSMENT

General Principles

Several types of juvenile firesetters have been described in the literature (U.S. Fire Administration, 2006). Categorization of these types of juvenile firesetters include the following: Curiosity/Experimental, Cognitively Impaired; Troubled/Crisis; Pathological/Emotionally Disturbed; Thought-Disordered; Compulsive; Disordered Coping; Delinquent/Criminal; Thrill-Seeker; and Revenge-Based Firestarters. Distinctive characteristics can be assigned to each of these 10 categories of firesetters. The following includes some characteristics for each category of juvenile firesetters.

Curiosity/Experimental

- Boys and girls usually ages 2 to 10
- Lack understanding of the destructive potential of fire

- Act typically lacks malice and was not intended to cause harm
- Ready access to lighters, matches, or open flame
- Firesetting behavior generally opportunistic, impulsive, and often accompanied by a lapse in adult supervision
- Are frightened by their acts; "learn their lesson from it"
- Low risk of future acts of firesetting

Cognitively Impaired

- Developmentally disabled or impaired children
- Lack good judgment but avoid intentional harm
- Significant property damage is common. Interventions may include special education, intensive fire education, and behavior management

Troubled/Crisis (also known as "cry for help" firesetters)

- Mostly boys of all ages
- Have set two or more fires
- Use fire to express emotion: anger, sadness, frustration, or powerless feelings concerning stress or major changes in their lives
- May not understand the consequences of uncontrolled fire
- Most likely will continue to set fires until needs are met or identified

Pathological/Emotionally Disturbed

- Involves a psychiatric diagnosis
- Fires may be random, ritualized, or with specific intent to destroy property
- Chronic history of school, behavioral, and social emotional problems
- Boys and girls of all ages
- Set multiple fires

This type can be said to include thought-disordered, compulsive, and disordered coping subtypes.

Thought-Disordered

- Set fire secondary to a delusional system; child often has targeted fire sites, such as churches or schools

- Fires set in direct response to disordered thinking, a misperception of reality and thinking errors that may revolve around religious, political, personal, or even counterintuitive agendas and result in related targets for firesetting

Compulsive

- Commonly known as pyromaniacs (falls under the diagnostic category of impulse control disorders), describing firesetting as a compulsive, anxiety-driven behavior

- Usually have a late-adolescent or adult-age onset and are far less common than other subtypes. Fires often set in clusters in and around an anniversary date of significance to them

- Appear to set fires approximately 4 weeks around the anniversary date and then the obsessive desire decreases and often disappears until the next year

- Have little regard for the possibility of apprehension and set fires even if the chances of discovery were imminent

- Fires are dangerous and unpredictable, as they are set seemingly at random with a wide range of seemingly counterintuitive targets

- Destruction from fire is much less important than the act of setting a fire

- Describe the increase in anxiety that precedes an act of firesetting with the immediate decrease in level of anxiety as soon as the fire has been set

- Expresses guilt and remorse for destructive behavior but often describes the need for firesetting as being beyond their ability to control

Disordered Coping

- Display an onset under age 6 as a learned, deliberate response to rage and a sense of disequilibrium in society

- Fire becomes the preferred method of responding to any assault on the ego that produces emotional discomfort

- Demonstrate rigid intrapsychic flexibility, poor interpersonal empathy, and do not understand the impact of their behavior on their arson victims

- Do not suffer guilt or remorse and cannot imaginatively identify another, more socially acceptable and adaptive behavior other than firesetting

- Targets of firesetting are often random and the crime is generally opportunistic

- Fires are conducted in secret from earliest childhood and may result in hundreds of fires over a lifetime

- Place little value on the size or outcome of the fire; rather, it is the fire itself that provides a method of release and a seeming method of coping

- Often self-report few friends from their earliest childhood memories and consider themselves social misfits

- Often describe the act of firesetting in positive terms and leave the scene as soon as they see the fire has started

- Highest risk for continued, deliberate firesetting behavior

Delinquent/Criminal

- Usually teens with a history of firesetting, gangs, truancy, antisocial behavior, or drug/alcohol abuse

- Targets are typically schools, open fields, dumpsters, or abandoned buildings

- Typically characterized by group-influenced behavior

- Often occurs while under the influence of drugs and/or alcohol

- Fires often serve as a cover-up for another crime such as vandalism or property destruction and is often only one of a number of delinquent or socially marginal acts committed by the youths

- Distinguished by the thoughtlessness of their actions, a disregard for consequences, and otherwise typical adult-centered activities such as smoking cigarettes and drinking at young ages

- Pose a risk for additional acts of arson until they grow up and out of delinquency or convert from offenses of a youthful nature into the adult justice system

Thrill-Seeker

- Begin in early to mid-adolescence and appear to have an attraction toward danger for its own sake

- Commit acts of firesetting for excitement and to experience the rush brought on by the peril and possibility of discovery and apprehension

- Enter into a "game" with fire investigators and police in which each fire is regarded as a triumph of the arsonist over authority

- Most likely type to collect trophies from the fire scene, including pieces of charred rubble; frequently keep scrapbooks of their fires and videotapes of news coverage from the fire scene. Almost exclusively male

- Often drawn to careers where there is an ever-present possibility of danger and where, as a bonus, they are required to wear uniforms

- Maintain an air of arrogance when arrested, generally resultant from their knowledge that they have successfully set many more fires than are known by authorities

- Typically have no compunction to confess and feel little guilt about their behavior

- Extreme risk for reoffending

Revenge-Based

- Usually begin experimenting with incendiaries and explosives during the school-age years and often "grow into" firebombing activity in addition to acts of arson

- Suspicious of the world at large and may believe that others must be taught a lesson about the consequences of real or fantasy-based insults

- Fueled by rage, they identify their targets in a methodical and purposeful manner and determine the type of havoc they wish to create

- Devoid of much emotion other than resentment, suspicion, or anger

- Feel little guilt or remorse because they feel justified for their actions

- Threat of discovery and/or arrest does not seem to deter revenge firesetters from their criminal behavior

- May have been raised in families that teach the concept of "getting even" for real or imagined slights

- Male revenge firesetters: enjoy collecting weapons; have often spent time in the military or participated in military-type activities with clear and intense systematic structure; pose an extremely high risk for recidivism because they are convinced of the appropriateness of their acts, reflective of psychopathy that fuels their destructive behavior. Adolescent boys who make specific threats to authority figures that include references to "burning something down" or "blowing something up" should be taken seriously.

- Female revenge firesetters: generally have a specific target; criminal act is typically directly related to intrapsychic trauma or perceived rejection; onset of the behavior is later, usually mid- to late adolescence or in adulthood; have a low rate of recidivist behavior and generally express guilt after an act of arson because the act was typically a "heat-of-the-moment" crime, caused by an overwhelming rush of emotion

The literature also shows associated pathology with firesetting. The most common associated disorder is conduct disorder, as well as attention deficit hyperactivity disorder and oppositional defiant disorder (all common disorders in delinquency). When the Minnesota Multiphasic Personality Inventory-Adolescent (MMPI-A) is administered, adolescent male firesetters were found to be more pathological, demonstrating higher scores on clinical scales of mania, psychasthenia (irrational fear, fascination, and obligation), and schizophrenia. The high mania scores are indicative of the juvenile being impulsive and challenging as well as hyperactive, while heightened psychasthenia suggests increased levels of anxiety and a tendency toward being compulsive and unsure of one's self. The schizophrenia scale includes psychotic tendencies; however, it also measures difficulties socializing and controlling behaviors, academic problems, and "intense, acute situational distress," which may be more relevant to characteristics of firesetters. Firesetters also had noticeably greater scores on several content scales, including depression, alienation, anger, conduct problems, family problems, school problems, and negative treatment indicators. Thus, adolescent male firesetters display a particular range of psychological difficulties as compared to nonfiresetters (Glancy, Spiers, Pitt, & Dvoskin, 2003).

History and Physical Assessment

Health care providers can screen children and adolescents to identify those who are at risk and assure that these children obtain appropriate interventions. Juveniles and their families can be described according to *three risk levels* that represent the likelihood that the child will become involved in future firesetting. Each level of risk represents a successively more severe form of firesetting behavior.

> *Little risk.* About 60%–70% of juveniles involved in unsupervised firestarting are motivated by curiosity and experimentation. Most of these children are at little risk for becoming involved in future firesetting if they receive the proper supervision and education. The majority of these children are young boys between the ages of 3 and 7 who come from all types of social and economic backgrounds. Young girls participate in unsupervised firestarts, but do so less frequently than young boys. Low-risk children do not exhibit significant psychological problems. Their family and peer relationships are intact and stable, and their school performance and behavior meets expectations. This risk group includes the curious and mild cognitively impaired firesetters.
>
> *Definite risk.* About 30%–40% of children and adolescents identified with firesetting histories fall into the definite risk category. These juveniles are very likely to engage in future firesetting incidents. The earlier they are identified, evaluated, and provided appropriate interventions, the better their chances of avoiding involvement in future firesetting. There are two major classes of definite risk juveniles, troubled/crisis and delinquent.
>
> - *Definite risk—troubled juveniles.* These juveniles can be described as the cry-for-help type that start fires to bring attention

to their psychological distress. In most cases, it is their emotional conflict that motivates their firesetting. The source of this emotional conflict can vary greatly, and can include such things as family turmoil, abuse, neglect, unresolved difficulties in school, and other recent or chronic stressful life events. Fire safety and prevention education may be helpful, but it will not address their primary psychological problems. Therefore, they should be referred to the appropriate mental health agencies. If these youth and their families receive the help they need in a timely fashion, the chances are reasonably good that their firesetting behavior will not recur.

■ *Definite risk—delinquent juveniles.* Delinquent juveniles exhibit a certain pattern of aggressive, deviant, and criminal behavior. These behaviors emerge at a young age, and occur with greater frequency and intensity as the juvenile matures. What begins as stubborn and disobedient behavior as a preschooler can lead to lying and stealing as a young child and to firesetting, petty theft, and vandalism as a teenager. Serious emotional or family dysfunction also may contribute to this pattern of antisocial behavior. The longer this delinquent behavior pattern continues, the harder it is to reverse. Therefore, early identification is critical. They can be referred to mental health, social service, and other community agencies, and, if their firesetting is classified as an arson crime, they can be referred to the juvenile justice system. These juveniles present one of the biggest and costliest challenges to their families and their communities.

Extreme risk. This group represents less than 1% of firesetting youth. These juveniles suffer from significant mental dysfunction, such as the psychotic disturbances of schizophrenia and affective disorders, as well as organically impaired disturbances of mental retardation and fetal alcoholic syndrome. These children are beyond most fire safety and prevention programs currently available and are a significant danger to themselves or others.

Diagnostic Testing

Some juvenile firesetting programs have identification instruments. However, these have not been developed for use by health care providers.

INTERVENTION

Intervention depends on the child's typology. Curious firesetters respond well to fire safety education, while cognitively impaired firesetters may need special education, intensive fire education, and behavior management. Thought-disordered firesetters require appropriate and aggressive treatment of their thinking errors while under therapeutic supervision to reduce the possibility of additional acts of firesetting. Resolution of their thought disorder generally causes the disappearance of firesetting as a high-risk behavior. Delinquent firesetters require interventions that include restitution and criminal punishment.

Health care providers should be aware of, and can become involved with, their community juvenile firesetting intervention program. According to the Pennsylvania Office of the State Fire Commissioner (n.d.), a juvenile firesetting intervention program should be part of a community- or regionally based network that offers a continuum of care. The program should be designed to provide a range of intervention services including prevention, education, immediate treatment, and graduated sanctions to juveniles and their families.

Community and regional intervention programs should be diverse in composition and include multiple disciplines that continually have contact with juveniles. These services include public and private school systems, fire service professionals, mental health professionals, school social workers and counselors, children and youth social service workers, juvenile justice probation officers, law enforcement, and other like team members. All of these professionals should be part of the planned and coordinated effort to reduce child-set fires.

At-risk children should also be referred for psychiatric evaluation and treatment. Treatment for firesetting usually occurs in the least restrictive environment; however, juveniles may need to be confined to a secure facility, residential treatment center, or hospital, depending on the seriousness of the offense and based on the needs of the juvenile. Although many juvenile firesetters can be maintained in the community with appropriate supervision, careful assessment is critical to provide the appropriate level of care. The assessment must consider the child, family, environment, facts about the fire and other fire history, as well as the child's reaction to the fire and sense of accountability. Consideration should also be given to ensure that the child does not pose a risk to others and that the public safety is protected.

The teaming up of mental health professionals and fire department professionals to treat juvenile firesetters is becoming an increasingly popular occurrence. Treatment programs that incorporate a collaborative and comprehensive approach to the treatment of juvenile firesetting are gaining popularity, and the outcomes of these programs show impressive potential to decrease the prevalence of juvenile firesetting behavior.

PREVENTION/PATIENT TEACHING

Primary Prevention

Health care providers should include age-appropriate fire-safety anticipatory guidance in their wellness visits and other forms of child injury prevention teachings, such as health fairs and other community programs.

Secondary Prevention

Health care providers can work with their community or regionally based juvenile firesetting prevention program to:

- Organize and coordinate community-based screening, assessment, and intervention programs.
- Identify and provide for the child's and family's needs (fire safety education, counseling, social services, etc.) using community resources.
- Assist parents/caregivers and all who work with children to better understand children's involvement with fire, along with when and where to go for help.

Tertiary Prevention

Tertiary prevention should aim at recidivism prevention for those children who are at risk for repeated firesetting. This is part of the continuum of a juvenile firesetting prevention program.

RESOURCES

The Burn Institute's Public Education Programs includes two age-appropriate curriculum guides: *The Burni The Dragon Curriculum Guide* is designed specifically for preschool through kindergarten and the *Fire Burns and You Guide* is designed for students in middle school through high school. To request a copy of any, or both of these guides, please call the Burn Institute at (858) 541–2277. www.burninstitute.org

Juvenile Firesetter Intervention Handbook: www.usfa.dhs.gov/downloads/pdf/publications/fa-210.pdf

National Association of State Fire Marshalls: www.firemarshals.org/mission/residential/human-behavior/juvenile-fire-setting

SOS Fires Youth Intervention Programs: www.sosfires.com/index.htm

REFERENCES

Federal Bureau of Investigation. (2006). *Arson.* Retrieved from http://www.fbi.gov/ucr/cius2006/offenses/property_crime/arson.html

Glancy, G., Spiers, E., Pitt, S., & Dvoskin, J. (2003). Commentary: Models and correlates of firesetting behavior. *Journal of the American Academy of Psychiatry & Law, 31,* 53–57.

Gliman, T., & Haden, S. (2006, Winter). Understanding and treating the juvenile firesetting: A review. *The Forensic Examiner.* Retrieved from http://findarticles.com/p/articles/mi_go1613/is_4_15/ai_n29310473/?tag=content;col1

Pennsylvania Office of the State Fire Commissioner. (n.d.). *Pennsylvania's Juvenile Firesetting Intervention Protocol.* Retrieved from www.portal.state.pa.us/portal/server.pt/community/juvenile_firesetter_intervention/11358/pennsylvania's_juvenile_firesetting_intervention_protocol/565686

Putnam, C., & Kirkpatrick, J. (2005). *Juvenile firesetting: A research overview.* Office of Juvenile Justice and Delinquency Prevention Juvenile Justice Bulletin NCJ 207606. Retrieved from www.ncjrs.gov/pdffiles1/ojjdp/207606.pdf

Root, C., MacKay, S., Henderson, J., DelBove, G., & Warling, D. (2008). The link between maltreatment and juvenile firesetting: Correlates and underlying mechanisms. *Child Abuse and Neglect, 32*(2), 161–176.

U.S. Fire Administration. (2006). Juvenile firesetting: A growing concern. Retrieved from http://www.usfa.dhs.gov/downloads/pdf/publications/fa_307.pdf

Williams, D., & Clements, P. (2007). Intrapsychic dynamics, behavioral manifestations, and related interventions with youthful fire setters. *Journal of Forensic Nursing, 3*(2), 67–83.

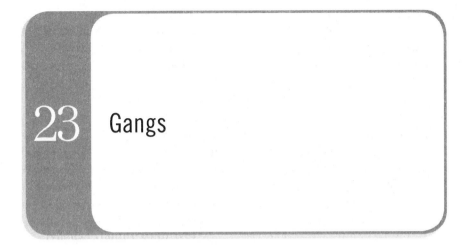

23 Gangs

DEFINITION

There is no set definition of a gang. Once thought to be an inner-city problem, *gang violence* has spread to communities throughout the United States. Gang problems have escalated since the 1960s, with most gangs comprising males with similar ethnic and racial backgrounds. Gang violence is particularly concentrated in Los Angeles and Chicago, where half of homicides are considered gang-related. Besides crime and violence, research frequently indicates that gang youth, in comparison with their nongang peers, are more likely to use drugs and alcohol, have mental health problems, and participate in early and unsafe sex. Gang youth are more likely than nongang youth to experience being victimized by violence and are at an increased risk of incarceration and recidivism. Thus, gang participation is an important indicator of a young person who is at an increased risk to the negative health outcomes (Hill, Lui, & Hawkins, 2001).

Gangs that support antisocial values and behaviors, such as intimidation, vandalism, extortion, and other acts of violence, create fear. If children affiliate with one of these groups, they are likely to adopt the gang's values and imitate their behaviors and behave in a violent manner. When teens become involved in gangs, they have higher incidences of violent and delinquent behaviors compared to when they are not active in a gang. Gang violence is intense, often resulting in injury and death.

The average age of gang members is from 14 to 21; however, they can be as young as 8 years old or as old as their mid-30s. Gang recruitment usually begins in the middle school where children are between ages 10 and 13, but some recruitment has also been seen in elementary school and into the early years of high school. Most gangs target children who are easily talked into doing work for the gang.

Gangs tend to have a leader or group of leaders who give orders and enjoy the fruits of the gang's labors. *Gangbangers* (gang members) wear their "colors," certain types of clothing, tattoos, brands, or likewise imprint their gang's name, logo, or other identifying marks on their bodies. Many gangs adopt specific hairdos and communicate through hand signals and graffiti. Organized graffiti is one of the first ways to know that a gang is taking hold in your community. Experts use graffiti to track gang growth, affiliation, and membership information.

The "three Rs" have a whole new meaning in gang mentality:

Reputation/Rep is a critical concern to gangbangers. The rep extends to each individual and the gang as a whole. Gang members gain status by having the most "juice" (power), based largely on one's rep. The manner in which one gains juice is important, so many members embellish their past gang activities to impress the listener, freely admitting to crimes. To even so much as gain membership, a person must be "jumped in" by being "beaten down" until the leader calls for it to end. Afterward, they all hug each other to further the "G thing," an action that bonds members together. Young members frequently talk of this fellowship as the reason they joined the gang.

Respect is something that they carry to the extreme for each member, the gang, their territory, and various other things, real or perceived. Some gangs require that members always show disrespect ("dis") for rival gangs through hand signals, graffiti, or a simple "mad dog" or stare down. If a member fails to dis a rival, causing a violation to his fellow posse (gang members), he will be "beaten down" by his own gang as punishment.

Revenge/Retaliation shows that no challenge goes unanswered in gang culture. Many drive-by shootings follow an event perceived as a dis. Typically, a confrontation takes place between a gang set and a single rival gangbanger. The gang member leaves, only to return with his "home boys" to complete the confrontation and keep his rep intact.

Youth gangs tend to be more heterogeneous and have less organized criminality than street gangs. But here are examples of street gangs in the United States since many have young members.

National Street Gangs (does not include outlaw motorcycle gangs or prison gangs)

18th Street. With membership estimated at 30,000 to 50,000, 18th Street is a group of loosely associated sets or cliques, each led by an influential member. The gang is active in 44 cities in 20 states. Eighty percent in California are illegal aliens from Mexico and Central America.

Almighty Latin King and Queen Nation. This gang was formed in Chicago in the 1960s and consisted predominantly of Mexican and Puerto Rican males. It operates throughout the United States under two umbrella factions—Motherland, also known as KMC (King Motherland Chicago), and Bloodline (New York)—but all members of the gang refer to themselves as Latin.

Asian Boyz. One of the largest Asian street gangs operating in the United States, the Asian Boyz gang was formed in southern California in the early 1970s and is currently estimated to have 1,300 to 2,000 members operating in at least 28 cities in 14 states. Members primarily are Vietnamese or Cambodian males.

Black P. Stone Nation. One of the largest and most violent associations of street gangs in the United States, this association consists of seven highly structured street gangs with a single leader and a common culture. There are an estimated 6,000 to 8,000 members, most of whom are African American males from the Chicago metropolitan area.

Bloods. Estimated to be 7,000 to 30,000 nationwide and active in 123 cities in 33 states, the Bloods is an association of structured and unstructured gangs that have adopted a single-gang culture. Membership is mostly African American males.

Crips. The Crips is also a collection of structured and unstructured gangs that have adopted a common gang culture. Membership is estimated at 30,000 to 35,000, consisting of mostly African American males.

Gangster Disciples. The Gangster Disciples gang was formed in Chicago in the mid-1960s and is structured like a corporation, led by a chairman of the board. Membership is estimated at 25,000 to 50,000 of mostly African American males.

Mara Salvatrucha. Also known as *MS 13*, this is one of the largest Hispanic street gangs in the country. The gang is estimated to have 8,000 to 10,000 members.

Tiny Rascal Gangsters. One of the largest and most violent Asian street gang associations in the United States, this group is composed of at least 60 structured and unstructured gangs, commonly referred to as sets, with an estimated 5,000 to 10,000 members and associates who have adopted a common gang culture. Most members are Asian American males.

Vice Lord Nation. Based in Chicago, this is a collection of structured gangs located in 74 cities in 28 states, primarily in the Great Lakes region. They are led by a national board and have an estimated 30,000 to 35,000 members, most of whom are African American males.

Skinhead Groups. Most skinhead groups are composed of White youths who often associate themselves with organizations like the Ku Klux Klan and other more organized hate groups.

PREVALENCE

The 2009 National Gang Threat Assessment (National Gang Intelligence Center, 2009) notes that there were approximately 1 million gang members belonging to more than 20,000 criminally active gangs within all 50 states and the District of Columbia as of September 2008. Gang members are migrating from urban areas to suburban and rural communities, expanding the gangs' influence; in most regions expansion is due to a number of reasons, including expanding drug distribution territories, increasing illicit revenue, recruiting new members, hiding from law enforcement, and escaping other gangs. Many suburban and rural communities are now experiencing increasing gang-related crime and violence.

The *National Youth Gang Survey Trends From 1996 to 2000 Report* (Egley & O'Donnell, 2008), which highlighted findings from five national surveys, showed that:

- Ninety-one percent of cities with a population of more than 250,000 reported at least one gang-related homicide from 1999 to 2000, as did 64% of cities with a population between 100,000 and 250,000; 55% of cities with a population between 50,000 and 100,000; and 32% of cities with a population between 25,000 and 50,000.

■ In 1996, 50% of gang members were younger than 18 and 50% were 18 and older. In 1999, these numbers were 37% and 63%, respectively.

■ In 1999, respondents reported that 47% of gang members were Hispanic, 31% African American, 13% White, 7% Asian, and 2% "other."

In 2004, the Federal Bureau of Investigation's (FBI) Uniform Crime Reporting (UCR) Program provided data on murder circumstances from 1999–2003 (FBI, 2004). Findings related to gangs from this study include the following statistics:

■ In 1999, there were 580 incidents of juvenile gang killings compared to the 819 in 2003.

■ In 2002, there were 75 incidents of gangland killings and a total 115 in 2003.

The *National Youth Gang Survey From 2006* (Egley & O'Donnell, 2008) noted that the proportion of respondents that reported youth gangs decreased in their jurisdiction (large cities, small cities, suburban counties, and rural counties). The *National Youth Gang Survey Trends From 1996 to 2000 Report* noted that 94% of gang members were male and 6% were female (39% of all youth gangs had female members; only 2% of gangs were identified as predominantly female).

ETIOLOGY

While some children are forced to join gangs, this is an unusual occurrence. More common reasons include the individual child's need for acceptance, for excitement; to follow the family tradition; for glamour, identity, or profit; response to peer pressure; or the need for protection or socialization.

Acceptance. When children feel that they are not getting the attention they feel they deserve at home, they start looking for love in other places and often find what they are looking for in a gang. The gang becomes their substitute family.

Excitement. Some children enjoy the high of committing crime and getting away with it. Many commit their crimes just to be chased by the police. These children are thrill seekers who live for the adrenaline rush of being in a gang.

Family tradition. Some join because another family member, usually a sibling, joined.

Glamour. Movies and music have glamorized gangs, making them attractive to children who are feeling chronically bored.

Identity. Being a gang member is better than being nothing.

Profit. It is becoming more common for gang members to turn toward using the gang to make a profit through illegal activities, such as selling narcotics, robberies, burglaries, auto thefts, and other property crimes. Many gangs specialize in a specific criminal activity.

Peer pressure. If children hang around gangs and gang members, it is almost guaranteed that they are being pressured to join the gang.

Protection. In bad neighborhoods, kids often have to join a gang just to survive because it is often easier to join the gang than to be victimized on a daily basis.

Socialization. The best parties are gang parties. Easy access to liquor, narcotics, and girls are attractive to potential young recruits, and young males who have a hard time socializing find that girls often like gang members.

ASSESSMENT

General Principles

Identifying gang members is not an easy task. The best place to identify and refer is in primary care or school health. However, at-risk youth and gang-involved youth may not attend school nor have primary care providers. Thus, the most realistic location may be the emergency department when gang members come in for treatment of trauma wounds, or though creative collaboration with law enforcement.

Health care providers may be able to assess where a juvenile is with regard to gang membership by reviewing the levels provided by the Durham (North Carolina) Police Department's *Guide for Parents, Teachers and Other Concerned Citizens.* This guide identifies five levels of involvement. They are:

Level I: Fantasy

Knows about gangs primarily from newspaper, newscasts, and movies

May or may not know about "real" gangs

May or may not know one or more gang members, but does not associate with them

May or may not like, respect, or admire a gang, gang member, or the gang lifestyle

See gang members "living out a fantasy"

Level II: Fringe

Knows about gangs and gang members firsthand

Occasionally casually associates with gang members

Lives in or near gang areas

May like or admire gangs or gang members as individuals

May like or admire the gang lifestyle, but not participate fully

Level III: Associate

Knows and likes gang members firsthand

Regularly associates with gang members

Considers gangs and related activity as normal, acceptable, and admirable

Finds many things in common with gang members

Is thinking seriously about joining a gang

Level IV: Member

   Is officially a gang member

   Associates almost exclusively with gang members to the exclusion of family and former friends

   Participates in gang crimes and most other related activities

   Is not considered hard-core by fellow gang members or others

   Has substantially rejected the authority or value system of family and society

Level V: Hard-Core Gang Member

   Totally committed to the gang and gang lifestyle

   Totally rejects anyone or any value system other than the gang

   Is considered hard-core by self, other gang-members, and authorities

   Will commit any act with the approval or a demand from the gang

   Does not accept any authority other than the gang

History and Physical Assessment

Gang members may be up-front with their involvement in a gang during the interview, especially if confidentiality is stressed. They may be identified by family members or on physical assessment when presenting with violence-inflicted injuries. Health care providers may also be able to identify gang members by their clothing, hand signals, tattoos, and graffiti.

Gang clothing. Gang members often wear clothing that is currently popular among all juveniles. Thus, "gansta" apparel does not automatically make that person a gang member. A combination of the clothing worn, along with a certain color scheme or the manner in which the clothing is worn, can indicate membership in a gang. However, as gang members realize their clothing is becoming too noticeable to people, they may change what they wear. And gang members like to be fashionable; thus, if it is no longer in vogue, it is no longer worn.

   Some gang members wear a gang-colored handkerchief on the head, often referred to as a "rag." Gangs often adopt a color that they will identify with. Many other gangs may use the same color rag and alliances between different gangs can often be recognized by the use of the same color rag. Pants may hang low, which is known as "sagging," to show off colored boxer shorts. Dickie work pants are popular among the gang culture, and they come in different colors, with tan usually being a neutral color worn by many different gangs. Colored beads are popular with gang members. The bead color is dependent on the color the gang has adopted for the gang. The beads can be made into a necklace, worn in the shoelaces, made into a key chain, worn in braids in the hair, or used in other fashions. Colored rubber bands worn in hair braids or around the wrists can also be indicators of gang membership. Some gang members use colored rosary beads and other religious articles because these are subtle indicators of gang membership and thus hard to notice if you are not looking for them.

Dress codes and school uniforms can be adapted into gang apparel. They may use colored shoelaces or certain types of sneakers. Popular styles include British Knights tennis shoes (the initials BK stand for Blood Killer); Columbia Knights tennis shoes (CK stands for Crip Killer); Nike tennis shoes (referred to as G-Nikes); and Converse canvas tennis shoes (the five-pointed star used on the Converse is the same as a gang symbol used by many gangs nationwide). Steel toe boots are popular, mainly with skinhead gangs, who like the Dr. Marten brand. T-shirts and baseball caps may be customized with the name or initials of the gang. Gang members will write gang graffiti on their clothing, shoes, baseball caps, wallets, or other articles of clothing or accessories. Many gangs adopt a popular sports team's style of apparel, especially if the color of that team is the same as their gang color or the team logo has some significant meaning to the gang.

Hand signs. Hand signs were first used by Chinese Triads several hundred years ago, but Black gang members introduced hand signs to the gang culture in the mid-1970s in Los Angeles. It is believed gangs copied their hand signs from family members who used secret hand signs in their fraternal societies and Masonic groups. Gang members have since developed hand signs unique to their particular gangs.

Hand signs represent gang nomenclature—using fingers to spell the word "blood," or to create the symbols found in gang graffiti, such as pitchforks and numbers. Hand signs have been quickly accepted and adopted by gangs across the nation and are a nonverbal form of communication much like American Sign Language. However, hand signs should not be confused with sign language. A quick flash of the hand is used as an announcement of gang affiliation or as a challenge, and has a very specific meaning to gang members. Gang members will even invert or modify the signs of a rival gang as an insult, known as "throwing down."

Tattoos. Nothing symbolizes gang loyalty like a tattoo. It is personal and permanent, written on the body itself. Tattoos are a way of asserting membership in the gang. The most common tattoo among gang members is one that demonstrates the gang they are in. Usually, only the most dedicated gang members will get a tattoo bearing the name of the gang, but many members will get tattoos depicting gang symbols. Crowns, Playboy bunnies, five- and six-pointed stars, and pitchforks are all common gang tattoos. A common tattoo among Hispanic gang members from many different gangs is the pachuco cross tattooed on the hand between the thumb and index finger. That same area is often embellished with three dots in a pyramid shape, a symbol that stands for *mi vida loca,* "my crazy life."

Often the gang name will be slightly disguised by giving it an assigned number. For example, the Nortenos will use 14, X4, XIV (all denoting the 14th letter of the alphabet, N) in their tattoos. The Vice Lords of Chicago are recognizable by their tattoos of the number 312, which is the Chicago area code. The 18th Street gang of Los Angeles uses the number 18. Gangs also find other ways to identify themselves without using their full gang names. The Nortenos use the Spanish word for "fourteen," *catorce,* while the Surenos sometimes use the Aztec language, Nahuatl, in their tattoos. They will also use Aztec numerology to denote the number 13.

Tattoos can tell other details about the bearer, including rank in the gang and the number of "hits" (kills) or other services performed on the gang's behalf. Tattoos can tell more personal details about gang members' lives, such as memorials to deceased loved ones, the names and birthdates of their children, what country or region they are from, and how many of their loved ones have died while they were incarcerated.

A common tattoo among gang members is a small teardrop below the eye. Some use this to mean that the bearer has killed someone; others use it to show that someone close to the bearer has died. Tombstones with "R.I.P." and a date are reserved for fellow gang members who were killed in gang-related violence.

Tattoos can appear anywhere on a gang members body. Traditionally, they are on the arm, with larger tattoos appearing on the chest or back. Tattoos may be found on the face, neck, and hands. Gang tattoos are usually fairly crude and crafted in blue or black ink. Serious gang members tend to have multiple tattoos that are displayed prominently, while juveniles may cover their tattoos with clothing, especially in the presence of law enforcement, parents, or school officials.

Graffiti. Community health care professional may notice graffiti while performing their duties, while other professionals may simply note it around their neighborhoods. Not all graffiti is gang graffiti. Taggers and tag crews use "tags" to gain notoriety and express their identity in what they consider to be a creative manner. Tags are usually multicolored and elaborate. Gangs use less elaborate graffiti as their "newspaper" or "bulletin board." It marks their turf and sends clear messages to rival gang members. Gang graffiti contains clear messages to mark territory, identify the gang's purpose, glorify the gang, advertise a "plan of attack," and disrespect or degrade a rival gang. Many times, it contains a roll call, or list of members in a particular gang or set.

Elements of gang graffiti include initials or symbols identifying the gang; street names or monikers to identify members; symbols or letters that identify the neighborhood or the area the gang is from; messages to rival gangs. Gang graffiti is often written in the gang's colors and is almost never meant for the general public. However, being able to read gang graffiti will help health care providers to know what is happening in a particular neighborhood.

INTERVENTION

Refer gang members to specialized programs specific for gang members, whenever possible. Contact your local or state police to find programs in your area.

PREVENTION/PATIENT TEACHING

Primary Prevention

Teach parents to:

- Spend quality time with your child and convey a strong sense of family.

- Supervise his activities, and know his whereabouts at all times.

- Know his friends and their families.

- Be a positive role model.

- Teach him values, and let him know why you think gangs are dangerous.

- Get involved in his activities.

- Stress the importance of schooling and encourage good study habits.

- Create rules, set limits, and be consistent, firm, and fair.

- Respect his feelings and attitudes.

- Foster healthy self-esteem.

- Help him develop self-control and deal effectively with problems.

Tell him not to:

- Associate with gang members or wannabe members.

- Communicate with gang members.

- Hang out near or where gangs hang out.

- Approach strangers in cars.

- Wear gang-related clothing.

- Wear gang-initialed clothing (BK [British Knights] also stands for Blood Killer)

- Use words like "slob" where gang members may be, like malls.

- Attend parties sponsored by gangs.

- Hang out near graffiti or take part in graffiti activity.

- Use any type of hand signal in public.

Teach him what to do if approached by a gang member. His best response is to walk away. Tell him not to respond with the same gesture, as a gang member could be "false flagging," using a sign of a rival gang, which could result in violence.

Contact your school if any gang activity takes place there. If they are not helpful, contact the police.

Look for signs of gang activity in your community, especially graffiti and young people hanging out on corners or near school property.

Secondary Prevention

Adolescents with preexisting psychopathic tendencies (i.e., a combination of high hyperactivity, low anxiety, and low prosociality as compared to national norms) appear to be vulnerable to join gangs, especially if they were raised in residentially unstable neighborhoods. However, good kids can be enticed into a gang, especially if they are unsupervised.

Warning signs of gang involvement (many of these can signal other problems, such as drug abuse):

Admits to being in gang

Obsesses with one particular color or logo

Wears excessive distinct jewelry; wears it on one side of the body

Obsesses with "gangsta" music

Withdraws from family

Associates with undesirables

Develops a strong desire for privacy

Uses hand signals at home

Has physical signs of being beaten and lies about events surrounding the injuries

Wears peculiar drawings or language on books or hands

Has unexplained cash or goods

Uses drugs and alcohol

Tertiary Prevention

Increase access to health care but take precautions so that youth is not attacked in retaliation by rival gangs or other gang members (a good approach is to treat rival gang members at different locations) and promote a healthy lifestyle.

Act as liaison between the youth, his family, and other agencies.

Teach about major causes of morbidity and mortality among youth, such as motor vehicle accidents, homicide, and suicide.

Teach about major health issues common to the participants' age group, such as drug use, obesity, mental health, and sexual health.

Refer for appropriate mental illness and substance abuse treatment, as well as social services.

RESOURCES

COPS Gang Tool Kit: www.cops.usdoj.gov/Default.asp?Item=1309
COPS Solutions to Address Gang Crime: www.cops.usdoj.gov/files/RIC/CDROMs/ GangCrime/index.html
Durham Police Department's *Guide for Parents, Teachers and Other Concerned Citizens:* www.durhampolice.com/pdf/gang_awareness_booklet.pdf
Facts for Teens: Youth Gangs: www.safeyouth.org
Female Gangs: A Focus on Research: www.ncjrs.gov/pdffiles1/ojjdp/186159.pdf
Gang Ink (gang tattoos): www.gangink.com
Parent's Guide to Gangs (printable brochure): www.iir.com/NYGC/publications/Parents Guide-EN.pdf
Parent's Quick Reference Card Recognizing and Preventing Gang Involvement: www. cops.usdoj.gov/files/ric/Publications/GangsCard_FBI.pdf

REFERENCES

Dupéré, V., Lacourse, E., Willms, J., Vitaro, F., & Tremblay, R. (2007). Affiliation to youth gangs during adolescence: The interaction between childhood psychopathic tendencies and neighborhood disadvantage. *Journal of Abnormal Child Psychology, 35,* 1035–1045.
Egley, A., & O'Donnell, C. (2008). *Highlights of the 2006 National Youth Gang Survey.* Office of Juvenile Justice and Delinquency Prevention. Retrieved from www.ncjrs. gov/pdffiles1/ojjdp/fs200805.pdf
Federal Bureau of Investigation (FBI). (2004). Crime in the United States, 2004. Retrieved from http://www.fbi.gov/ucr/cius_04/
Hill, K., Lui, K., & Hawkins, D. (2001). Early precursors of gang membership: A study of Seattle youth. Office of Juvenile Justice and Delinquency Prevention. *Juvenile Justice Bulletin.* NCJ 190106. Retrieved from http://www.ncjrs.gov/pdffiles1/ojjdp/190106. pdf
National Gang Intelligence Center. (2009). *National gang threat assessment 2009.* Retrieved from www.fbi.gov/publications/ngta2009.pdf

San Antonio Police Department Youth Crime Service Unit. (n.d.). *Gang awareness: A handbook for parents, teachers, and concerned citizens.* Retrieved from http://sanan tonio.gov/sapd/pdf/Awareness.pdf

Sanders, B., Schneiderman, J., Loken, A., Lankenau, S., & Bloom, J. (2009). Gang youth as a vulnerable population for nursing intervention. *Public Health Nursing, 26*(4), 346–352.

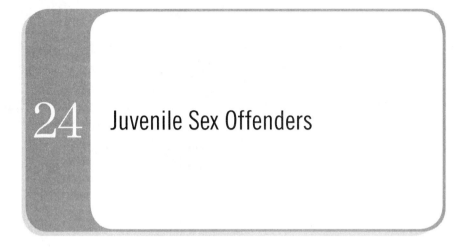

24 Juvenile Sex Offenders

DEFINITION

Juvenile sex offenders (JSOs) are youths under the age of 18 who commit illegal sexual behavior as defined by the sex crime statutes of the jurisdiction in which their offense(s) occurred. Juveniles who have committed sex offenses are a heterogeneous group. Some are otherwise well functioning with limited behavioral or psychological problems; some have multiple nonsexual behavior problems or prior nonsexual juvenile offenses; some have major psychiatric disorders. Many come from well-functioning families; others come from highly chaotic or abusive backgrounds. Contrary to common belief, most adolescent sex offenders have not been victims of childhood sexual abuse. Juvenile sexual offenders under age 12 are more likely to have been victims of sexual and/or physical abuse.

Juvenile sex offenders differ according to victim and offense characteristics and a wide range of other variables, including types of offending behaviors, sexual knowledge and experiences, academic and cognitive functioning, and mental health issues.

Their sexually abusive behaviors range from noncontact offenses to penetrative acts, and their offense characteristics include factors such as the age and sex of the victim, the relationship between victim and offender, and the degree of coercion and violence used for the offense.

Many juvenile sex offenders also engage in nonsexual criminal and antisocial behavior.

Juveniles who sexually offend are distinct from their adult counterparts. Youth who commit sexual offenses are not necessarily "just small adults." Many will not continue to offend sexually. Adolescent sex offenders are significantly different from adult sex offenders in a number of ways:

- Adolescent sex offenders have fewer numbers of victims than adult offenders and tend to engage in less serious and aggressive behaviors.

- Most adolescents do not have deviant sexual arousal and/or deviant sexual fantasies.

- Most adolescents are not sexual predators, nor do most meet the accepted criteria for pedophilia.

- Adolescent sex offenders are thought to be more responsive to treatment than adult sex offenders.

- Adolescent sex offenders do not appear to continue reoffending into adulthood, especially when provided with appropriate treatment.

- The overall sexual recidivism rate for adolescent sex offenders who receive treatment is low. Adolescents who offend against young children tend to have slightly lower sexual recidivism rates than adolescents who sexually offend against other teens.

The onset of sexual offending behavior in these youth can be linked to numerous factors reflected in their experiences, exposure, and/or developmental deficits. The literature suggests that a distinction can be made between youth who target peers or adults and those who offend against children (Center for Sex Offender Management, 1999).

Juvenile Offenders Who Sexually Offend Against Peers or Adults

- Predominantly assault females and strangers or casual acquaintances

- Are more likely to commit sexual assaults in association with other types of criminal activity (e.g., burglary)

- Are more likely to have histories of nonsexual criminal offenses, and appear more generally delinquent and conduct-disordered

- Are more likely to commit their offenses in public areas

- Generally display higher levels of aggression and violence in the commission of their sexual crimes

- Are more likely to use weapons and to cause injuries to their victims

Juvenile Offenders Who Sexually Offend Against Children

- Have both a higher number of male victims and female victims

- Have female victim rates that are slightly higher rates than males; however, almost 50% of this group of juvenile sex offenders has at least one male victim

- Have as many as 40% of their victims being either siblings or other relatives

- Commit sexual crimes that tend to reflect a greater reliance on opportunity and guile than injurious force, particularly when their victim is related to them

- May "trick" the child into complying with the molestation, use bribes, or threaten the child with loss of the relationship—all forms of grooming

- May display high levels of aggression and violence; generally, these are youths who display more severe levels of personality and/or psychosexual disturbances (e.g., psychopathy, sexual sadism, etc.)

- Have often been characterized as suffering from deficits in self-esteem and social competency

- May show evidence of depression

- May have impaired ability to form and maintain healthy peer relationships and successfully resolve interpersonal conflict

- Generally show less emotional indifference to the needs of others than peer/adult offenders

Laws regarding juvenile sexual offending vary per state. Many jurisdictions and the federal government have enacted laws aimed at preventing recidivism and protecting the public from future victimization once sex offenders are released from custody. These laws allow information gathered from juvenile sex offenders to be used to determine a juvenile's status for referral to a sex-offender registry or to a civil commitment process commonly known as sexually violent offender (SVO) or sexually violent predator (SVP) commitment.

That information can include the presence of sexual disorders (i.e., paraphilia), conduct disorder, other mental illness, or prior sexual assaults not known to the criminal justice system. As of 2008, 38 states include the registration of juvenile sex offenders in their sex offender registries without restrictions. Alaska, Florida, and Maine will register juveniles if they are tried as an adult; Indiana registers juveniles age 14 and older; South Dakota registers juveniles age 15 and older. Mississippi registers juveniles with two sexual offense convictions. New Hampshire, New Mexico, Utah, and Wyoming only register individuals age 18 and older, and Alabama only registers individuals 20 years and older. Links to state sex offender registries can be found at www.prevent-abuse-now.com/register.htm.

Female Juvenile Sex Offenders

The average female juvenile sex offender is 14 years old and exhibits greater variability in her sexual arousal and behavior patterns than adult male/female sex offenders. The most common sexual offenses committed by female adolescents are nonaggressive acts, such as mutual fondling, that occur during a caregiving activity such as babysitting. They rarely commit sex offenses against adults. Their victims are typically young acquaintances or relatives, with male and female children equally at risk for sexual victimization by female adolescents.

Female juvenile sex offenders are similar to their male juvenile sex offenders in the level of diversity that exists within their population. They commit a wide range of illegal sexual behaviors, ranging from limited exploratory behaviors committed largely out of curiosity to repeated aggressive acts. Some have histories of multiple nonsexual behavior problems or prior nonsexual juvenile offenses, but many are otherwise well-functioning youth with limited behavioral problems. While some female juvenile sex offenders experience high levels of individual and family psychopathology, others have limited psychological problems and minimal family dysfunction. Female juvenile sex offenders differ from male juvenile sex offenders with regard to physical and sexual abuse history. On average, female juvenile sex offenders have experienced more extensive and severe physical and sexual maltreatment during their childhood than male juvenile sex offenders. Female juvenile sex offenders are also sexually victimized at younger ages and are more likely to have had multiple perpetrators.

Juvenile Sex Offenders Under Age 13

Research in the area of prepubertal sex offenders area is still in its infancy, but one literature review (Araji, 1997) revealed that some children are sexually aggressive as early as age 3 or 4, although the most common age of onset appears to be between 6 and 9. Contrary to findings regarding adolescent sex offenders, girls were represented in much greater numbers among preadolescent offenders. Furthermore, these girls often engaged in behaviors that were just as aggressive as the boys' actions. Victims of child sex offenders range in ages from 1 to 9, and many offenders have multiple victims.

Sexting

Sexting is the sending of sexually charged messages or images via cell phone. The National Campaign to Prevent Teen and Unplanned Pregnancy and Cosmogirl.com (2008) conducted a survey of 653 teens (ages 13–19) and 637 young adults (ages 20–26) to better understand the connection between sex and cyberspace. They found that 20% of teens (22% of girls and 18% of boys) electronically sent or posted online nude or seminude photos or videos of themselves. Eleven percent of young teens, ages 13–16, electronically sent nude/seminude photos. Even more teens sent out sexually suggestive test messages, e-mails, or instant messages: 39% overall, 37% of teen girls, and 40% of teen boys. Forty-eight percent of teens stated they received sexually explicit messages. The numbers were higher in all areas for young adults. Possessing and distributing nude/seminude photos of minors constitute child pornography crimes in most jurisdictions, and these crimes often constitute felonies.

A felony is a serious crime that may be punishable by incarceration in a state correctional facility if the teen is convicted as an adult. Incarceration is bad enough, but a felony conviction can haunt a teen for life. State laws vary, but convicted felons may have difficulty finding a job, or receiving government clearance for security jobs; be unable to enter some foreign countries; be disqualified from serving as jurors; forfeit their right to vote, be a candidate for public office, or hold public office; be unable to qualify for federal assistance including loans, grants, and work study; be disallowed to possess firearms; and may be disallowed from obtaining licensure in certain professions.

They may also be denied becoming a foster or adoptive parent, especially once branded a sex offender. Sex offenders convicted of child pornography charges typically must register as sex offenders for a term that can be 10 years, 20 years, or even life. Depending on the state, their photo may be posted on the state's Sex Offender Registry Web site for the whole world to see, and they may be assessed to determine if they meet their state's criteria to be deemed a sexually violent predator.

PREVALENCE

Adults commit the majority of sexual offences; however, juveniles commit a significant percentage:

One in every five sexual assaults is committed by a juvenile.

About one-third of sexual offenses against children are committed by juveniles.

The average age of onset of juvenile sexual offending is 12 to 15.

Somewhere between 90% and 97% of juvenile sex offenders are male.

Victims are often relatives or acquaintances.

ETIOLOGY

A number of etiological factors (casual influences) have been identified that are believed to help explain the developmental origin of juvenile sex offending. Factors that have received the most attention to date include maltreatment experiences, exposure to pornography, substance abuse, and exposure to aggressive role models.

While sexual aggression may emerge early in the developmental process, there is no compelling evidence to suggest that the majority of juvenile sex offenders are likely to become adult sex offenders. The estimated risk of juvenile sex offending leading to adult offending may have been exaggerated by an overreliance on retrospective research studies. Existent longitudinal studies suggest that aggressive behavior in youths is not always continuous, and that juveniles who engage in sexual aggression frequently cease such behavior by the time they reach adulthood (Center for Sex Offender Management, 1999).

ASSESSMENT

General Principles

The focus of assessment in juvenile sexual offending is recidivism risk assessment. Risk assessment can be useful for informing many key decisions with juvenile sex offenders, such as disposition or sentencing, the type of placement or required level of care, release from facilities, and the application of registration and community notification policies. Assessing risk is particularly helpful for guiding treatment decisions.

Risk assessment includes the identification of static and dynamic risk factors. Historical characteristics that cannot be altered, such as age of the offender, gender of the victims, relationship between the offender and the victims, and prior offense history, are referred to as *static factors*. Attitudes and characteristics that can change throughout a person's life are termed *dynamic factors*. Dynamic factors include not accepting responsibility for offense(s), lack of internal motivation for change, not understanding risk factors, lack of empathy, lack of remorse and guilt, and cognitive distortions.

History and Physical Assessment

Health care professionals need to obtain detailed sexual histories on all adolescents to ascertain whether they are exhibiting unhealthy sexual behaviors. Harassing behaviors such as repeated obscene phone calls, "flashing," and "peeping" are sex offenses, as are coercive or forcible sexual behaviors, including touching breasts, genitals, and buttocks over one's clothing. Health care professionals should also ask about sexually precocious, coercive, and forcible behavior in younger children who are exhibiting conduct-disordered behaviors and/or who have been observed, usually by a parent or teacher, engaging in unusual sexual behavior.

Adjudicated juvenile sex offenders require the same psychosocial and physiological assessment as other adjudicated juvenile offenders (see

Chapter 16, "Juvenile Delinquency"). Health care providers should also have an understanding of risk assessment, treatment, and reentry issues (including the sex offender registration laws in their jurisdiction with regard to juvenile sex offenders) so that they can provide proper health care for these youths and so that they can work with other involved professionals to decrease the chances of recidivism.

Screening Tools

Child Sexual Behavior Inventory, Version 2 (CSAI-2). The CSBI-2 is a 35-item instrument that is completed by a parent or caregiver to determine the presence and intensity of a range of sexual behaviors in children ages 2 to 12 over a 6-month period. It assesses the child's sexual behaviors on a continuum ranging from mild to aggressive and provides separate clinical scores based on the child's age and gender. It can be found at www. childwelfare.gov/pubs/usermanuals/sexabuse/sexabuse1.cfm.

Risk Assessment Tools

At present, there no empirically validated, actuarial instruments that can be used to accurately estimate the risk of adolescent sexual reoffending. However, the following tools can be used to aid in the assessment of risk in this population.

Juvenile Sex Offender Assessment Protocol-II (J-SOAP-II). The J-SOAP-II is a checklist whose purpose is to aid in the systematic review of risk factors that have been identified in the professional literature as being associated with sexual and criminal offending. The J-SOAP-II items are scored using a 0 to 2 scale, with 0 always associated with the apparent absence of the item and 2 always associated with the clear presence of the item. Thus, "0" implies the apparent absence of the risk factor described by the item, and "2" implies the clear presence of the risk factor as described by the item. A score of "1" implies the presence of some information that suggests the presence of the item, but the information is insufficient, unclear, or too sketchy to justify a score of "2." There are four factors utilized to assess risk: Factor 1—Sexual Drive/Preoccupation Factor and Factor 2—Impulsive and Antisocial Behavior. These are static (unchangeable) factors that are based solely on the history of the youth. Factor 3—Intervention and Factor 4—Community Stability/Adjustment are dynamic (changeable) factors based on the present choices made by the youth. The overall J-SOAP-II score is divided by the total possible score to determine the relative proportion of risk to reoffend sexually or criminally. The JSOAP-II is available at www.csom.org/pubs/juvenile sex offenderAP.pdf.

The Estimate of Risk of Adolescent Sexual Offense Recidivism (ERASOR). The ERASOR is an empirically guided checklist used to estimate the short-term risk of a sexual reoffense for youth aged 12–18 years of age. The ERASOR provides objective coding instructions for 25 risk factors (16 dynamic and 9 static). The ERASOR is available at www.dshs. wa.gov/pdf/ca/ERASOR.pdf.

Nonsex offense–specific instruments for youth can be useful for evaluating juvenile sex offenders to explore multiple areas of risk and needs. These include the *Structured Assessment of Violence Risk in Youth (SAVRY)* and the *Psychopathy Checklist–Youth Version (PCL–YV)*, which can be used to estimate violent recidivism (not specific to sexual recidivism) and to identify the presence of psychopathic traits among juveniles, respectively.

Other Testing Measures Sometimes Used in Evaluation and Treatment

The *Abel Assessment for Sexual Interest (AASI-2)*, a screening tool for deviant sexual interests that measures visual reaction time, requires a test subject to view slides of clothed persons of varying ages and sexes, so that the person's level of sexual attraction can be rated. The length of time an individual views a particular slide determines the individual's sexual interest for different groups of people, both adults and children. The AASI-2 is widely mandated by U.S. courts as a condition of sex offender supervised release. Abel, penile plethysmography (PPG), and polygraph examinations are used to determine whether a sex offender is at heightened risk of reoffending.

Penile plethysmography (PPG) measures increments of erection of the penis via a small device on the penis. The device is attached to a computer operated by an evaluator in another room. The offender listens to audiotape descriptions of various kinds of sexual behavior, or views slides that depict males and females of various ages, typically photographs of individual nudes, while the plethysmograph detects blood flow to his penis, a measure of his erotic arousal to these various stimuli. The test is intrusive and costly and not completely accurate because some offenders can distract themselves sufficiently so that they do not exhibit arousal in the laboratory when, in fact, they do have arousal in ordinary circumstances.

The *polygraph* assesses whether sex offenders are being deceptive, and this tool is regarded as a valuable tool in sex offender treatment. Determining whether an offender is being deceptive can be critically important in the treatment process. The polygraph assesses whether or not sex offenders have knowingly withheld any information from their sexual history. This can result in significantly increased disclosures of sexual misconduct, even prior to the actual administration of the polygraph examination.

INTERVENTION

The *Center for Sex Offender Management (CSOM)* notes that sex offender treatment is a field where the stakes are high, the dynamics are complex, the interventions are specialized, and the literature is evolving; therefore, it is essential that treatment providers be equipped with the necessary knowledge and skills to provide ethically sound and quality treatment. They strongly suggest specialized education, training, experience, and supervision, and note that some states (e.g., Colorado, Illinois, Texas, and Utah) require that those wishing to provide treatment for sex offenders meet established criteria or undergo a formal certification process. Many of the criteria used for these purposes are based on published practice standards from the *Association for the Treatment of Sexual Abusers (ATSA)*.

Commonalities and Differences of Sex Offender Treatment

Sex offender treatment has similarities to other psychiatric treatments. Clients should understand the interventions and procedures that will be utilized, as well as any associated risks and benefits. Thus, informed consent should be provided. Interventions should be guided by formal assessments and appropriately individualized to the needs of each client. A therapeutic rapport must be established and maintained. Treatment goals should be specific and measurable, and progress (lack of progress) must be accurately and thoroughly documented.

Some aspects of treatment are qualitatively different than approaches to intervention for other populations:

- Treatment is defined as the delivery of prescribed interventions as a means of managing crime-producing factors and promoting positive and meaningful goal attainment for participants. This is in the interest of enhancing public safety.

- Treatment is often involuntary. Sex offenders tend to enter specialized treatment as a result of external pressures or legal mandates, rather than being driven solely by internal motivation.
- Treatment goals are not solely driven by the client's desires. Many of the broad goals of sex offender treatment are largely predetermined to include relatively "standard" goals, such as addressing denial, identifying and managing risk factors, enhancing empathy for victims, and developing prosocial skills.
- Confidentiality is limited because treatment takes place within the context of the justice system. The routine involvement of the courts and multiple agencies often necessitates collaboration and critical information sharing in order to support accountability, enhance management strategies, and ultimately promote public safety.
- With treatment for those who commit sex offenses, the potential impact of failed interventions is more far-reaching than treatment failure in other venues. Beside the impact on the offender and his family, public safety may be compromised. The result of treatment failure can be additional sexual victimization and the associated impact on the victim, victim's family, and the community.
- Working with sex offenders increases the potential for vicarious trauma and burnout for treatment providers. Those who provide treatment to sex offenders are regularly exposed to very detailed descriptions of abusive sexual behaviors, the attitudes and statements that support or minimize these behaviors, and the readily apparent harm to victims. This cumulative exposure, especially when combined with other influences, such as professional isolation, a high volume of cases, intense public scrutiny, and limited healthy coping responses, can lead treatment providers to experience vicarious or secondary trauma.

Most adjudicated juvenile sex offenders reside at some point in the community, thus requiring a comprehensive and collaborative sex offender management program that combines treatment with supervision to enable the offenders to control their sexually abusive behaviors. The desired outcome of treatment is the prevention of future sexual victimization. In general, most sex offender treatment has the following goals:

- Accept responsibility.
- Learn to understand their patterns (cycles) of criminal behavior.

- Modify cognitive distortions.
- Learn attitudes, cognitive skills, and behaviors needed to safely live in the community.
- Develop victim empathy.
- Control deviant sexual arousal, interests, preferences, and behaviors.
- Improve social competence.
- Reduce impulsivity and develop self-regulation.
- Manage negative emotions.
- Develop healthy relationships and correct intimacy deficits.
- Establish supervision conditions and networks.
- Develop an effective relapse prevention plan.

Treatment is also individualized and aimed at underlying disorders (e.g., conduct disorder) and associated problems (substance abuse, mood disorders, developmental disability, etc.). Treatment may take place in a detention, forensic psychiatric unit, or the community. Offenders can be terminated from treatment for noncompliance or failure to make adequate progress in treatment, sexual behavior, assaults and fighting, violating confidentiality of others in the program, or being placed in a high-security category.

Treatment of young and preadolescent children. Very young sex offenders (under age 13) require alternate treatment modalities. One suggestion is to target risk factors that predispose a child to sexual behavior problems or that precipitate or perpetuate the problems. Many programs include cognitive-behavioral approaches; treatment modalities involved with individual, group, pair, and family therapy. Important intervention factors include addressing developmental issues and involving parents and other caregivers.

Treatment of juveniles with cognitive or developmental disabilities. Special interventions may be warranted for juveniles with intellectual and cognitive impairments since they may not respond well to traditional therapies. Unfortunately, this is a highly understudied area. However, it can be assumed that treatment needs to be tailored to meet the juveniles' cognitive developmental status.

PREVENTION/PATIENT TEACHING

Primary Prevention

ATSA takes the position that primary prevention programs should target modifiable risk factors identified by research. Since it is generally easier to alter developing behaviors as compared to behaviors that are ingrained, ATSA also supports the development of early intervention programs.

Secondary Prevention

Health care providers need to differentiate unusual sexual behaviors in children from offending behaviors, and should be able to identify early problematic behavior and refer these children for appropriate early interventions. A classification system for problematic sexual behaviors in children has been proposed by Berliner, Manaois, and Monastersky (1986):

1. *Precocious sexual behavior* involves actions such as oral-genital contact or intercourse between preadolescents with no evidence of force or coercion. This may be a temporary, unsocialized response to victimization or a response to exposure to sexually explicit behavior. These children should have further assessment to determine the necessity and level of appropriate intervention. Their behavior may cease upon disclosure, increased supervision, or therapeutic intervention.

2. *Inappropriate sexual behavior* includes actions such as persistent and/or public masturbation, excessive interest or preoccupation with sexual matters, and highly sexualized behavior or play. These children may be in the initial process of developing a deviant sexual arousal pattern. Intervention depends on the frequency, persistence, and consequences of the behavior.

3. *Coercive sexual behavior* refers to sexual acts in which force is used or threatened, or where a significant disparity in development or size exists. These children may engage in sexually aggressive behavior with other antisocial activity. The sexual behavior may be reflective of anger and hostility rather than an attempt at gratification. These children require immediate, intensive intervention.

Tertiary Prevention

The goals of tertiary prevention are recidivism prevention and successful reentry back into society.

RESOURCES

The Association for the Treatment of Sexual Abusers: www.atsa.com
Center for Sex Offender Management: www.csom.org

The National Guidelines for Sex Offender Registration and Notification: www.ojp.usdoj. gov/smart/pdfs/final_sornaguidelines.pdf

REFERENCES

Araji, S. (1997). *Sexually aggressive children: Coming to understand them.* Thousand Oaks, CA: Sage Publications.

Berliner, L., Manaois, O., & Monastersky, C. (1986). *Child sexual behavior disturbance: An assessment and treatment model.* Seattle, WA: Harborview Medical Center.

Center for Sex Offender Management. (1999). Understanding juvenile sexual offending behavior: Emerging research, treatment approaches and management practices. Retrieved from http://www.csom.org/pubs/juvbrf10.html

Center for Sex Offender Management, U.S. Department of Justice, Office of Justice Programs. (2006). *Understanding treatment for adults and juveniles who have committed sex offenses.* Retrieved from www.csom.org/pubs/treatment_brief.pdf

Criminal Info Network. (2007). *How will pleading guilty to a felony affect your life?* Retrieved from www.criminalinfonetwork.com/pleading-guilty.htm

Friedrich, W., Fisher, J., Dittner, C., Acton, R., Berliner, L., Butler, J., et al. (1992). Child Sexual Behavior Inventory: Normative and clinical comparisons. *Psychological Assessment, 4,* 303–311.

Frierson, R., Bell, C., & Williamson, J. (2008). The mandatory registration of juvenile sex offenders and commitment of juveniles as sexually violent predators: Controversies and recommendations. *Adolescent Psychiatry.* Retrieved from http://findarticles. com/p/articles/mi_qa3882/is_200801/ai_n27901318/?tag=content;col1

Muscari, M. (2009). *Sexting: New technology, old problem.* Medscape Public Health. Retrieved from www.medscape.com/viewarticle/702078

National Campaign to Prevent Teen and Unplanned Pregnancy, and Cosmogirl.com. (2008). *Sex and tech: Results from a survey of teens and young adults.* Retrieved from www.thenationalcampaign.org/sextech/PDF/SexTech_Summary.pdf

National Center on Sexual Behavior of Youth. (2003, July). *Fact sheet. What research shows about adolescent sex offenders.* #1. Retrieved from www.ncsby.org/pages/publications/ What%20Research%20Shows%20About%20Adolescent%20Sex%20Offenders%20 060404.pdf

Reinhart, C. (2003). *Consequences of a felony conviction.* State of Connecticut General Assembly. Retrieved from www.cga.ct.gov/2003/olrdata/jud/rpt/2003-R-0333.htm

Righthand, S., & Welch, C. (2001). *Juveniles who have sexually offended: A review of the professional literature.* Office of Juvenile Justice and Delinquency Prevention. Retrieved from www.ncjrs.gov/html/ojjdp/report_juvsex_offend/index.html

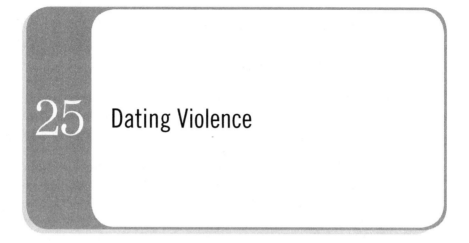

25   Dating Violence

DEFINITION

The U.S. Department of Justice defines *dating violence* as the act or threat of an act of violence by at least one member of an unmarried couple on the other member within the context of dating or courtship. Dating violence crosses all socioeconomic groups, and most victims are female. Although nothing new, dating violence has developed some worrisome trends with possessive dating behavior extending into even younger ages, and some teens believing that dating violence is acceptable.

    Violence in a dating situation can be defined as physical, emotional, financial, sexual, or all of these. Health care providers often confine their thinking about dating violence to physical violence. However, physical violence is a small percentage of the violent behavior that occurs in this population. Dating violence can include:

Physical: shoving, hitting, punching

Verbal: yelling, screaming, put-downs, name calling

Emotional: spreading rumors, lying, possessiveness, and other sexual behaviors

Sexual: unwanted touching

Psychological: manipulation, mind games, guilt tripping, controlling

Financial: perpetrator takes control over victim's money

Adolescent female victims of dating violence have an elevated risk for a broad range of serious health concerns. They are more likely to use alcohol, tobacco, and cocaine; engage in unhealthy weight control; engage in sexual health risk behavior, including first intercourse before the age of 15 years and multiple partnering; have been pregnant; and seriously consider or attempt suicide. Many of these risks associated with experiences of either physical or sexual dating violence are heightened for adolescent girls who reported both forms of abuse. It is not clear, however, whether dating violence increases the risk for these problems, whether these problem behaviors place girls at greater vulnerability to dating violence, or whether other factors place them at greater risk for dating violence and these other concerns. What is clear is that, regardless of directionality or mechanism, adolescent females who experience dating violence engage in a number of problem behaviors that put them at risk for negative outcomes ranging from contracting HIV to pregnancy and suicide.

All 50 states and the District of Columbia have laws against dating violence behaviors such as sexual assault, domestic violence, and stalking, but the term "dating violence" is almost never used in these laws. Numerous states and the District of Columbia allow victims of dating violence to apply for protective orders against the perpetrator. Age requirements and the language of the laws vary by state.

PREVALENCE

The differences in estimates of the incidence and prevalence of teen dating violence range from 9% to 57%, depending on the study. Some estimates note that women ages 16 to 24 experience the highest per capita rates of intimate violence—nearly 20 per 1,000 women. According to the Centers for Disease Control and Prevention:

- 1 in 11 adolescents reports being a victim of physical dating violence
- 1 in 4 adolescents reports verbal, physical, emotional, or sexual violence each year

- 1 in 5 adolescents reports being a victim of emotional violence
- 1 in 5 high school girls has been physically or sexually abused by a dating partner
- Dating violence occurs more frequently among Black students (13.9%) than among Hispanic (9.3%) or White (7.0%) students
- 72% of 8th and 9th graders reportedly "date," and by the time they are in high school, 54% of students report dating violence among their peers

Studies, such as those by Malik, Sorenson, and Aneshensel (1997) and O'Keefe (1997), show that nonsexual violence in teen dating relationships involves the reciprocal use of violence by both partners, referred to as *mutual aggression*. Several studies have found that girls inflict more physical violence than boys. However, gender differences are pronounced in motivations for using violence and the consequences of being a victim of teen dating violence. Both boys and girls report that anger is the primary motivating factor for using violence, but girls also commonly report self-defense as a motivating factor, and boys commonly cite the need to exert control. Boys are more likely to react with laughter when their partner is physically aggressive, and girls are more likely than boys to suffer long-term negative behavioral and health consequences, including suicide attempts, depression, cigarette smoking, and marijuana use. Dramatic differences exist when sexual violence is examined, with females sustaining significantly more sexual violence than males.

Since girls engage in high levels of physical aggression and psychological abuse, and since most abusive adolescent relationships are characterized by mutual aggression, prevention efforts must be directed toward both boys and girls. Interventions also must distinguish between severe forms of violence that produce injury and fear and other, more common abuse. Providers must respond with appropriate safety planning, mental health services, and criminal or juvenile justice involvement.

ETIOLOGY

Teen dating violence only recently has been recognized as a public health problem; thus, the complex nature of this phenomenon is not fully understood. The etiology of dating violence is unknown and most likely multifactorial. Several correlate factors have been associated with being either a victim or perpetrator of adolescent relationship violence.

Dating violence may be associated with families in which violence is used as conflict resolution, where low levels of parental control and supervision are present, and where poor parent-child relationships exist. Tenuous parent-child attachments may lead to a life course of violence, including dating violence. A childhood history of sexual, physical, or emotional abuse serves as a strong risk factor for both victimization and perpetration of dating violence, and risk may increase with the length of time the child is abused. Individuals who experience sexual intercourse as part of the abuse also demonstrate higher rates of interpersonal violence.

Both victims and perpetrators bear several common personality traits, including feelings of betrayal, jealousy, insecurity, and hostility. Those who commit dating violence often are found to have a high response to social pressures, have difficulty with anger management, have a previous history of peer violence, and exemplify poor interpersonal skills. They also are prone to substance use and abuse, and a high proportion of dating violence incidents is connected with alcohol use. Victims often perpetrate violence on others, further perpetuating the contagious nature of violent acts. Self-defense may relate to the escalation of violence, which can impact the individuals involved and perceptions of the event. Another variable contributing to the victimization is pregnancy. A pregnancy during the teen years increases a young woman's chance of being victimized fivefold.

ASSESSMENT

General Principles

The National Youth Violence Prevention Resource Center notes that teens rarely report dating violence and may even view it as a normal part of a relationship, thus health care professionals need to take an active approach and screen all adolescents for dating violence. This is best preformed during wellness visits, as well as episodic exams when presenting manifestations suggest the possibility of assault. One approach to screening begins with an open-ended question about relationships with peers, narrows the focus by asking how they resolve conflicts with peers, followed by direct questions about specific behaviors, such as pushing, hitting, being afraid, being hurt, or being forced to have sexual contact.

Practitioners should avoid using emotionally loaded terms such as abuse, rape, or violence.

History and Physical Assessment

Health care professionals should be alert for signs, symptoms, or contextual factors that suggest an adolescent is at high risk for dating violence. Health care professionals should assess for:

- General signs and symptoms of distress that may or may not be related to dating violence such as depression, anxiety, mood swings, abdominal pain, pelvic pain, sudden changes in relationships with family and friends or in functioning at school, and drug and alcohol abuse. Other possible indicators include school failure, truancy, dropping out of school, substance abuse, pregnancy, isolation, and withdrawal.
- Signs and symptoms that are more specific to intentional injury, including dating violence, such as contusions; abrasions; lacerations to the torso, breasts, face, and genital or anal area; fractures; burns; multiple sites of injury; and a pattern of injury over time. Suspect abuse if the stated explanation for injury is inconsistent with the apparent mechanism of injury.

Other specific signs of dating violence victimization include:

- Signs that the individual is afraid of his or her boyfriend or girlfriend
- The boyfriend or girlfriend seem to try to control the individual's behavior, making all of the decisions, checking up on his or her behavior, demanding to know who the individual has been with, and acting jealous and possessive
- The boyfriend or girlfriend lashes out, criticizes, or insults the individual
- The individual apologizes for the boyfriend or girlfriend's behavior to you and others
- The individual casually mentioned the boyfriend or girlfriend's temper or violent behavior, but then laughed it off as a joke
- The boyfriend or girlfriend is observed acting abusive toward other people or things

Herrman (2009) suggests directive and probing questions that can be asked during assessments.

Examples of directive questions include:

- "During the past year, did your boy friend or girlfriend do anything physically to you that made you feel very uneasy or uncomfortable?"
- "Do you feel safe at home?"
- "Do you feel safe in your relationship?"
- "Have you experienced threats of violence?"
- "Does your partner seem jealous, controlling, or possessive?"
- "Have you been forced to have sex?"
- "Have weapons been used against you?"

Examples of probing questions include:

- "Tell me about a time when you have felt unsafe in your home."
- "Tell me about a time when you have felt unsafe in your relationship."
- "To what types of violent behaviors have you been subjected?"
- "Tell me about your partner's behaviors related to jealousy, control, or possessiveness."
- "Tell me about your experiences when forced to have sex."
- "Tell me about your experience when weapons were used against you."

Health care providers should also monitor for signs of dating violence perpetration as noted by the Alabama Coalition Against Domestic Violence (ACADV), including:

Extreme jealousy

Controlling behavior

Quick involvement

Unpredictable mood swings

Alcohol and drug use

Explosive anger

Isolation from friends and family

Uses force during an argument

Shows hypersensitivity

Believes in rigid sex roles

Blames others for his or her problems or feelings

Cruel to animals or children

Verbally abusive

Abused former partners

Threatens violence

Cell phones can become "leashes" in dating violence situations, whereby the perpetrator keeps tabs on the victim with constant phone calls and/or text messages. Asking about cell phone usage, particularly how often they speak to their partner, may be a clue to a controlling situation. Signs of sleep deprivation may also be red flags since abusers may call often during the night.

INTERVENTIONS

Interventions are warranted when clients are victims or perpetrators of dating violence. Victims should receive support, as well as care for injuries, and should be referred to an appropriate therapist and community support group. Most counties have women's or victims' resource centers. Victims may need assistance to end the relationship due to dependence and/or fear, some may need to obtain an order of protection, and some may benefit from the interventions suggested for victims of stalking, such as keeping diaries. The following precautions are also suggested:

- Obtain an unlisted telephone number, caller ID, voice mail, and cellular phone.
- Install and utilize quality deadbolt locks, solid core doors, and security systems.
- Install adequate outdoor lighting; trim bushes and shrubs to avoid hiding places.
- Notify family, friends, and trusted neighbors of stalking. Provide them with a photo and the vehicle information of the stalker, if possible.

- Create a contingency plan should going to or staying home not be possible; keep a suitcase packed with necessary supplies.
- Stay alert and be aware of surroundings.
- Vary routes of travel to and from work.
- Park in secure and well-lit areas. Ask a trusted person for an escort to the car.
- Do not dismiss threats. Report them immediately to the authorities.
- Encourage the victim to collect evidence of stalking:
- Document all incidents.

  - Keep a stalking journal or log (the Stalking Resource Center has a Stalking Incident and Behavior Log that can be downloaded from its Web site: http://www.ncvc.org/src). Since this information can possibly be used as evidence or inadvertently shared with the stalker at a future time, encourage the victim to not include any information that they do not want the offender to see.
  - Take photographs.
  - Obtain affidavits from witnesses.
  - Videotape stalker in action, if possible.
  - Keep phone answering machine messages.
  - Keep a list of potential witnesses.

- Carefully preserve all evidence:

  - Letters, notes, e-mails
  - Gifts
  - Damaged property

Perpetrators should also be referred for counseling, as well as to programs for juvenile batterers. In some jurisdictions, health care providers may also be required to report dating violence to law enforcement.

Health care providers should also provide safety tips for victims of dating violence:

Keep a journal describing your partner's behavior.

Keep your parents or another trustworthy adult informed of what is happening.

Consider changing your school locker or lock.

Consider changing your route to/from school.

Use a buddy system for going to school, classes, and after-school activities.

Have a back-up plan whenever getting a ride home in case you are stranded.

Get rid of or change the number to any beepers, pagers, or cell phones the abuser gave you.

Keep spare change, calling cards, number of the local shelter, number of someone who could help you, and restraining orders with you at all times.

Have safe places to go, such as on your route from home to school.

Keep a cell phone handy in case you need to call your parents or 911.

Orders of Protection

Several states and the District of Columbia allow victims of dating violence to obtain an order of protection. An order of protection is a legally binding court order that restrains an individual who has committed an act of violence against a person from further acts against that person. Protective orders vary state by state and are called by various names (restraining orders, protection from abuse orders [PFAs], etc.). Most are used to protect against family/intimate partner violence; some jurisdictions use them for strangers. There are different types of protective orders, demonstrated by the three stages of Protection from Abuse (PFA) orders issued in Pennsylvania:

An *emergency order* is issued by District Justice when the Court of Common Pleas is closed. It is in effect until the next business day at the Court of Common Pleas.

A *temporary order* is issued on a daily basis by the Court of Common Pleas in Media and is in effect until the hearing for a Permanent PFA is held.

A *permanent order* is issued for up to 18 months at a hearing before the Court of Common Pleas. The hearing date is scheduled when you receive the temporary PFA.

Health care providers can contact the police, district attorney's office, or victim advocate center to learn how victims may obtain protective orders in their areas. However, it is best they do this before a situation occurs and keep the information readily available for emergent purposes.

The protection order can prohibit the abuser from committing acts of violence; exclude the abuser from the residence shared by the petitioner and abuser; prohibit the abuser from harassing or contacting the petitioner by mail, telephone, or in person; award temporary custody of minor children; establish temporary visitation and restrain the abuser from interfering with custody; prohibit the abuser from removing the children from the jurisdiction of the court; and order the abuser to participate in treatment or counseling. Some states, including New York, include pets in the protective orders. Although seemingly powerful, protective orders are nothing more than pieces of paper—they are not bulletproof. They seem to work best on those offenders who have something to lose if they disobey them, and, in some cases, may aggravate the situation. Therefore, victims still need to take precautions to keep themselves safe. No matter how good they are, orders of protection are not bulletproof.

PREVENTION/PATIENT TEACHING

Primary Prevention

Primary prevention of dating violence would include teaching and discussion forums in middle schools and high schools. Health care providers may want to become involved in school projects, as well as church and community projects aimed at prevention of dating violence. The content of primary prevention projects includes explanations of the dynamics of abusive relationships and discussion about avoidance of involvement in violent relationships.

Health care providers can also teach about healthy relationships, as well as safe dating. A safe dating teaching plan can include the recommendation to adopt the following strategies when dating:

Double-date or "mall" date for the first few dates.

Know exact plans before leaving for a date, and make sure parents know these plans, as well as the time the teen is expected home.

Avoid drugs and alcohol, which decrease reaction abilities.

Carry a cell phone with a charged battery.

Do not leave a party alone with someone you do not know.

Assert yourself when necessary.

Be straightforward in relationships.

Trust your instincts.

If a situation arises, remain calm and remove yourself from the situation.

Secondary Prevention

Secondary prevention promotes early identification and intervention of teens at risk. Projects should target young people involved in a violent relationship so that they do not repeat the observed pattern.

Tertiary Prevention

Altering or ending the relationship requires counseling to increase self-esteem and planning to end or alter the relationship. It is of importance that the health care provider who recognizes dating violence does not recommend that the young person "just leave" the relationship. Further evaluation prior to any recommendation is necessary. Leaving a violent dating relationship can be very dangerous to the victim. Interpersonal violence offenders have been known to attack their victims when they attempt to leave the relationship.

RESOURCES

Community United Against Violence (CUAV): www.cuav.org
Dating Violence Brochure: www.ncvc.org/ncvc/AGP.Net/Components/documentViewer/
    Download.aspxnz?DocumentID=38561
Empower Program: www.empowered.org
Girls Incorporated National Resource Center: www.girlsinc.org/index.html
Loveisnotabuse.com: www.loveisnotabuse.com
Loveisrespect.org: www.loveisrespect.org
National Center for Victims of Crime: www.ncvc.org
Pennsylvania Coalition Against Domestic Violence: Teen Dating Violence: www.pcadv.
    org/Domestic-Violence-Information-Center/Children-and-Teens/Teen-Dating-
    Violence.asp
Teen Dating Violence Prevention Recommendations: www.abanet.org/unmet/teendat
    ing/preventionrecommendations.pdf

REFERENCES

Centers for Disease Control and Prevention. (2006). Physical dating violence among high school students—United States, 2003. *Morbidity and Mortality Weekly Report, MMWR, 55*, 532–535.

Chan, K., & Strauss, M. (2008). Prevalence of dating partner violence and suicidal ideation among male and female university students worldwide. *Journal of Midwifery and Women's Health, 53*(1), 529–537.

English, D. (2009). At risk and maltreated children exposed to interpersonal violence: What the conflict looks like and its relationship to child outcomes. *Child Maltreatment, 14*(2), 157–171.

Grover, A., Kekkonen, C., & Fox, K. (2008). The relationship between violence in the family of origin and dating violence among college students. *Journal of Interpersonal Violence, 23*(12), 667–693.

Hamberger, L. K., & Ambuel, B. (1998). Dating violence. *Pediatric Clinics of North America, 45*, 381–390.

Herrman, J. (2009). There's a fine line . . . adolescent dating violence and prevention. *Pediatric Nursing, 35*(3), 164–170.

Malik, S., Sorenson, S. B., & Aneshensel, C. S. (1997). Community and dating violence among adolescents: Prepetration and victimization. *Journal of Adolescent Health, 21*(5), 291–302.

Mulford, C., & Giordano, P. (2008). *Teen dating violence: A closer look at adolescent romantic relationships.* National Institutes of Justice, NCJ 224089, 261, 34–41. Retrieved from www.ncjrs.gov/pdffiles1/nij/224089.pdf

Muscari, M. (2005, April). *What should I tell clients about teen dating violence?* Medscape for Nurses. Retrieved from www.medscape.com/viewarticle/502450

O'Keefe, M. (1997). Predictors of dating violence among high school students. *Journal of Interpersonal Violence, 12*, 546–568.

Rennison, C., & Welchans, S. (2000). *Intimate partner violence.* Bureau of Justice Statistics Special Report NCJ 178247. Retrieved from www.ojp.usdoj.gov/bjs/pub/pdf/ipv.pdf

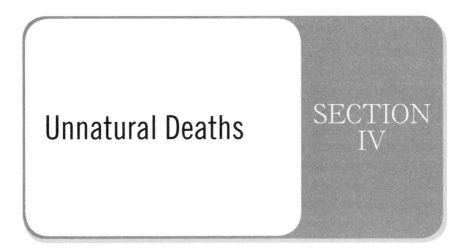

Unnatural Deaths

SECTION IV

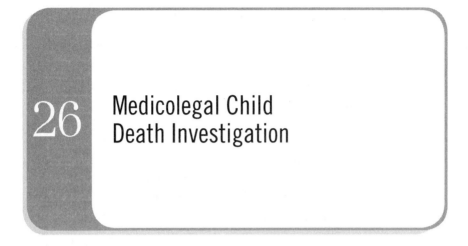

26 Medicolegal Child Death Investigation

The purpose of all death investigations is to determine the cause and manner of death. The process involves the systematic collection and analysis of interview data and physical evidence. Not all deaths warrant investigation. Those that do include, but are not limited to, deaths in which there are unexplained, unusual, or suspicious circumstances; homicides; deaths due to poisoning, accidents, suicides; maternal deaths due to abortion; deaths of inmates in public institutions; deaths of persons in custody of law enforcement; deaths associated with diagnostic, therapeutic, or anesthetic procedures; deaths from neglect; sudden unexpected infant death; natural deaths where the decedent does not have a physician familiar with the case, or when the decedent's physician refuses to sign the death certificate. Some jurisdictions require investigation and/or autopsy of infants less than 1 year of age.

DEFINITIONS

- *Cause of death* is the injury, disease, or combination of the two responsible for initiating the sequence of disturbances that produce the fatal termination. The term "initiating" is critical because causes may not be immediately fatal, such as carcinoma or gunshot wounds.

■ *Manner of death* is the circumstance in which the cause of death arose.

■ *Natural:* Death is directly related to a natural disease (cancer, arteriosclerotic heart disease)

■ *Accident:* Death is the result of the unintentional actions of the decedent or another person (motor vehicle accident, drowning)

■ *Homicide:* Death results from the intentional act of another, whether lawfully or unlawfully (intentional gunshot, death penalty)

■ *Suicide:* Death results from intentional act by the decedent who anticipates dying (self-inflicted gunshot, intentional drug overdose)

■ *Undetermined:* Circumstances surrounding the death cannot be determined with reasonable certainty (cannot tell if overdose was accidental or suicide)

■ *Mechanism of death* is the physiologic change or biochemical disturbance incompatible with life initiated by the cause of death.

Families may be unsure as to why an investigation is needed, especially when a loved one dies of natural causes, so it helps to know the benefits of death investigation: obtaining life insurance benefits, discovery of genetic/inherited disorders, provide evidence for prosecution or exoneration, provide evidence for civil matters, identify infectious diseases, identify defective products, identify medical errors, and evaluate transplant donors.

The death of any child is difficult; however, when a child dies suddenly and unexpectedly, it becomes the responsibility of law enforcement and death investigators to determine whether any criminal activity may have been involved. Professional investigations of child fatalities in which abuse or neglect is in question ensure that the innocent are not falsely accused and that the guilty are held accountable for their crimes. Child homicides differ from typical homicides in many ways, including the causes of death, the offender's motivations and legal culpability for the crime, the methods used to inflict the fatal injuries, the types of injuries that the victim sustained, the forensic and physical evidence involved, and the investigative techniques used. Child abuse deaths may differ because they often involve a delay between the time the child sustains the fatal injury and the subsequent death of the child.

CORONER AND MEDICAL EXAMINER SYSTEMS

Deaths are investigated by coroners, medical examiners, and/or death investigators. Death investigation varies among jurisdictions (state, county, district, or city). The most noticeable difference among jurisdictions is that some jurisdictions use the medical examiner system and others use the coroner system. Medical examiners are usually appointed and usually must be licensed physicians. Coroners are usually elected, may not need to be physicians, and usually only have be of a minimum age (often 18) and a resident of the county or district. There are approximately 2,000 medical examiners and coroners' offices in the United States. These offices are responsible for the medicolegal investigation of death.

Medicolegal investigations include the following activities: conducting death scene investigations, performing autopsies, and determining the cause and manner of death when a person has died as a result of violence, under suspicious circumstances, without a physician in attendance, or for other reasons. States function differently when it comes to having coroner- or medical examiner–based systems. Each has one of the following: centralized statewide medical examiner system, county coroner system, county medical examiner system, mixed county medical examiner and coroner system, or a decentralized death investigation system.

Medical examiners and coroners are responsible for investigating sudden, unexpected, and violent deaths and for providing accurate, legally defensible determinations of the causes of these deaths. Information provided by medical examiners and coroners plays a critical role in the judicial system and in decisions made by public safety and public health agencies. Coroner and medical examiner records provide vital information about patterns and trends of mortality in the United States and are excellent sources of data for public health studies and surveillance.

SIGNS OF DEATH

When a person dies, the pupils dilate and become unresponsive. The corneal reflexes are absent and the cornea becomes cloudy. Other changes include the following.

Rigor mortis. The muscles become flaccid after death, but within 1 to 3 hours, they become increasingly rigid and the joints freeze. Rigor is affected by body temperature—the higher the temperature, the faster rigor occurs. Thus, someone with a fever or who exercised vigorously before death will develop rigor faster. Conversely, rigor is slowed by cooling, as in death from exposure in winter. The body appears to stiffen from the head down, from the jaws to the elbows and then to the knees. A body is in complete rigor when the jaw, elbows, and knees are immovable, a process that takes 10 to 12 hours in an environmental temperature of 70 °F to 75 °F. A body remains rigid for 24 to 36 hours before muscles start to loosen in the same order it stiffened. Rigor develops more rapidly in children due to their small muscle mass. Rigor may also be incomplete in infants and cases where there is decreased muscle mass such as severe malnutrition.

Livor mortis. This discoloration is due to the settling of blood no longer being circulated through the body. Blood settles in vessels by gravity in dependent areas and colors the skin purple red; however, the skin may not discolor if it is pressed against a bony prominence. Livor is noticeable 1 hour after death. The color increases intensity and becomes fixed (does not blanche under pressure) in 8 hours. Fixed blood in nondependent areas means the body was moved after death. Color variations may occur depending on the cause of death. Carbon monoxide or cyanide poisoning may cause bright cherry red livor, while extensive blood loss may have a very light or nonexistent livor. Livor can be difficult to determine in dark-skinned persons.

Algor mortis. The body cools after death to the surrounding environmental temperature. Liver temperature and environmental temperature can give a very crude estimate of the time of death. In children, rapid antemortem temperature instability can occur during resuscitation, especially in cases of severe shock.

Decomposition. As rigor passes, the body first turns green in the abdomen, and the color spreads to the rest of the trunk. The body swells due to bacterial methane gas production. Rates and types of decomposition depend on the environment. Bodies buried in dirt, submerged in water, left in the hot sun, or placed in a cool basement all look different after the same postmortem period.

SCENE INVESTIGATION

The sudden or unexplained death of a loved one has a profound impact on families and friends and places significant responsibility on the agencies tasked with determining the cause of death. Adherence to clear and well-grounded protocols aids investigators in carefully assessing and analyzing the death. The following is from the U.S. Department of Justice Office of Justice Programs National Institute of Justice (1999) *Death Investigation: A Guide for the Scene Investigator.*

Arriving at the Scene

1. Introduce and identify self and role: Introductions aid in establishing a collaborative investigative effort.
2. Exercise scene safety: The safety of all investigative personnel is essential to the investigative process. Risks of environmental and physical injury (e.g., hostile crowds, collapsing structures, traffic, and environmental and chemical threats) must be removed prior to initiating a scene investigation.
3. Confirm or pronounce death: Appropriate personnel must make a determination of death prior to the initiation of the death investigation. Confirmation determines jurisdictional responsibilities.
4. Participate in scene briefing with attending agency representatives: Scene investigators must recognize jurisdictional and statutory responsibilities that apply to each agency representatives (e.g., law enforcement, fire, EMT, death investigator). Determining each agency's responsibility is essential in planning the scope and depth of each scene investigation and the release of information to the public.
5. Conduct scene "walk through": The walk through provides an overview of the entire scene and gives the investigator the first opportunity to locate and view the body, identify valuable and fragile evidence, and determine initial investigative procedures that will allow for systematic examination and documentation of the scene and body.
6. Establish chain of custody: This ensures the integrity of the evidence and safeguards against subsequent allegations of tampering, theft, planting, and contamination of evidence.
7. Follow laws of evidence: All agencies must follow local, state, and federal laws for the collection of evidence to ensure its admissibility. The death investigator works with law enforcement and the legal authorities to determine laws regarding collection of evidence.

Documenting and Evaluating the Scene

1. Photograph the scene: Photographic documentation creates a permanent historical record of the scene. Photographs provide detailed corroborating evidence that constructs a system of redundancy should questions arise concerning the report, witness statements, or position of evidence at the scene.
2. Develop descriptive documentation of the scene: The narrative report provides a permanent record that may be used to correlate with and enhance photographic documentation, refresh recollections, and record observations.
3. Establish probable location of injury or illness: The death scene may not be the actual location where the injury/illness that contributed to the death occurred. It is imperative that the investigator attempt to determine the locations of any and all injuries/illnesses that may have contributed to the death. Physical evidence at these locations may be pertinent in establishing the cause, manner, and circumstances of death.
4. Collect, inventory, and safeguard property and evidence: The investigator must safeguard the decedent's valuables/ property to ensure proper processing and eventual return to next of kin.
5. Interview witnesses at the scene: Documented comments of witnesses allow the investigator to obtain primary source data regarding discovery of the body, witness corroboration, and terminal history.

Documenting and Evaluating the Body

1. Photograph the body: Photographic documentation of the body creates a permanent record that preserves essential details of body position, appearance, identity, and final movements. Photographs also allow sharing of information with other agencies investigating the death.
2. Conduct superficial external body examination: This provides the investigator with objective data regarding the single most important piece of evidence at the scene, the body, by giving detailed information regarding the decedent's physical attributes, the person's relationship to the scene, and possible

cause, manner, and circumstances of death. This examination is performed in a manner that does not contaminate or destroy evidence.

3. Preserve evidence on the body: Photographic and narrative documentation of evidence on the body allows the investigator to obtain a permanent historical record of that evidence. Evidence must be collected, preserved, and transported properly, and the chain of custody maintained. All of the physical evidence visible on the body (such as blood and other body fluids) must be photographed and documented prior to collection and transport. Fragile evidence (that which can be easily contaminated, lost, or altered) must also be collected and preserved, and the chain of custody maintained.

4. Establish decedent identification: Confirmation of the decedent's identity is paramount to the death investigation to allow notification of next of kin, settlement of estates, resolution of criminal and civil litigation, and the proper completion of the death certificate.

5. Document postmortem changes: Documenting postmortem changes assists the investigator in explaining body appearance in the interval following death. Inconsistencies between postmortem changes and body location may indicate movement of the body and validate or invalidate witness statements. Postmortem changes to the body, when correlated with circumstantial information, can also assist the investigators in estimating the approximate time of death.

6. Participate in scene debriefing: Scene debriefing helps investigators from all agencies to establish postscene responsibilities. Scene debriefing provides each agency the opportunity for input regarding special requests for assistance, additional information, special examinations, and other requests requiring interagency communication, cooperation, and education.

7. Determine notification procedures (next of kin): Every reasonable effort should be made to notify the next of kin as soon as possible. This helps initiate closure for the family and disposition of remains, and facilitates the collection of additional information relative to the case.

8. Ensure security of the remains: Ensuring security of the body requires the investigator to supervise the labeling, packaging, and removal of the remains. An appropriate identification tag is placed on the body to preclude misidentification upon receipt at the examining agency. This function also includes safeguarding all potential physical evidence and/or property and clothing that remains on the body.

Establishing and Recording Decedent Profile Information

1. Document the discovery history: The decedent profile includes documenting a discovery history and circumstances surrounding the discovery. The basic profile will dictate subsequent levels of investigation, jurisdiction, and authority, as well as the focus (breadth/depth) of further investigation.
2. Determine terminal episode history: Preterminal circumstances play a significant role in determining cause and manner of death. Documentation of medical intervention and/or procurement of antemortem specimens help to establish the decedent's condition prior to death.
3. Document decedent medical history: Most deaths referred to the medical examiner/coroner are natural deaths. Establishing the decedent's medical history helps focus the investigation. Documenting the decedent's medical signs or symptoms prior to death determines the need for subsequent examinations, since the relationship between disease and injury may play a role in the cause, manner, and circumstances of death.
4. Document decedent mental health history: The decedent's mental health history can provide insight into his or her behavior/state of mind. That insight may produce clues that will aid in establishing the cause, manner, and circumstances of the death.
5. Document social history: Social history includes marital, family, sexual, educational, employment, and financial information, just as it does in the social history of the living. Daily routines, habits and activities, and friends and associates of the decedent help develop the decedent's profile and aid in establishing the cause, manner, and circumstances of death.

Completing the Scene Investigation

1. Maintain jurisdiction over the body: This helps the investigator to protect the chain of custody as the body is transported from the scene for autopsy, specimen collection, or storage.
2. Release jurisdiction of the body: Prior to releasing jurisdiction of the body to an authorized receiving agent or funeral director, it is necessary to determine the person responsible for certification of the death. Information to complete the death certificate includes demographic information and the date, time, and location of death.
3. Perform exit procedures: Bringing closure to the scene investigation ensures that important evidence has been collected and the scene has been fully processed. A systematic review of the scene ensures that artifacts or equipment are not inadvertently left behind and that any dangerous materials or conditions have been reported.
4. Assist the family: The death investigator provides the family with a timetable so they can arrange for final disposition. The death investigator also provides information on available community and professional resources that may assist the family.

CONDUCTING THE CHILD DEATH INVESTIGATION

Most sudden and unexpected deaths of children are not caused by abuse and neglect; however, death investigators should approach every such death with the hypothesis that the child may have been a victim of maltreatment. This position should be maintained until the investigation is completed and the evidence proves otherwise.

Child death investigation usually begins when a law enforcement or CPS agency receives notification of a child's death or life-threatening injury. At that point, it is very important that investigators from all appropriate agencies coordinate their efforts. Agencies conducting joint investigations must follow any state law regarding cross-reporting (the exchange of initial reports of suspected abuse and neglect that each agency receives). They must also observe any investigative protocol specific for investigating abuse and neglect.

Law enforcement should determine if a search warrant is necessary to search the scene. Law enforcement usually is responsible for the scene, and death investigators are responsible for the body, but assure that the following principles are followed:

- Ensure that scale diagrams are made of the layout and that photographs and/or a video are taken. Photographs should show the general location and progress to specific items of interest.
- Consider as evidence prescription or over-the-counter medicine the child was taking and other medicine or substances the child may have ingested. If it is not practical to remove such medicine from the scene, document the information on the label.
- If it appears that the child may have died of malnourishment, take an inventory of the amount of baby food or formula that is present. Document and photograph what you find.
- If you find evidence of the caretaker's alcohol and/or substance abuse, carefully document and photograph your findings. Take appropriate legal action if you find illegal drugs or drug paraphernalia.
- Search trash cans for possible evidence, such as bloodstained clothing; items used to clean up blood, vomit, urine, or feces; and implements used to injure the child, such as wooden spoons, belts, and electrical extension cords.
- Conduct timely, thorough interviews of witnesses, which may include the deceased child's siblings and parents; the child's caretakers immediately prior to the death or during the time the child appeared to be in medical distress; neighbors; law enforcement first responders; paramedics; medical providers; and anyone else who may have relevant information about the child or the events leading to the injury or death.
- Conduct interviews as early in the investigation as practical.
- Whenever possible, interview witnesses separately.
- Distinguish between what a witness actually observed and knows firsthand from what someone else may have told that witness.
- Do not make assumptions based on a witness's attitude, behavior, or emotional state during the interview. People react differently in a situation as emotionally charged as the death of a child.
- Do not share what you have learned with the witnesses because that can influence their statements and willingness to cooperate. They could also share any information you give them with someone who is later identified as the suspect.

- Allow the witness to provide a narrative account of what he or she actually knows about the event under investigation.
- Every child fatality investigation benefits from having as much background information as possible.

Sources of potentially important background information include the following:

- Prior CPS reports or investigations involving the child, siblings, parents, and caretakers. CPS records for a child are often filed under the mother's name. Check records in all states where the involved parties have previously lived. A witness's involvement in an abuse case in another state could be very important information for your current case.
- Medical records for the deceased child's entire life. Secure the records and have a medical professional review them for any signs of prior abuse or neglect and any preexisting medical problems. Members of child death review teams (medical examiners, coroners, doctors, and prosecutors) may be of assistance in reviewing medical records. Look at birth records, growth charts, X rays, regular pediatrician checkups, and any records of emergency room treatment. Remember that access to medical records is governed by both state law and federal law (the Health Insurance Portability and Accountability Act, known as HIPAA). Consult with your legal advisor or prosecutor regarding court orders, subpoenas, or search warrants required to obtain medical records.
- Law enforcement will look into previous law enforcement records and insurance policies.

THE FORENSIC AUTOPSY

The forensic autopsy, which should be performed by a forensic pathologist, is performed chiefly for legal purposes to determine the cause and manner of death. Forensic autopsies protect the public interest and provide the information necessary to address legal, public health, and public safety issues in each case.

The pathologist can provide information about the child's injuries, including those related to the death and those previously inflicted, and about the child's general state of health prior to death. It is important to ascertain whether a single event or multiple factors caused or contributed to the death. Additionally, the pathologist or a pediatric health care provider may be able to say how the child would have reacted after being injured (e.g., whether the child would have been able to walk or talk, been in obvious pain, or lost consciousness). Another important question to ask is when the child's symptoms would have first appeared. The answers to these questions may help determine whether witness accounts are truthful. In turn, the death investigator can tell the pathologist what was learned from your interviews and investigation. In many cases, the pathologist can offer an opinion regarding the possibility that the child's injuries occurred in the manner described by witnesses, and may also be able to estimate the time of death, based on stomach contents, your notes about the child's last meal, and other factors.

CULTURE AND DEATH RITUALS

Death rituals vary across cultures and frequently are influenced by religion, the country of origin, and the level of acculturation. The duration, frequency, and intensity of the grief process may also vary based on the manner of death and the individual family's cultural beliefs. Rituals may be performed so that family members can be with the body and prepare the body for viewing. These rituals are critical and in many cases provide closure for the family. Some religions require that the body be buried on the day of death, which is not feasible in many cases when the death is being investigated. This and other beliefs may warrant certain considerations in the investigative process. Other beliefs may include the following:

- Many Native American cultures are not concerned with body preservation, so embalming is not common. Dismemberment and mutilation outside the natural deterioration of the body is taboo, which may impact on the need for autopsy.
- Muslims require that the body be washed with certain rituals before the funeral ceremony begins. This typically takes place at a special section of the mosque or in the morgue.
- In Catholicism, the Sacraments of the Sick are performed as the person is dying. However, if a person dies before the sacraments are given, the priest will anoint the deceased conditionally within 3 hours of the time of death.

FAMILY NOTIFICATION

The office of the coroner or medical examiner is responsible for family notification of the death. Sudden, unexpected, or violent death creates significant stress for the families of the decedent. Child deaths caused by accidents, suicides, murders, natural disasters, sudden illness, and other unexpected events trigger painful and profound emotional grief reactions in family members, and for emergency care providers. Homicide bereavement is typically intense, persistent, and inescapable, and the cruel and purposeful nature of murder compounds the rage, grief, and despair of the survivors. Unlike the loss of a relative with a progressive illness, bereavement by homicide does not allow anticipatory psychological inoculation to soften the traumatic impact. Survivors are also confronted with their own mortality and vulnerability as their vision of safety and order in the world is shattered. Therefore, it is critical that the death investigator be well educated in bereavement and crisis intervention.

- Preparation
    - Obtain specialized training to perform death notification.
    - Assure that you have the correct name of the decedent, as well as the correct name and address of the family members who are being notified.
    - Rehearse what will be said and discuss anticipated reactions and problems with your team; create a sample script of what to say.
    - Talk about your reactions to the death with your team to enhance your focusing on the family when you arrive.
- Initial Contact
    - Go in person. If there is no alternative to a phone call, arrange for a professional, neighbor, or a friend to be with the next of kin at the time of your call.
    - Do not take any possessions of the victim to the notification.
    - Take someone who is experienced in dealing with shock and/ or trained in CPR/medical emergency (next of kin have been known to suffer heart attacks when notified). The additional person may also be needed to create a diversion for children when they are present.
    - If a large group is to be notified, bring a team of notifiers.
    - Identify yourself, present credentials, and ask for permission to enter.

- Ask if there are any other family members in the house that need to hear this information. Conversely, ascertain if some family members (e.g., young children, frail elderly) may be better off not being present during the notification.
- Sit down, ask them to sit down, and be sure you have the nearest next of kin—do not notify siblings before notifying parents or spouse; do not notify a minor child, and do not use a child as a translator.
- Be compassionate but direct with your notification; avoid euphemisms.
- Use the victim's name.
- Allow time for the family to comprehend the news; repeat information as necessary.
- Answer all questions tactfully and truthfully, but don't reveal more information than is necessary during initial contact; if the family member requests more information, provide it at an appropriate pace and level.
- Do not give unsolicited and unnecessary advice, and do not encourage a quick recovery from their grief.
- Encourage them to verbalize their feelings, but do not attempt to falsely identify with them.
- Offer to make phone calls to family, friends, neighbors, employers, clergy, doctors, child care, and so on. Provide them with a list of the calls you make as they will have difficulty remembering what you have told them.
- Ask family members if they want you to get someone to stay with them.
- Respect the family's privacy, but don't leave a family member alone unless you're sure the person is safe.
- High emotionality can impair memory, so give pertinent information and instructions in writing.
- Provide family members with the names and telephone numbers of appropriate agency contacts: a victim advocate, prosecutor, medical examiner, social service agency, and/or hospital. It helps to have preprinted cards with this information.
- Determine if the family members require some means of traveling to the coroner/medical examiner's office, hospital, or police station. Offer to drive them or arrange for a ride if they have no transportation, but be sure to arrange for a ride back home.

■ Follow-up

   ■ When leaving, let them know you will check back the next day to see how they are doing and if there is anything else you can do for them.
   ■ Call and visit again the next day.
   ■ If the family does not want you to visit, spend some time on the phone and reexpress willingness to answer all questions.
   ■ Ask the family if they are ready to receive their loved one's possessions (if appropriate); honor their wishes.
   ■ Debrief your personal reactions with your team after the notification and regularly with qualified mental health personnel on a frequent and regular basis.

BODY IDENTIFICATION

Bodies are identified through DNA and possibly dental records. But families may be asked to identify the bodies of their deceased loved one (or the family members may ask to view the body). The finality of identifying the deceased's body can have a paradoxical effect. Viewing the body shatters any hope that decedent may still be alive, but it also often provides a strange sort of reassuring confirmation that the decedent's death agonies may have fallen short of the survivor's imagined horrors or that the decedent's suffering is finally over. Families may want to touch the decedent to say a final good-bye. Allow them time to do so, unless there is a reason the body is not to be disturbed, such as when further evidence is being collected. This is a difficult time, so provide appropriate support.

When the victim's body is significantly mutilated, dismembered, burned, decomposed, or disintegrated, try to arrange to have the viewing area as clean as possible. Major wounds should be dressed or covered and the viewing area should be reasonably free of blood spills, body fluids, and other debris. However, law enforcement may insist on keeping the body as it was found if evidence is yet to be collected, and the family should be notified of same for these cases. At times the visual sight of a finger or a relatively intact portion of the face can solidify the reality of the death for the family member and allow a final goodbye.

CHILD DEATH REVIEW TEAMS

The first child death review team was created in California in 1978. According to the National MCH Center for Child Death Review, the purpose of child death (fatality) review teams is to conduct a comprehensive, multidisciplinary review of child deaths, to better understand how and why children die, and use the findings to take action that can prevent other deaths and improve the health and safety of children. The objectives of the review process are complex and will meet the needs of many different agencies, ranging from the investigation of deaths to their prevention. Primary objectives of the Child Death Review include the following:

- Ensure the accurate identification and uniform, consistent reporting of the cause and manner of every child death.
- Improve communication and linkages among local and state agencies and enhance coordination of efforts.
- Improve agency responses in the investigation of child deaths.
- Improve agency response to protect siblings and other children in the homes of deceased children.
- Improve criminal investigations and the prosecution of child homicides.
- Improve delivery of services to children, families, providers, and community members.
- Identify specific barriers and system issues involved in the deaths of children.
- Identify significant risk factors and trends in child deaths.
- Identify and advocate for needed changes in legislation, policy and practices, and expanded efforts in child health and safety to prevent child deaths.
- Increase public awareness and advocacy for the issues that affect the health and safety of children.

RESOURCES

American Board of Medicolegal Death Investigators: http://medschool.slu.edu/abmdi/index.php

International Association of Coroners and Medical Examiners: http://theiacme.com/iacme/index.aspx

Medline Bereavement: www.nlm.nih.gov/medlineplus/bereavement.html

National Association of Medical Examiners: http://thename.org/

National Association of Medical Examiners Forensic Autopsy Performance Standards (2006): http://thename.org/index2.php?option=com_docman& task=doc_view& gid=18&Itemid=26

National Center for Child Death Review. Phone: (800) 656-2434. E-mail: info@child deathreview.org. Web site: www.childdeathreview.org

The National Center for Child Death Review is a national resource center for state and local CDR programs, established and funded since 2002 by the Maternal and Child Health Bureau of the U.S. Department of Health and Human Services.

National Center on Child Fatality Review. Phone: (626) 455-4586. Web site: www.ican ncfr.org

The National Center on Child Fatality Review (NCFR) is a clearinghouse for the collection and dissemination of information and resources related to child deaths. NCFR is dedicated to providing training and technical assistance to CDR teams throughout the world.

REFERENCES

Hickman, M., Hughes, K., Strom, K., & Ropero-Miller, J. (2007). *Medical examiners and coroners' offices, 2004.* Bureau of Justice Statistics NCJ 216756. Retrieved from www. ojp.usdoj.gov/bjs/pub/pdf/meco04.pdf

Miller, L. (2008). Death investigation for families of homicide victims: Healing dimensions of a complex process. *Omega, 57*(4), 367–380.

U.S. Department of Justice Office of Justice Programs National Institute of Justice. (1999). *Death investigation: A guide for the scene investigator.* Retrieved from www. ncjrs.gov/pdffiles/167568.pdf

Walsh, B. (2005). *Investigating child fatalities. Portable guides to investigating child abuse.* Office of Justice Programs Partnerships for Safer Communities; Office of Juvenile Justice and Delinquency Prevention. Retrieved from www.ncjrs.gov/pdffiles1/ojjdp/ 209764.pdf

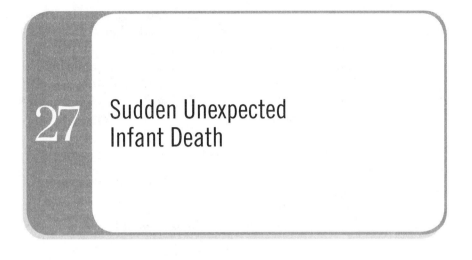

27 Sudden Unexpected Infant Death

DEFINITION

Sudden unexpected infant deaths (SUID) are infant deaths that occur suddenly and unexpectedly, and whose manner and cause of death are not immediately obvious prior to investigation.

Sudden infant death syndrome (SIDS) is the sudden death of an infant less than 1 year of age that cannot be explained after a thorough investigation is conducted, including a complete autopsy, examination of the death scene, and review of the clinical history.

The Sudden Unexpected Infant Death Investigation (SUIDI) Initiative

According to the Centers for Disease Control and Prevention (CDC), many SUID cases are not investigated. When they are investigated, cause-of-death data are not always collected and reported consistently. The inaccurate classification of cause and manner of death hampers prevention efforts and researchers are unable to adequately monitor national trends, identify risk factors, or evaluate intervention programs. The CDC's Division of Reproductive Health (DRH) and its partners implemented activities aimed at improving the accuracy and consistency of the reporting and classification of SUID deaths (CDC, n.d.). These activities included the development of a new standard investigation reporting form, training curriculum materials for conducting a thorough SUID death scene investigation, a planned effort to disseminate and promote the use of these SUID investigations tools and materials, and the development of a SUID case registry. The goals of this initiative are to develop tools and protocols to:

Standardize and improve data collected at infant death scenes.

Promote consistent diagnosis and reporting of cause and manner of death for SUID cases.

Prevent SUIDs by using improved data to monitor trends and identify those at risk.

Improve national reporting of SUID.

PREVALENCE

More than 4,500 infants die suddenly of no obvious cause each year in the United States. Half of these sudden unexpected infant deaths (SUID) are due to sudden infant death syndrome (SIDS), the leading cause of SUID and of all deaths among infants aged 1–12 months (Centers for Disease Control and Prevention, n.d.).

SIDS remains the leading cause of death among infants aged 1–12 months, and is the third leading cause overall of infant mortality in the United States. The overall rate of SIDS in the United States has been cut in half since 1990, but rates have declined less among non-Hispanic Black and American Indian/Alaska Native infants. Preventing SIDS remains an important public health priority. SIDS is rare during the first month of life. It increases to a peak between 2 and 3 months of age, and then decreases.

ETIOLOGY

Despite extensive research, the cause(s) of SIDS remains unknown. Abnormalities in the arcuate nucleus of the brainstems of some SIDS victims suggest delayed development of arousal, cardiorespiratory control, or cardiovascular control. When the physiologic stability of these infants is compromised during sleep, they may not arouse sufficiently to avoid the problem causing the compromise. While SIDS remains the leading cause of death in infants, other causes must be considered, including fatal child abuse:

Unintentional suffocation

Poisoning

Unintentional head injury

Inborn errors of metabolism

Hypothermia or hyperthermia

Neglect (failure to thrive)

Abuse

According the American Academy of Pediatrics (Hymel, The American Academy of Pediatrics Committee on Child Abuse and Neglect, & The National Association of Medical Examiners, 2006), it is difficult, if not impossible, to distinguish at autopsy between SIDS and accidental or deliberate suffocation with a soft object. However, the academy notes that there are certain circumstances that could indicate the possibility of intentional suffocation, including:

- Age at death older than 6 months
- Recurrent cyanosis, apnea, or apparent life-threatening events (ALTEs) occurring only while in the care of the same person
- Previous unexpected or unexplained deaths of one or more siblings
- Simultaneous or nearly simultaneous death of twins
- Evidence of previous pulmonary hemorrhage (such as marked siderophages in the lung)
- Previous death of infants under the care of the same unrelated person

Health care providers should be aware that these circumstances alone are not adequate to determine fatal child abuse. For example, previous unexplained deaths of one or more siblings may be attributed to undiagnosed inborn error of metabolism. The only thing worse than a parent killing his or her own child is a parent wrongly accused of killing his or her own child. Therefore, it is critical that those involved in the investigation of sudden unexplained infant deaths utilize the SUIDI protocols.

The American Academy of Pediatrics and the National Association of Medical Examiners (NAME) endorse universal performance of autopsies by forensic pathologists experienced in the diagnosis of SIDS on infants who die suddenly and unexpectedly. Postmortem findings in infant victims of fatal child abuse usually reveal cranial injuries, abdominal trauma, burns, or drowning as the cause of death. Cytomegalovirus inclusion bodies have been identified in some infants who died suddenly and unexpectedly; however, a definitive causal link between cytomegalovirus infection and SIDS has not been established. Forensic pathologists establish the diagnosis of SIDS only when, after a thorough investigation including a complete autopsy, they are unable to identify a specific cause for a child's death.

INFANT DEATH SCENE INVESTIGATION

Death-scene investigations are critical in differentiating SIDS from other sudden infant deaths. Bass and colleagues (1986) conducted death-scene investigations in 26 consecutive cases brought to the emergency department in which the presumptive diagnosis was SIDS. They found that 6 were accidental and 18 had causes of death other than SIDS, leaving only 2 remaining deaths. They concluded that many sudden infant deaths have a definable cause that can be revealed by careful investigation of the death scene. A similar conclusion was reached by Meadow (1999) based on the review of 81 cases in England. However, the extent of the use of death scene investigations in the diagnosis and differentiation of SIDS remains uncertain.

The CDC's SUIDI *Guidelines for the Scene Investigator* (www.cdc. gov/sids/PDF/508SUIDIGuidelinesSingles.pdf), developed in conjunction with leading experts in the field, provides step-by-step instructions on infant death investigation. While it is similar to the process outlined in Chapter 26, "Medicolegal Child Death Investigation," it also contains some differences specific to infant death investigation.

Arriving at the Scene

Introduce and identify self and role. Introductions allow the investigator to establish formal contact with all official agency representatives. Infant deaths can create multiple scenes, and each requires the investigator to communicate with people who have different roles and responsibilities. The investigator must ascertain if artifacts or contamination may have been introduced to, or removed from, the death scene. Investigators work with other official personnel to ensure all scenes and key witnesses are identified before starting the investigation.

Exercise scene safety. Determining scene safety is essential to the investigative process. Risks of environmental and physical injury must be removed before starting the investigation.

Confirm or pronounce death. Depending upon jurisdictional statutes, appropriate personnel make a determination of death before the death investigation is initiated. The confirmation or pronouncement of death also determines jurisdictional responsibilities.

Participate in scene briefing. Infant death investigations can involve multiple medical, legal, social, as well as public and private family health agency representatives. Scene investigators must recognize the varying jurisdictional and statutory responsibilities that apply to these representatives and the role of each of the child-focused organizations involved with infant deaths. Determining roles in the investigation and eventual follow-up is essential to planning the scope and depth of each scene investigation and the release of information to the public.

Conduct scene "walk through." The "walk through" provides an overview of the entire scene and allows the first opportunity to locate and view the environment where the infant was placed, last known alive, and found dead or unresponsive. Items of evidentiary value may be identified, and initial investigative procedures can be established to ensure a systematic examination of the scene and body.

Establish chain of custody. Ensuring the integrity of the evidence by establishing and maintaining a chain of custody is vital to an investigation. Documenting the collection and handling of all evidence and property will safeguard against subsequent allegations of tampering, theft, planting, and contamination of evidence.

Follow evidence-collection laws. The investigator follows local, state, and federal laws for the collection of evidence to ensure its admissibility, and works collaboratively with all agency representatives to determine which agency has the legal authority to perform specific tasks related to collecting evidence.

Documenting and Evaluating the Scene

Photograph scene. Photographic documentation creates a permanent historical record, and scene photographs are required to begin an autopsy. Photographs provide forensic scientists with the details required to correlate scene findings with physical findings, and provide corroborating evidence that constructs a system of redundancy, especially if questions arise concerning the report, witness statements, or evidence.

Develop descriptive documentation of scene. The written narrative documentation of the scene(s) provides a permanent record that may be used to correlate with and enhance photographic documentation, refresh recollections, and record observations.

Establish probable location of injury or illness. The location where the infant is first viewed by the investigator may not be the actual location where the injury/illness that contributed to the death occurred. Thus, the investigator must attempt to determine the locations of any and all injury/illness that may have contributed to the death. Physical and environmental evidence at any and all scenes visited within 24 hours of death may be pertinent in establishing the cause, manner, and circumstances of an infant's death.

Collect, inventory, and safeguard property and evidence. Evidence must be safeguarded by a chain of custody to ensure proper processing and availability for further evaluation. Property removed from the scene must be properly inventoried to ensure its eventual return to the parents or guardians.

Interview witness(es) at scene. Witness statements and their nonverbal behavior observed at the scene allow the investigator to obtain primary data regarding placement and discovery of the infant, as well as witness corroboration and history.

Documenting and Evaluating the Body

Photograph body and doll reenactment. Photographic documentation of the infant at the scene creates a permanent historical record of the body, the infant's terminal position, appearance, and any external trauma. In cases where the infant's body has been moved, doll reenactments allow for the visualization and documentation of the infant's initial placed position, and discovered position.

Conduct the external body examination. Conducting the superficial external examination documents the infant's physical characteristics, relationship to the scene, and injuries (if present). The photographic and graphic (body diagram) documentation provides detailed information about the possible cause, manner, and circumstances of death.

Preserve evidence. To maintain chain of custody, evidence must be collected, preserved, and transported properly. Physical evidence visible on the body and bedding, blood and other body fluids present must be photographed and documented before collection and transport. Fragile evidence (that which can be easily contaminated, lost, or altered) must also be documented.

Establish infant identification. Establishing or confirming the identification of an infant and his or her parents or guardians is paramount to the death investigation. Proper identification allows notification of the next of kin, aids in the investigation, and allows the death certificate to be completed properly.

Document postmortem changes. Documented postmortem changes, when correlated with circumstantial information, can assist investigators in estimating the approximate time of death and is essential to the pathologist before the autopsy begins. Inconsistencies between postmortem changes and body location may indicate movement of the body and validate or invalidate witness statements.

Participate in scene debriefing. Scene debriefing helps investigators from all participating agencies to establish postscene responsibilities by sharing data regarding particular scene findings. It also provides each agency the opportunity for input, special requests for assistance, additional information, special examinations, and other requests requiring interagency communication, cooperation, and education.

Determine next-of-kin notification procedures. Parents or guardians are not always present at the scene of an infant death, and every reasonable effort should be made to notify them as soon as possible. Investigators may wish to enlist the support of a local bereavement agency and use a "team" approach for the actual notification. The notification initiates the closure process for the family, helps determine disposition of remains, and facilitates the collection of additional information relative to the case.

Ensure security of remains. The investigator performs or supervises the removal of the infant from the scene in a sensitive and caring manner. Appropriate chain of custody is maintained to preclude misidentification upon receipt at the examining agency and to safeguard all potential physical evidence and/or property and clothing that remain on the body.

Establishing Infant Profile Information

Document discovery history. Infant death investigation begins with the circumstances of the discovery history. This information dictates the direction of the subsequent investigation, jurisdiction, and authority, as well as the focus (breadth/depth) of any further investigation.

Document terminal episode history. The circumstances and events that surround the infant's death play a critical role in determining cause and manner of death. Documenting medical interventions or procuring antemortem specimens from emergency medical personnel help establish the infant's medical condition or activities before death.

Document infant medical history. The infant's medical records and history frequently contain information important to the investigation because they may assist in identifying elements that may have caused the death. Signs and symptoms of medical illness, as well as previous exposures to illnesses, may assist the pathologist in determining the cause of death.

Document caregiver mental health history. The mental health of the caregiver may be a factor in the infant's death. Therefore, insight into the caregiver's state of mind and ability to care for an infant may produce clues that will aid in establishing the cause, manner, and circumstances of the death.

Document caregiver social history. Caregiver social history includes marital, family, educational, employment, and financial information of the infant's primary caregiver(s). The caregiver's daily routines, habits, activities, friends, and associates help develop a caregiver profile, which may assist the investigator in establishing cause, manner, and circumstances of an infant's death.

Completing the Scene Investigation

Maintain jurisdiction over body. Maintaining jurisdiction of the infant's body allows the investigator to protect the chain of custody when the infant is transported from the scene for autopsy, specimen collection, or storage.

Release jurisdiction of body. The investigator releases jurisdiction of the body after examination by the pathologist. But before releasing jurisdiction of the infant to the family or funeral director, the investigator contacts the person responsible for certifying the death to review the circumstances of the death and verifies all information required to complete the death certificate, including demographic information, date, time, and location of death.

Perform exit procedures. Bringing formal closure to the scene investigation ensures that important evidence has been collected and the scene has been processed. The investigator performs a systematic review of the scene to ensure that artifacts or equipment are not inadvertently left behind, dangerous materials or conditions have been reported, and that the family or caregiver has a support network available before they are left alone.

Assist family. The investigator gives the family a timetable so they can arrange for final disposition of the infant. They also provide the family with information on available community resources that may assist the family.

The CDC Program also outlines the "SUIDI Top 25." Forensic pathologists consider these details critical to determining the cause and manner of death in the investigation of sudden, unexplained infant death, and all should be collected and provided to the pathologist before the autopsy:

1. Case information
2. Evidence of asphyxia
3. Sharing sleep surfaces
4. Change in sleep conditions
5. Evidence of hyperthermia/hypothermia
6. Environmental scene hazards

7. Unsafe sleeping conditions
8. Diet or recent change in diet
9. Recent hospitalizations
10. Previous medical diagnosis
11. History of acute life-threatening events
12. History of medical care—without diagnosis
13. Recent fall or other injury
14. History of religious, cultural, or ethnic remedies
15. Death due to natural causes other than SIDS
16. Prior sibling deaths
17. Previous encounters with police or social service agencies
18. Request for tissue or organ donation
19. Objection to autopsy
20. Preterminal resuscitative treatment
21. Death due to trauma (injury), poisoning, or intoxication
22. Suspicious circumstances
23. Other alerts for pathologist's attention
24. Description of the circumstances surrounding the death
25. Pathologist contact information

Designed for both novice and veteran death investigators, the eight-page Sudden, Unexplained Infant Death Initiative Reporting Form (SUIDI RF) is designed to ensure that all information is collected in a consistent, sensitive manner. The form can be downloaded from www.cdc.gov/sids/PDF/SUIDIforms.pdf.

PREVENTION/PATIENT TEACHING

Health care providers can decrease the incidence of SUID by teaching parents about safe sleep for their infants. Follow the recommendations by the National Institutes of Health Eunice Kennedy Shriver National Institute of Child Health and Human Development as outlined in its Safe Sleep Top 10:

1. Always place your baby on his or her back to sleep, for naps and at nighttime. The back sleep position is the safest, so every sleep time counts.
2. Place your baby on a firm sleep surface, such as on a safety-approved crib mattress, covered by a fitted sheet. Never place

your baby to sleep on pillows, quilts, sheepskins, or other soft surfaces. (For information on crib safety guidelines, contact the Consumer Product Safety Commission at 1-800-638-2772.)

3. Keep soft objects, toys, and loose bedding out of your baby's sleep area. Don't use pillows, blankets, quilts, sheepskins, and pillow-like crib bumpers in your baby's sleep area, and keep any other items away from your baby's face.

4. Do not allow smoking around your baby. Don't smoke before or after the birth of your baby, and don't let others smoke around your baby.

5. Keep your baby's sleep area close to, but separate from, where you and others sleep. Your baby should not sleep in a bed or on a couch or armchair with adults or other children, but he or she can sleep in the same room as you. If you bring the baby into bed with you to breastfeed, put him or her back in a separate sleep area, such as a bassinet, crib, cradle, or a bedside cosleeper (infant bed that attaches to an adult bed) when finished.

6. Think about using a clean, dry pacifier when placing the infant down to sleep, but don't force the baby to take it. (If you are breastfeeding your baby, wait until your child is 1 month old or is used to breastfeeding before using a pacifier.)

7. Do not let your baby overheat during sleep. Dress your baby in light sleep clothing, and keep the room at a temperature that is comfortable for an adult.

8. Avoid products that claim to reduce the risk of SIDS because most have not been tested for effectiveness or safety.

9. Do not use home monitors to reduce the risk of SIDS. If you have questions about using monitors for other conditions, talk to your health care provider.

10. Reduce the chance that flat spots will develop on your baby's head: provide "tummy time" when your baby is awake and someone is watching; change the direction that your baby lies in the crib from one week to the next; and avoid too much time in car seats, carriers, and bouncers.

FAMILY SUPPORT

As mentioned in the previous chapter, the death of a child is a difficult experience for any parent. For a parent who has suddenly and unexpectedly lost an otherwise healthy infant, the loss can be especially devastating. Health care providers can refer grieving parents to programs that provide professional case management, counseling, referral, and support services. In some areas, a community health nurse, social worker, or trained community outreach worker visits the family in their home. In others, the program works with the medical examiner or coroner and contacts the family immediately after the death.

RESOURCES

Appendix A: "Infant Developmental Milestones Important for SUID Investigations."

Centers for Disease Control and Prevention. Sudden Infant Death Syndrome (SIDS) and Sudden Unexpected Infant Death (SUID): Sudden, Unexpected Infant Death (SUID) Initiative: www.cdc.gov/sids/SUID.htm

National Sudden and Unexpected Infant/Child Death and Pregnancy Loss Resource Center: www.sidscenter.org

State Laws Regarding SIDS: www.ncsl.org/IssuesResearch/Health/SuddenInfantDeath SyndromeLaws/tabid/14371/Default.aspx

Association of SIDS and Infant Mortality Programs (ASIP)
8280 Greensboro Drive
Suite 300
McLean, VA 22102
Phone (800) 930-7437
Fax: (703) 902-1230
http://www.ASIP1.org

The Compassionate Friends
PO Box 3696
Oak Brook, IL 60522-3696
Phone: (877) 969-0010
http://www.compassionatefriends.org

First Candle/SIDS Alliance
Suite 210
1314 Bedford Avenue
Baltimore, MD 21208
Phone: (800) 221-7437
http://www.firstcandle.org

National SIDS and Infant Death Program Support Center (NSIDPSC)
Suite 210
1314 Bedford Avenue
Baltimore, MD 21208
Phone: (800) 221-7437
Fax: (410) 415-5093
http://www.sids-id-psc.org

SHARE Pregnancy and Infant Loss Support, Inc.
National Share Office
St. Joseph Health Center
300 First Capitol Drive
St. Charles, MO 63301-2893
Phone: (800) 821-6819
Fax: (636) 947-7486
E-mail: share@nationalshareoffice.com
http://www.nationalshareoffice.com

REFERENCES

American Academy of Pediatrics Task Force on Sudden Infant Death Syndrome. (2005). The changing concept of sudden infant death syndrome: Diagnostic coding shifts, controversies regarding the sleeping environment, and new variables to consider in reducing risk. *Pediatrics, 115,* 1247–1253.

Bass, M., Kravath, R., & Glass, L. (1986). Death-scene investigation in sudden infant death. *New England Journal of Medicine, 315,* 100–105.

Centers for Disease Control and Prevention. (n.d.). *Sudden infant death syndrome (SIDS) and sudden unexpected infant death (SUID): Sudden, unexpected infant death (SUID) initiative.* Retrieved from www.cdc.gov/sids/SUID.htm

Hymel, K., The American Academy of Pediatrics Committee on Child Abuse and Neglect, & The National Association of Medical Examiners. (2006). Distinguishing sudden infant death syndrome from child abuse fatalities. *Pediatrics, 118*(1), 421–427.

Meadow, R. (1999). Unnatural sudden infant death. *Archive of Diseases in Children, 80,* 7–14.

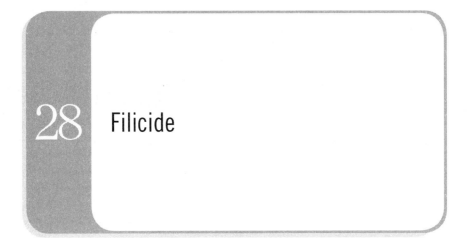

28 Filicide

DEFINITION

The United States has the highest rate of child homicide among developed countries, and when a young child is murdered, the most likely perpetrator is the child's parent or stepparent. Many child abuse specialists believe child fatalities due to abuse and neglect are still underreported. However, not all child homicides are the result of abuse or neglect. Some are intentional acts aimed at killing the child. *Filicide* is the killing of a child by its parents. Subcategories of filicide are *neonaticide,* when the victim does not survive the first 24 hours of life, and *infanticide* when the child is less than 1 year at the time of death. Filicide may also occur within the context of *filicide/suicide,* whereby the offending parent also kills himself or herself or in the context of *familicide,* which is the extermination of the entire family.

PREVALENCE

The United States has the highest rates of child homicide (8.0/100,000 for infants; 2.5/100,000 for preschool-aged children; and 1.5/100,000 for school-aged children) (Finkelhor, 1997). These rates of child murder are probably underestimates, due to problems such as inaccurate coroner rulings and some bodies never being discovered. The homicides of young children are also difficult to document because they often resemble deaths resulting from accidents and other causes. A child who dies from SIDS (sudden infant death syndrome) is difficult to distinguish from one who has been smothered, and a child who has been thrown or intentionally dropped may have injuries similar to those of one who died from an accidental fall.

Other important occurrence factors are:

- Filicide had been considered a female crime; however, men have become increasingly likely to be convicted of killing their child.
- Over the past four decades, approximately 50% of parents who murdered their children also made a nonfatal or fatal attempt at suicide.
- Approximately 60% of the child victims of filicide-suicide are between 1 and 6 years old and, unlike fatal child abuse, this percent tends to remain stable across time and countries.
- Homicides of young children are committed primarily by the common use of "personal weapons" (i.e., hands and feet) to batter, strangle, or suffocate victims.

ETIOLOGY

Fatal Child Abuse

The second largest group of filicidal mothers is that comprised of those who accidentally batter their children to death. Deaths from accidental filicide occur in the context of psychosocial stress and limited support. There is no clear impulse to kill, but instead a sudden impulsive act characterized by a loss of temper. In several studies of large groups of filicidal mothers, these battering mothers suffered the highest rates of social and family stress, such as marital stress and housing and financial problems.

Neonaticide

Neonaticide is virtually exclusively committed by women. The mothers are younger, rarely married, poorly educated, have a low level of psychiatric disorders and psychosocial stressors, no history of criminal behavior, and do not attempt suicide after the murders. The women generally

do not seek out abortions, and conceal or do not acknowledge their pregnancies, and they are apparently chiefly motivated by extreme shame
and guilt over pregnancy and childrearing out of marriage. Women who
commit neonaticide make no plans for the birth and care of their child,
and their decisions are mostly based in denial and dissociation.

Infanticide

FBI homicide data do not identify infanticides as a distinct subgroup. Maternal infanticide studies found a predominance of unemployed mothers in their early 20s. Many cases occurred in the context of child abuse,
though some mothers had associated suicide attempts. Many experienced
psychiatric disorders.

Postpartum (puerperal) psychosis is a relatively rare disorder that affects approximately 1 to 2 per 1,000 women and that occurs within 1 to
4 weeks from delivery. Data suggest that postpartum psychosis is a presentation of bipolar disorder that coincides with tremendous hormonal
shifts after delivery. Results from a study by Valdimarsdo, Hultman, Harlow, and Cnattingius (2009) suggested that the immediate time period
following childbirth entailed a substantially increased risk of psychotic
illness of the first-time mother. This also held true for mothers without
any previous psychiatric hospitalization, who account for almost half of
the psychosis cases during the first 90 days postpartum. Among women
without any previous psychiatric hospitalization, greater maternal age
and lower infant birth weight increase the risk of psychoses during the
postpartum period, while maternal diabetes and high birth weight of
the infant appear to be protective. Presentation is often dramatic, with
rapid onset of symptoms as early as the first 48 to 72 hours after delivery.
Manifestations resemble those of a rapidly evolving manic (or mixed)
episode with the earliest signs being restlessness, irritability, and insomnia. Women may exhibit a rapidly shifting depressed or elated mood,
disorientation or confusion, erratic or disorganized behavior, delusional
beliefs that often center on the infant, and auditory hallucinations that
instruct the mother to harm herself or her infant. The risk for infanticide, as well as suicide, is significant.

Filicide-Suicide

Research on filicide-suicide using psychological autopsies demonstrates
that most filicide-suicide parents were functioning well in all social roles

prior to the incident (Gross, 2008). They were not abusive and did not have a diagnosable problem with substance abuse. While they do not manifest more obvious psychiatric illness, filicide-suicide parents generally do suffer from depression and anxiety that is exclusive of a thought disorder. A qualitative study of 30 families' files from a county coroner's office showed that parental motives for filicide-suicide included altruistic and acutely psychotic motives. Twice as many fathers as mothers committed filicide-suicide, and older children were more often victims than infants. Parents frequently showed evidence of depression or psychosis and had prior mental health care. The data support the researchers' hypothesis that traditional risk factors for violence appear different from commonly occurring factors in filicide-suicide (Friedman, Hrouda, Holden, Noffsinger, & Resnick, 2005).

Most of the extensive retrospective research has been conducted on filicide-suicide mothers. Gross (2008) noted that this body of work reveals certain personality traits and trends that can serve as risk factors or indicators of vulnerability for filicide-suicide. Some personality traits shared by these mothers include the following:

- They have chronic symptoms of depression and anxiety that result from an overwhelming sensitivity to real and perceived rejection.
- They are unrealistically afraid of not being able to meet the real or perceived standards of others, creating paralyzing performance anxiety. Filicide-suicide mothers dread their perceived shortcomings will be exposed, causing them to be rejected and stigmatized. In an effort to avoid being "found out," they tend to be overly responsible, very orderly, and given to following the rules.
- These mothers often had difficult childhoods that may have included emotional and/or sexual abuse, and their own mothers may have been incapable of providing nurturance or unconditional acceptance. Thus, their fear of rejection dates back to early age and may have made their adolescence especially painful. Over time, they developed a profound sense of guilt over essentially "normal" behaviors that they perceive as shameful, and they live with the fear that these "secrets" will be discovered and bring disgrace to their family.
- They view themselves as "damaged goods" and fear their weaknesses and limitations will be passed on to their children. The guilt is exacerbated if their child is in any way disabled due to both rejection fears and the demands of parenting a special needs child.

- Despite appearances, they find every aspect of life hard. They have a limited ability to cope with stress and change. When stressed, their fear of impending doom and disaster can become absolutely overwhelming. Events that should be happy and filled with positive anticipation, including a child's birthday party or first day of school, can be agonizing for these mothers.
- To survive their turmoil, filicide-suicide mothers essentially "shut off" their thinking and awareness and focus on tasks. Although emotionally numb and detached, they can give an appearance of normality. When they can no longer suppress fear and anxiety, these mothers may see no way to protect themselves and their children from current and future misery other than filicide-suicide.

Familicide

Liem and Koenraadt (2005) found that familicide perpetrators were more likely than filicide perpetrators to be male, older, more educated, and more likely to commit the offense with physical violence. They were more likely than uxoricide (intimate partner homicide) perpetrators to be married and less likely to have committed a previous violent offense. They were more likely to suffer from a personality disorder and more likely to attempt suicide following the homicide.

Though well-publicized, familicide is a rare and isolated event. Unfortunately, rarity makes finding trends difficult. The greatest risk factor for familicide appears to be a prior history of domestic violence. However, some of the male perpetrators do not fit any stereotype associated with abusers and do not have histories or records. Typically, there is a gradual build-up of tensions and conflicts after which one event may trigger the event—a sense of a loss of control over finances, unemployment, or, more frequently, when the wife announces that she is leaving. However, in other cases, threats of violence become more frequent and more specific over time until the man acts on his threats. Access to a gun is a major risk factor since it is easier to be impulsive when a gun is nearby.

ASSESSMENT

General Principles

Children may die as the result of abuse, but there are also times when the parent intentionally kills the child. There is no single profile of a perpetrator of fatal child abuse, although certain characteristics exist. The perpetrator is often a young adult in his or her mid-20s, without a high school diploma, living at or below the poverty level, depressed, and who may have difficulty coping with stressful situations. The perpetrator often has experienced violence firsthand. Most physical abuse fatalities are caused by fathers and other male caregivers, while deaths from neglect are most often caused by the mother. While this chapter focuses on abusive parents, it is critical for health care providers to realize that at least one study showed that being a biologically unrelated caregiver is the strongest predictor of fatal child maltreatment (Yampolskaya, Greenbaum, & Berson, 2009).

Resnick (1969) organized maternal filicide perpetrators into five major categories:

Altruistic. These mothers kill their children out of love to relieve real or imagined suffering of their children. They believe death to be in the child's best interest. A suicidal mother may not wish to leave her motherless child to face an intolerable world, while a psychotic mother may believe that she is saving her child from a fate worse than death. Altruistic filicide may be associated with suicide.

Acutely psychotic. Psychotic or delirious mothers kill their children without any comprehensible motive (e.g., a mother may follow command hallucinations to kill).

Fatal maltreatment filicide. When fatal child abuse occurs, death is usually not the anticipated outcome. Instead, it results from cumulative child abuse, neglect, or Münchausen syndrome by proxy.

Unwanted child filicide. These mothers think that their children are a hindrance.

Spouse revenge filicide. This fortunately rare event occurs when a mother kills her child specifically to emotionally harm that child's father.

History and Physical Assessment and Diagnostic Testing

As many as 60% of parents who committed filicide were in contact with a health care provider prior to the crime, indicating a strong need for empirically based assessment and intervention strategies.

While there are no definitive assessment strategies, there are suggestions. Health care providers must be alert to the filicide potential of depressed mothers contemplating suicide. Consider phenotypic vulnerabilities, current and past illness variables, psychosocial stressors, and the quality and stability of key interpersonal relationships of a mother. Psychotic symptoms coupled with agitation, hypochondriasis, delusions of sinfulness and self-guilt, and fear are prominent signs of risk and indicate a need for hospitalization. Hospitalization should be considered if a mother expresses fear of harming her offspring, has delusions associated with the suffering or health of her child, or demonstrates enmity toward the favorite child of a spouse. In addition, the mother may be at risk in the following situations:

- Mothers who come to psychiatric attention because of severe mental illnesses, personality disorders, or substance use disorders may be abusing or neglecting their children. Ask about childrearing practices, parenting problems, and feelings of being overwhelmed.
- Depressed mothers who have the potential to kill in extended suicides should be identified early. Mothers contemplating suicide should be asked directly about the fate of their children if they were to take their own lives.
- Query about thoughts or fears of harming their children and take threats seriously.
- Consider hospitalization for mentally ill mothers of young children due to the possibility of multiple deaths from a filicide-suicide.
- Maternal fears of harming their child, delusions of their child's suffering, improbable concerns about their child's health, and hostility toward a despised partner's favorite child: The presence of these factors may merit psychiatric hospitalization of the mother.
- Psychotic mothers who fear that their children may suffer a fate worse than death due to persecutory delusions. These mothers should either be hospitalized or separated from their children. They may be reluctant to share their delusional ideas, and thus delusions may need to be elicited through a sympathetic exploration of their concerns for the safety of their children.
- Too-frequent checking by the mother on the health and safety of her children. Sometimes this is the only evidence of concern.
- Psychotic mothers who may have less warning about filicide; however, health care providers can ask about hallucinations or delusional thoughts regarding the children.

Postpartum Psychosis. Health care providers caring for pregnant and puerperal women should maintain a high index of suspicion for postpartum mood disorders and should ask all mothers about their postpartum adjustments. Useful tools to screen for depression and mania/hypomania include the Edinburgh Postnatal Depression Scale (EPDS; www.fresno. ucsf.edu/pediatrics/downloads/edinburghscale.pdf) and the Mood Disorder Questionnaire (MDQ; www.dbsalliance.org/pdfs/MDQ.pdf).

The EPDS is a self-rating instrument that uncovers the presence of persistent low mood, anhedonia, guilt, anxiety, and thoughts of self-harm, while the MDQ assesses past and current symptoms of high, hyper, or irritable mood; excess energy; racing thoughts; pressured speech; and symptoms that are linked with mania/hypomania. The initial evaluation requires a thorough history, physical examination with complete neurological assessment, and laboratory investigations to exclude an organic cause for acute psychosis, which include cerebral vascular accident, systemic lupus erythematosus, metabolic and nutritional disorders, neurological infections, substance abuse, and medication effects. Diagnostic tests may include complete blood count (CBC), electrolytes, blood urea nitrogen (BUN), creatinine, glucose, vitamin B12, folate, thyroid function tests, calcium, urinalysis and urine culture in the patient with fever, and a urine drug screen. The client may warrant a head CT or MRI scan to rule out the presence of a stroke related to ischemia (vascular occlusion) or hemorrhage (uncontrolled hypertension, ruptured arteriovenous malformation, or aneurysm). Clients who report confusion, threats to harm self or others, difficulty caring for their children, or poor self-care warrant immediate psychiatric referral.

INTERVENTION AND PREVENTION

Postpartum psychosis (PP). Lack of treatment increases the risk for mortality. These patients respond best to pharmacotherapy with atypical antipsychotic drugs; however, if the health care provider suspects the presence of comorbid depression, the addition of an antidepressant medication is highly recommended. Another option for treatment is the use of antidepressants and a mood stabilizer, such as lithium, valproic acid, and carbamazepine, in combination with antipsychotics. Mothers taking lithium and antipsychotics should be advised to not breast-feed due to the risks of toxicity to the infant. If medication treatment fails or in cases where rapid stabilization is required, electroconvulsive therapy

(ECT) is a possible course of treatment. ECT also has the benefit of avoiding infant exposure to medications excreted in breast milk.

Other intervention/prevention strategies may include immediate access to psychiatric care and prompt intervention by health care providers, law enforcement, and social agencies at the first report of an abused or unwanted child. Strategies include the following:

- Community education is critical. Support services for mothers and accessible psychiatric services for at-risk populations should be identified.
- Parenting classes, emotional support, and 24-hour emergency numbers for overwhelmed mothers can be helpful in preventing fatal maltreatment filicides.
- Maternal substance abuse must be treated.
- Mothers diagnosed with Münchausen syndrome should be evaluated to see if they have engaged in Münchausen syndrome by proxy (MSBP) behaviors.
- Child factors such as colic or autism may increase risk.
- Child protective agencies must remove children who are at risk of serious abuse.
- Child protective agencies should be receptive to accepting children into their care who are unwanted, even if no abuse or neglect has yet occurred.

Prevention of spousal revenge filicide is difficult because there is usually little warning. However, it most often occurs after the perpetrator learns of spousal infidelity or during child custody disputes. Evaluators of child custody disputes should be alert for this potential.

RESOURCES

Brandon's House: www.brandonshouse.org
Stop Family Violence: www.stopfamilyviolence.org/tags?id=filicide

REFERENCES

Cylc, L. (n.d.). *Classifications and descriptions of parents who commit filicide.* Retrieved from www.publications.villanova.edu/Concept/2005/Filicide.pdf
Finkelhor D. (1997). The homicides of children and youth: A developmental perspective. In G. K. Kantor & J. L. Jasinski (Ed.), *Out of the darkness: Contemporary perspectives on family violence* (pp. 17–34). Thousand Oaks, CA: Sage.

Finkelhor, D., & Ormrod, R. (2001). *Homicides of children and youth*. Office of Juvenile Justice and Delinquency Prevention Juvenile Justice Bulletin NCJ18723. Retrieved from www.ncjrs.gov/pdffiles1/ojjdp/187239.pdf

Friedman, S., Horowitz, S., & Resnick, P. (2005). Child murder by mothers: A critical analysis of the current state of knowledge and a research agenda. *American Journal of Psychiatry, 162*(9), 1578–1587.

Friedman, S., Hrouda, D., Holden, C., Noffsinger, S., & Resnick, P. (2005). Filicide-suicide: Common factors in parents who kill their children and themselves. *Journal of the American Academy of Psychiatry and Law, 33,* 496–504.

Freidman, S., & Resnick, P. (2007). Child murder by mothers: Patterns and prevention. *World Psychiatry, 6,* 137–141.

Gilbert, R., Spatz Widom, C., Browne, K., Fergusson, D., Webb, E., & Janson, S. (2009). Burden and consequences of child maltreatment in high-income countries. *The Lancet, 373,* 68–81.

Gross, B. (2008). Identifying clients at risk for filicide-suicide. *Annals of the American Psychotherapy Association.* Retrieved from http://findarticles.com/p/articles/mi_hb013/is_2_11/ai_n29445898/?tag=content;col1

Guileyardo, J., Prahlow, J., & Barnard, J. (1999). Familial filicide and filicide classification. *American Journal of Forensic Medicine and Pathology, 20*(3), 286–292.

Herman-Giddens, M., Brown, G., Verbiest, S., Carlson, P., Hooten, E., Howell, E., et al. (1999). Underascertainment of child abuse mortality in the United States. *Journal of the American Medical Association, 282*(5), 463–467.

Liem, M., & Koenraadt, F. (2005). Familicide: A comparison with spousal and child homicide by mentally disordered perpetrators. *Criminal Behaviour and Mental Health, 18*(5), 306–318.

Mugavin, M. (2005). A meta-synthesis of filicide classification systems: Psychosocial and psychodynamic issues in women who kill their children. *Journal of Forensic Nursing, 1*(2), 65–72.

Office of Community Oriented Policing Services (COPS). (2009). *National Institute of Justice panel explores familicide phenomenon.* Retrieved from www.corrections.com/news/article/21981

Papapietro, D., & Barbo, E. (2005). Toward a psychodynamic understanding of filicide—beyond psychosis and into the heart of darkness. *Journal of the American Academy of Psychiatry Law, 33*(4), 505–508.

Resnick, P. (1969). Child murder by parents: A psychiatric review of filicide. *American Journal of Psychiatry, 126*(3), 325–334.

U.S. Department of Health and Human Services, Administration on Children, Youth and Families. (2005). *Child maltreatment 2003.* Washington, DC: U.S. Government Printing Office.

Valdimarsdo, Y., Hultman, C., Harlow, B., & Cnattingius, S. (2009). Psychotic illness in first-time mothers with no previous psychiatric hospitalizations: A population-based study. *PLOS Medicine, 6*(2), 0194–0201. Retrieved from http://www.plosmedicine.org/article/info:doi%2F10.1371%2Fjournal.pmed.1000013

Yampolskaya, S., Greenbaum, P., & Berson, I. (2009). Profiles of child maltreatment perpetrators and risk for fatal assault: A latent class analysis. *Journal of Family Violence, 24*(5), 337–348.

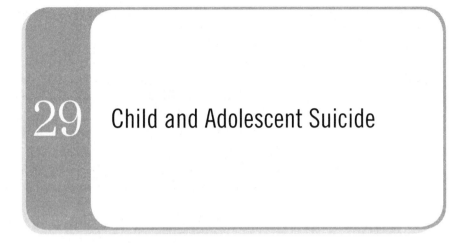

29 Child and Adolescent Suicide

DEFINITIONS

Suicide describes the destructive, self-inflicted actions that result in actual or attempted self-harm or death, the intentional ending of one's life. *Suicidal ideation* is defined as having thoughts of wanting to end one's own life. Clinicians usually view the severity of suicide risk along a continuum, ranging from suicidal ideation alone (relatively less severe) to suicidal ideation with plan (highest severity). The latter is a significant risk factor for suicide attempts. *Suicide attempts* are the self-initiated acts with the intention of ending one's own life and are less frequent than suicidal ideation. In adolescents, overdose is the most common method of attempt, whereas firearms, jumping, and hanging are more common methods in completed suicides.

PREVALENCE

Suicide is the third leading cause of death for 15- to 24-year-olds, and the sixth leading cause of death for 5- to 14-year-olds. In 2004, suicide was the third leading cause of death among youths and young adults aged 10–24 years in the United States, accounting for 4,599 deaths; however, the true number of youth suicide deaths may be higher, because some of these deaths are recorded as accidental (Centers for Disease Control and Prevention, 2007).

Completed suicides are only part of the problem. Many young people survive suicide attempts, more than those who actually die. According to the Centers for Disease Control and Prevention (2007), a survey of youth in Grades 9–12 in public and private schools in the United States found that 15% of students reported seriously considering suicide, 11% reported creating a plan, and 7% reported trying to take their own lives in the 12 months preceding the survey. Approximately 149,000 youth between the ages of 10 and 24 receive medical care for self-inflicted injuries at emergency departments across the United States each year.

Suicide affects all youths; however, some are at higher risk than others. Boys are more likely than girls to die from suicide—in the 10 to 24 age group, 83% of the deaths were males and 17% were females. Girls are more likely to report attempting suicide than boys. Cultural variations also exist, with Latino and Native American/Alaskan Native youths having the highest rates of suicide-related fatalities. Latino youth were more likely to report attempting suicide than their Black and White, non-Latino peers.

ETIOLOGY

Most of the research on adolescent suicide has focused on the relationship between depression and suicide. The common stressors of adolescence, compounded by limited problem-solving abilities, can sometimes lead to harmful, life-threatening behaviors. Common contributing factors include:

- *Historical factors:* Previous suicide attempts, family member or friend who has made an attempt, history of physical or sexual abuse, chronic or debilitating physical disorders, physical ailments (including hypochondriacal preoccupation), breakup of a relationship, school difficulties or failure, legal difficulties, and death of a parent when the child was young.
- *Family factors:* Conflict, paternal rejection or hostility, divorce and separation, relocation, unrealistic parental expectations, and parental indifference.
- *Adolescent factors:* Hopelessness, social isolation, depression, substance abuse, impulsivity, difficulty tolerating frustration, feelings

of self-loathing or guilt, thought disorder, physical or body image problems, gender-identify concerns, gay and bisexual orientation, and a perfectionist personality.

■ *Socioeconomical factors:* Access to firearms; isolation; ineffective support systems; incarceration; living out of the home (in a correctional facility or group home); limited social, economic, or vocational opportunities; high levels of community violence; and exposure to the suicides of others.

Health care professionals should become familiar with affective disorders in childhood:

■ *Major depressive disorder* is characterized by one or more major depressive episodes. In children and adolescents, episodes last from 7 to 9 months and have many features similar to those seen in adults. Depressed children are sad. They lose interest in pleasurable activities, and they criticize themselves and feel that others criticize them. They feel unloved, pessimistic, or even hopeless about the future. Some think that life is not worth living and have thoughts of suicide. Depressed children and adolescents are often irritable and sometimes aggressive. They may be indecisive, have problems concentrating, lack energy or motivation, neglect their appearance and hygiene, and have abnormal sleep patterns. Childhood depression also differs in important ways from adult depression. Psychotic features do not occur as often in children and adolescents, and associated anxiety and somatic symptoms are more common in depressed children and adolescents than in adults with depression.

■ *Dysthymic disorder,* with fewer symptoms than major depression, is more chronic. Its persistent nature is likely to interfere with normal adjustment. Affected youth are depressed for most of the day, on most days, and symptoms continue for several years. Children may be depressed for so long that they do not recognize their mood as out of the ordinary and thus may not complain of feeling depressed.

■ *Bipolar disorder* is a mood disorder in which episodes of mania usually alternate with episodes of depression. The first manifestation of bipolar illness may be a depressive episode, and the first manic features may not occur for months or even years thereafter.

Adolescents with mania or hypomania feel energetic, confident, and special. They usually have difficulty sleeping but do not tire; and they talk a great deal, often speaking very rapidly or loudly. They may complain that their thoughts are racing and may do school-work in a quick, creative, but disorganized and chaotic fashion. Manic adolescents may have exaggerated or even delusional ideas about their capabilities and importance, may become overconfident, and may start numerous projects that they do not finish. They may engage in reckless or risky behavior, such as fast driving or unsafe sex.

■ *Reactive depression* is the most common form of mood problem in children and adolescents. Depressed feelings are short-lived and usually occur in response to some adverse experience, such as the loss of a loved one. Children may feel sad or lethargic and appear preoccupied for periods as short as a few hours or as long as 2 weeks; however, mood improves with a change in activity or an interesting or pleasant event. These transient mood swings in reaction to minor environmental adversities are not regarded as a form of mental disorder.

ASSESSMENT

General Principles

Suicide risk often goes undetected in health care settings. Unrecognized suicidality in emergency departments (EDs) is an important problem for several reasons: increasing numbers of children and adolescents now present to hospital EDs with mental health concerns, particularly self-destructive behavior; ED staff are increasingly being given the responsibility of triaging children and adolescents with mental health problems to crisis intervention and appropriate follow-up treatments; unrecognized suicidality in the ED is associated with substantial morbidity, possible mortality, and increased health care utilization and costs. Approximately one-half to two-thirds of individuals who commit suicide visit health care providers less than 1 month before taking their lives; 10% to 40% visit in the week before. Yet, despite the substantial proportion of primary care providers who encountered suicidal adolescent patients, most providers do not routinely screen their patients for suicidality or associated risk factors.

Most of what is known pertains to adolescent suicide; however, with regard to child suicide, the primary risk factor for girls is depression, second only to previous suicide attempts. For boys, previous suicide attempts is the primary risk factor for suicide, followed by depression, disruptive behavior, and substance abuse.

History and Physical Assessment

History

Suicide assessment should be performed on all adolescents as part of their routine wellness exams, and on all youth with the following problems:

- Vegetative symptoms of depression that are relatively uncommon in adolescents
- Somatic complaints
- Acting out behaviors
- Substance abuse
- Running away from home
- Decreased concentration, academic difficulty
- Unusual boredom

Assess for risk factors:

- Severe depression accompanied by a recent romantic breakup or assault (highest risk for attempts)
- Previous attempt
- Suicide of family member or close friend
- History of abuse, neglect, or psychiatric hospitalization
- Substance abuse
- Preoccupation with death themes, such as in music, art, films, or television shows
- Gives away valued possessions
- Makes statements like, "You won't have to worry about me anymore."
- Talks about death, especially own
- Reckless or antisocial behavior
- Rapid change in school performance
- Sudden cheerfulness after being depressed
- Dramatic changes in everyday behaviors, such as sleeping and eating

- Chain smoking
- Sense of worthlessness or hopelessness

Explore suicidal ideation:

- Ask if they ever thought of hurting or killing themselves (hurting is different than killing).
- If the answer is yes, ask when they thought of killing themselves.
- Ask how they planned to kill themselves.
- Ask if they ever tried to kill themselves before and if they received help that time.
- Ask if they believe that they have any other options beside suicide to resolve their problems.

Children/adolescents who verbalize planned, lethal means to commit suicide and who feel that they do not have any other options are at extreme risk of carrying out their plan, especially if they have attempted it in the past.

Physical Examination

- Assess for signs of underlying medical disorders.
- Inspect for signs of self-abusive behaviors (unusual scars, death-themed body art).

Diagnostic Testing

The U.S. Preventive Services Task Force (USPSTF, 2004) found no evidence that screening for suicide risk reduces suicide attempts or mortality and that there is limited evidence on the accuracy of screening tools to identify suicide risk in the primary care setting, including tools to identify those at high risk. As a result, the USPSTF could not determine the balance of benefits and harms of screening for suicide risk in the primary care setting.

INTERVENTION

Suicidal youth should be referred for appropriate evaluation and treatment. Those who verbalize significant ideation or other high risk factors should be transferred to mental health immediately.

PREVENTION/PATIENT TEACHING

Primary Prevention

Promote overall mental health among school-aged children by reducing early risk factors for depression, substance abuse, and aggressive behaviors and building resiliency. Youths will also benefit from an overall enhancement of academic performance and a reduction in peer and family conflict.

Secondary Prevention

There are many paths to suicide, thus prevention must address psychological, biological, and social factors if it is to be effective. Collaboration across a broad array of agencies, institutions, and groups—from schools to faith-based organizations to health care associations—is a way to ensure that prevention efforts are comprehensive. Collaboration can also generate greater and more effective attention to suicide prevention than can these groups working alone.

One way to prevent youth suicide is to identify youth at risk and to engage them in treatments that are effective in reducing the personal and situational factors associated with suicidal behavior, such as depressed mood, hopelessness, helplessness, low academic achievement, alcohol and other drug abuse, among others. Another way to prevent youth suicide is to promote and support the presence of protective factors, including such tools as learning skills in problem solving, conflict resolution, and nonviolent handling of disputes.

Tertiary Prevention

Assure that suicidal youth have access to adequate mental health and substance abuse treatment programs that can decrease suicidality and its underlying factors.

RESOURCES

CDC Youth Suicide Prevention Programs: www.cdc.gov/ncipc/pub-res/youthsui.htm
National Association of School Psychologists: Suicide Prevention: http://www.nasponline.org/resources/crisis_safety/suicideprevention.aspx
National Youth Violence Prevention Resource Center: Suicide: www.safeyouth.org/scripts/topics/suicide.asp
School-Based Youth Suicide Prevention Guide: http://theguide.fmhi.usf.edu

REFERENCES

Centers for Disease Control and Prevention. (2007). Suicide trends among youths and young adults aged 10–24 years—United States, 1990–2004. *Morbidity and Mortality Weekly Report, 56*(35), 905–906.

Fordwood, S., Asarnow, D., Huizar, D., & Reise, S. (2007). Suicide attempts among depressed adolescents in primary care. *Journal of Clinical Child and Adolescent Psychology, 36*(3), 392–404.

Horowitz, L., Wang, P., Koocher, G., Burr, B., Smith, M., Klavon, S., et al. (2001). Detecting suicide risk in a pediatric emergency department: Development of a brief screening tool. *Pediatrics, 107,* 1133–1137.

Pennsylvania Youth Suicide Prevention Plan. (n.d.). Retrieved from www.sap.state.pa.us/uploadedfiles/PA%20Youth%20Suicide%20Prevention%20Plan%20Final.pdf

U.S. Preventive Services Task Force (USPSTF). (2004). *Screening for suicide risk: Recommendation and rationale.* Retrieved from www.ahrq.gov/clinic/3rduspstf/suicide/suiciderr.htm

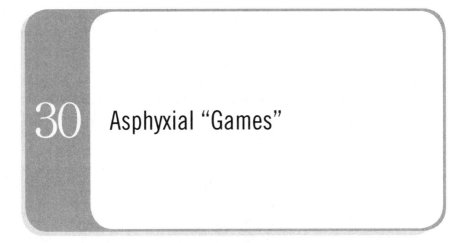

30 Asphyxial "Games"

DEFINITION

Asphyxial activities involve strangulation and are known by various names such as "the choking game" and "autoerotic asphyxia." They are not a new phenomena. However, there has been an increase in lethality due to these activities that has been introduced by the increased use of ligatures and "playing" the game alone. Many young people see these games as a way to get high without drugs.

Various techniques are used to obtain the desired effect, but the general goals are strangulation and self-induced hypoxia.

- *Strangulation* restricts the blood flow to the brain through compression of the carotid arteries. The participant achieves this by either pressing the thumbs against the arteries on both sides of the neck simultaneously or by the use of a ligature or constricting band.

- *Self-induced hypocapnia* requires hyperventilation causing light-headedness or dizziness, then followed by a breath-hold. This alone causes a blackout, but often a number of other actions are used for enhancement, such as a bear hug given from behind or pressure applied to the chest by another person.

377

The *choking game* refers to self-strangulation or strangulation by another person. It is performed alone, in pairs, or in groups. The hands or a ligature are used to produce a euphoric state caused by cerebral hypoxia. Some versions of this "game" involve breath holding and/or compression of the abdomen or thorax. The object is to release the pressure just before loss of consciousness. Unfortunately, failure to do so can result in death, particularly when the activity is performed alone using ligatures. There are numerous other names for this activity. Terms usually depend on geographical location and age of the children. Alternate names include airplaning, American dream, blacking out/blackout, California choke, cloud nine, dream game, fainting game, flat liner, hang-man, purple dragon, purple hazing, scarf game, something dreaming game, space cowboy, space monkey, suffocation roulette, pass-out game, and tap-out.

Autoerotic asphyxia involves choking oneself during sexual stimulation to heighten sexual pleasure. Sometimes referred to as scarfing, bagging, or breath play, autoerotic asphyxia may involve elaborate bindings, sophisticated escape mechanisms, sexual images, or cross-dressing, although these are said to be more common in adults than adolescents. Death can occur if loss of consciousness leads to inability to reverse or stop the means of strangulation. Autoerotic death is usually associated with a constrictive cervical ligature tied to other parts of the victim's body or to an inanimate object such as a door. Other modalities include ligature around the thorax or abdomen, plastic bags covering the face, electrical current, inhalation of a toxic gas or chemicals, or partial or total submersion, known as *aquaerotic asphyxiation.* Sexual asphyxia can also be practiced as part of a consensual sadomasochistic activity between two or more people, and can still result in fatality.

Persistent autoerotic asphyxia is classified as a Paraphilia Not Otherwise Specified in the *Diagnostic and Statistical Manual of Mental Disorders* (American Psychiatric Association, 2000). *Hypoxyphilia* or *asphyxiophilia* is a form of sexual masochism that involves sexual arousal by oxygen deprivation via strangulation, chest compression, plastic bag, mask, or chemicals (typically a volatile nitrate). *Paraphilias* are disorders characterized by recurrent, intense sexually arousing fantasies, sexual urges, or behaviors that generally involve nonhuman objects, the suffering or humiliation of oneself or one's partner, or children or other nonconsenting persons, over a period of at least 6 months.

Participants of asphyxia activities are at risk for short-term memory loss, hemorrhage, and retinal damage, as well as head injuries from falling when unconscious, stroke, seizures, permanent brain damage, coma, and death. Death can be caused by prolonged asphyxia or nerve pressure that causes the heart to stop.

PREVALENCE

Choking Game

In a study of 8 middle and high schools in Texas (6) and Ontario (2) by Cannon and associates (n.d.), results revealed that of 2,504 respondents with a mean age of 13.7 years (*SD* 2.2), 68% of children had heard about the game, 45% knew somebody who played it, and 6.6% had tried it. Forty percent of children perceived no risk. According to the Centers for Disease Control and Prevention's Injury Center (2008), at least 82 children and adolescents have died as a result of playing "the choking game" since 1995. These children were aged 6 through 19, with a peak at 13.3 years. Eighty-seven percent were male. The majority of these deaths occurred when the children were playing alone.

Autoerotic Asphyxia

Most participants are older adolescent and adult males under age 30. The number of deaths from autoerotic asphyxia is unknown since it is most often practiced in secrecy and solitude. Most cases become apparent when the results are fatal. However, approximately 500 to 1,000 autoerotic fatalities are reported each year in the United States and Canada. Adolescents at risk are especially vulnerable to a fatal outcome because they often do not understand the risks associated with this behavior.

ETIOLOGY

Asphyxia activities involve cutting off the oxygen supply to the brain causing a euphoric rush, or high, as the blood rushes to the brain once the oxygen flow is resumed. Cutting off blood flow to the brain (the first high) and then allowing it to resume in a rush (the second high) are perceived by some as pleasurable. Youth do it for the euphoric rush, sexual pleasure, as a dare, or as a bullying tactic. Some youths find it amusing to watch others losing consciousness or behaving erratically, while others find the prospect of an altered state of consciousness, the experience of a brownout, or copycatting elements of the film *Flatliners* attractive.

A brownout (also called grey-out) is a transient loss of vision characterized by a perceived dimming of light accompanied by a brown hue and a loss of peripheral vision. The brownout is a precursor to fainting or a blackout and is caused by hypoxia, a loss of blood pressure or restriction of blood flow to the brain. Participants can become unconscious in seconds. Within 3 minutes of continued strangulation, basic functions such as memory, balance, and the central nervous system start to fail, and death occurs shortly thereafter.

Deaths from autoerotic asphyxia often occur when their rescue method/mechanism fails. Loss of consciousness caused by partial asphyxia leads to loss of control over the means of strangulation, resulting in continued asphyxia and death. In some cases, the body is discovered naked surrounded by signs of masturbatory activity and/or sexual paraphernalia, which can include pornography, fetishistic materials, bondage materials, sex toys, and other equipment. However, family members often clean up the death scene to preserve the victim's dignity and/or minimize their own embarrassment. This can lead death investigators to suspect suicide unless they perform a careful history and assessment.

ASSESSMENT

General Principles

Death investigators should consider asphyxia activities when investigating asphyxia deaths, particularly those that appear to be suicide. Health care providers should assess for signs of autoerotic activities in their clients.

History and Physical Assessment

Most children involved in the asphyxial activities are well-adjusted youths with positive family and peer relationships. Health care providers should be cognizant of these activities and discuss it at wellness visits. Asphyxial activities should also be added to the differential diagnosis when assessing headaches, behavior changes, head injuries, or abnormal marks around the neck or neck area in youth.

The following signs indicate that a child may be involved in asphyxia activities:

Discussion of the game or its aliases (for the choking game)

Bloodshot eyes

Marks on the neck

Wearing high-necked shirts, even in warm weather

Frequent, severe headaches

Disorientation after spending time alone

Increased and uncharacteristic irritability or hostility

Ropes, scarves, and belts tied to bedroom furniture or doorknobs or found knotted on the floor

Wear marks on furniture (bunk beds, curtain rods) from previous incidences

The unexplained presence of dog leashes, choke collars, bungee cords, etc.

Petechiae under the skin of the face, especially the eyelids, or the conjunctiva

Health care professionals may become involved in the death investigation of an adolescent who had unknowingly been participating in autoerotic asphyxia. Health care professionals can assist the investigation on determining the manner of death. Hazelwood and colleagues (1981) have developed five criteria for determining an autoerotic death:

1. Well-defined self-rescue mechanism
2. A solitary activity
3. Employment of sexual fantasy aids
4. Previous autoerotic behavior
5. No suicidal ideation

Protective padding around the neck to prevent ligature marks and a distinct release mechanism may confirm the accidental and "typical" nature of this activity. However, these findings may be lacking at the scene. Investigators should also consider gender differences when evaluating the scene, and realize that most of what is known about autoerotic asphyxia is known about adult victims. Review of the literature (Hazelwood, Burgess, & Groth, 1981) suggests the following characteristics:

■ Male victims are more likely to be involved in atypical autoerotic asphyxia, resorting to gas masks, plastic bags, anesthetic gases, and binding the body with plastic or chains. Males often engage in cross-dressing and enjoy pornographic materials such as videos, magazines, or mirrors to a greater extent during their autoerotic experience.

■ Females are more inclined to use a ligature about the neck, which is controlled by movements of body position. They tend to be found naked without excessive paraphernalia. Female autoerotic death poses a greater challenge to investigators, usually because of the subtle findings at the scene, which may create an appearance of suicide. This subtleness may suggest that women are more cautious in their secretive behavior, or that their deaths may be misinterpreted as sexual homicides if the female utilized elaborate bondage mechanisms during the activity.

INTERVENTION

Intervention focuses on consequences of the asphyxia injuries and on preventative teaching. Adolescents who participate in autoerotic asphyxia are usually experimenting and have few if any paraphilic behaviors. Thus, adolescents suspected of having paraphilic behavior should be referred to an appropriate therapist. Most persons with paraphilias have multiple paraphilias, and asphyxiophilia can be deadly.

PREVENTION/PATIENT TEACHING

Research is not available on the best strategies to prevent asphyxia activities. Parents, educators, and health care providers should be made aware of this public health threat and the warning signs that children and adolescents may be involved in asphyxial games.

RESOURCES

Butler County Drug and Alcohol Program Fact Sheet: The Choking Game: www.co. butler.pa.us/butler/lib/butler/drugalc/FS_Choking_Game.pdf
Centers for Disease Control and Prevention: www.cdc.gov/ncipc/duip/research/chok ing_game.htm (Contains podcast on Choking Game)
The Choking Game: http://www.chokinggame.net

REFERENCES

American Psychiatric Association. (2000). *Diagnostic and statistical manual of mental disorders* (4th ed., text rev.). Washington, DC: Author.

Cannon, W., Macnab, A., Deevske, M., Gagnon, F., Jain, R., & Thanboo, A. (n.d.) *The choking game: Risk-taking behavior in children and adolescents.* Injury Research and Prevention Unit. Retrieved from www.injuryresearch.bc.ca/admin/DocUpload/ 3_20081104_220324Wendy%20Cannon%20-%20Abstract.pdf

Centers for Disease Control and Prevention. (2008). Unintentional strangulation deaths from the "choking game" among youths aged 6–19 years—United States, 1995–2007. *Morbidity and Mortality Weekly Report, 57,* 141–144.

Hazelwood, R., Burgess, A., & Groth, A. (1981). Death during dangerous autoerotic practice. *Social Science Medicine, 15E,* 129–133.

Macnab, A., Deevska, M., Gagnon, F., Cannon, W., & Andrew, T. (2009). Asphyxial games or "the choking game": A potentially fatal risk behavior. *Injury Prevention, 15,* 45–49.

Shields, L., Hunsaker, D., Hunsaker, J., Wetli, C., Hutchins, K., & Holmes, R. (2005). Atypical autoerotic death: Part II. *American Journal of Forensic Medicine and Pathology, 26*(1), 53–62.

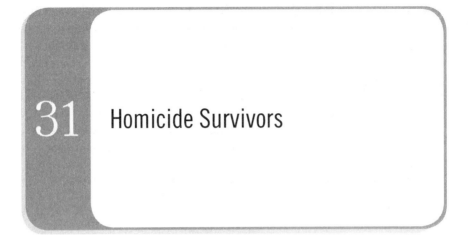

31 Homicide Survivors

DEFINITION

Losing a family member to homicide is one of the most traumatic experiences that a person can have. There is no way to prepare for this tragic event, which leaves tremendous pain and upheaval in its wake. The impact crosses all cultures, races, and genders. Homicide grief experts estimate that there are 7 to 10 close relatives for each victim, and this does not count significant others, friends, neighbors, and co-workers (Redmond, 1989).

Those left behind after homicide are called *homicide survivors*. No amount of justice, restitution, prayer, or compassion will bring their loved one back. However, health care professionals need to assist these survivors in moving through the grieving process so that they do not succumb to complications.

When a person is murdered, the death is sudden, violent, final, and completely incomprehensible. Shared plans and dreams are suddenly shattered and no longer possible. The loss will be grieved in different ways by all those who felt close to the victim, and grief reactions may be manifested long after the incident. Family members may have had a conflicted relationship with the victim, and the death means that these issues or bad feelings will remain unresolved, leaving the survivor with the additional loss of hope that things could have been worked out while the victim lived. The turmoil and shock is manifested by an array of emotional reactions to trauma, including shock, anger, grief, and guilt. Homicide survivors often experience financial hardship due to expenses related to planning funerals, medical fees, and mental health counseling. They may have feelings of loss of self, helplessness, loss of control, loss of religion, and loss of safety and security, because homicide leaves survivors feeling victimized physically, socially, and spiritually. This chapter focuses on parents who have lost a child to homicide and children who have lost a parent to homicide.

ETIOLOGY

The concept of "stages of grief" is no longer accepted; however, grief reactions and the tasks of grieving have been identified. Homicide survivors may also experience symptoms of posttraumatic stress disorder (PTSD). Grief usually follows any loss. The violence, suddenness, unexpectedness, and sometimes randomness of the death create anger, self-blame, and guilt that may place family members at risk for what has been termed "complicated mourning."

Grief Reactions

Redmond (1989) described factors that may affect the grieving process for homicide survivors: the ages of the survivor and the victim at the time of the homicide; the survivors' physical and/or emotional state before the murder; their prior history of trauma; the way in which their loved one died; and whether or not the survivor has, and can make use of, social support systems. Social and cultural factors can also have great impact on the grieving process.

Initially homicide survivors may experience shock and disbelief, numbness, changes in appetite or sleeping patterns, difficulty concentrating, confusion, anger, fear, and anxiety. In cases where family members have not been able to view the deceased's body (either because it was not permitted or they felt unable to do so), it is often difficult for them to accept the reality of the death. Thus, some urge that family members be permitted to go through this viewing process, as painful as it may be at the time. Homicide survivors sometimes feel like the whole world has stopped, and they cannot understand how everyone else is able to go on about their daily routine.

Later reactions usually include feelings of isolation, helplessness, fear and vulnerability, guilt or self-blame, nightmares, and a desire for revenge. They may experience heightened anxiety or phobic reactions. Their anguish may seem intense and sometimes overwhelming. Some describe a physical pain (lump in the throat) that they could feel for several years after the murder.

It is not unusual for homicide survivors to have tremendous feelings of rage toward the perpetrator, and some experience anger toward the victim for getting killed. Depression and hopelessness can lead some to feel that they will never be happy again. Some may experience suicidal ideation, which warrants immediate attention.

Survivors may find themselves suddenly crying over their loss years after the event. These feelings reflect the depth of the pain of the loss. Many say that they know they are doing better when they begin to have more good days than bad days.

Tasks of Grieving

Worden (1991) described four "tasks" of grieving: accepting the reality of the loss; feeling the grief; adjusting to a life in which the deceased is no longer present; and emotionally relocating the deceased so that life can go on.

First task. The survivor acknowledges and accepts the reality that the loved one is dead. Some survivors often report a sense that they will still see the deceased; others report feeling compelled to follow someone who looked like the deceased. It is difficult for homicide survivors who have not viewed the body to know that their loved one is really dead.

Second task. Survivors must acknowledge and experience the physical and/or emotional pain associated with losing their loved one. This is a difficult task, even under the most supportive of circumstances. Homicide survivors may have to put their feelings on hold through court hearings, trials, and numerous appeals. However, no matter how quickly the pain is put aside, the survivors must experience these feelings or they may carry the pain of the loss for the rest of their lives.

Third task. Survivors must adjust to life without the deceased. They must begin to make personal or lifestyle changes that might take them in a very different direction than that planned while their loved one was still alive. Survivors may feel some guilt around these decisions and may feel they are being disloyal to the deceased; however, it is important for survivors to recognize and come to terms with these reactions and feelings.

Last task. Survivors must somehow find a place for their loved one within their emotional life and still realize that their own lives can and do go on.

Posttraumatic Stress Reactions

Families of homicide victims may be at risk for developing posttraumatic stress disorder (PTSD). When a family member is murdered, the survivors often react with intense feelings of helplessness, fear, and horror. PTSD in parents is described in the next section, while traumatic stress disorders of childhood are found in Chapter 14, "Psychological Effects of Victimization."

PARENTS WHO LOSE THEIR CHILD TO HOMICIDE

Parents may find that they reexperience feelings of loss many years later, such as when they see friends of their murdered child graduate from high school or college, get a job, or start a family.

Parents may have believed that, in the natural order of life, the older generation should die first; if so, they may have great difficulty with the fact that their young or grown children were killed while they themselves still live, thus violating this expectation.

Compassionate Friends notes that there are several unique issues that may complicate the grief process for the parents and family left behind. These may include:

- The child's body may be evidence, and the investigation and autopsy may cause a lengthy delay in the release of the child's body to the parents.

- The child's body may not be found.

- The child's body may not be viewable.

- The family may be viewed as suspects, creating a revictimization of those very survivors feeling the most acute pain.

- The child may have been killed by one of the family members, possibly one of the parents.

- Information on new developments may come slowly, and sometimes weeks and months may pass without contact unless initiated by the family.

- If the child was murdered in another country, the family may be forced to deal with that country's law enforcement and legal system. They may also need to deal with language and communication barriers and untold costly and frustrating trips.

- The child may become dehumanized as the police, the press, prosecutors, and others refer to "the victim," "the body," and "the deceased."

- The perpetrator may never be caught or may choose suicide or death rather than capture.

- The perpetrator may go free for any number of reasons or receive a sentence far lighter than the family expected.

- The child may be blamed by some for contributing to the murder.

- The media may take away any hopes of privacy the family may normally value.

Posttraumatic stress disorder (PTSD) often presents in primary and community care, but goes unrecognized. Failure to identify and treat PTSD has adverse effects on client health since PTSD is associated with increased health complaints, health services utilization, morbidity, and mortality. Persons with PTSD have persistent frightening thoughts and memories of the incident and feel emotionally numb, especially with people they were once close to. They may experience sleep disturbances, feel numb or detached, or be easily startled.

The American Psychiatric Association (APA, 2000) revised the diagnostic criteria for PTSD in the *DSM–IV–TR*. The diagnostic criteria include a history of exposure to a traumatic event meeting two criteria and symptoms from each of three symptom clusters: intrusive recollections, avoidant/numbing symptoms, and hyperarousal symptoms. A fifth criterion concerns duration of symptoms and a sixth assesses functioning. The stressor criterion requires that the person experienced, witnessed, or was confronted with an event(s) that involve actual or threatened death or serious injury to oneself or others and the person's response involved intense fear, helplessness, or horror.

The person must have at least one intrusive recollection criterion: recurrent and intrusive distressing recollections of the event, including images, thoughts, or perceptions; recurrent distressing dreams of the event; acting or feeling as if the traumatic event were recurring, including a sense of reliving the experience, illusions, hallucinations, or dissociative flashback; intense psychological distress at exposure to cues that symbolize or resemble an aspect of the traumatic event; or physiologic reaction when exposed to cues that symbolize or resemble an aspect of the traumatic event.

The person must exhibit at least three of the following avoidant/ numbing criteria: efforts to avoid thoughts, feelings, or conversations associated with the trauma; efforts to avoid activities, places, or people that arouse recollections of the trauma; inability to recall an important aspect of the trauma; markedly diminished interest or participation in significant activities; feeling of detachment or estrangement from others; restricted range of affect; and/or a sense of foreshortened future. The person must exhibit at least two of the following hyperarousal criteria: difficulty falling or staying asleep; irritability or outbursts of anger; difficulty concentrating; hypervigilance; and/or exaggerated startle response. The duration of the symptom criteria must be more than 1 month, and the disturbance must cause clinically significant distress or impairment in social, occupational, or other important areas of functioning.

The National Center for PTSD provides links to a number of *PTSD screening tools* (www.ptsd.va.gov/professional/pages/assessments/list-screening-instruments.asp). This site includes training resources as well as information on multiple assessment instruments used to measure trauma exposure and PTSD. The information for each measure includes descriptions, references, contacts, and sample items. There are also charts that list the instruments by category to help compare various measures and select the one most suitable for your practice. Screening tools include:

Primary Care PTSD Screen (PC-PTSD). The PC-PTSD is a 4-item screen designed for use in primary care and other medical settings. It is currently used to screen for PTSD in veterans at the VA. The screen includes an introductory sentence to cue respondents to traumatic events, and, in most circumstances, its results should be considered "positive" if a client answers "yes" to any 3 items. Those screening positive should then be assessed with a structured interview for PTSD. This screening tool may be found at Prins et al. (2003).

Trauma Screening Questionnaire (TSQ). The TSQ is a 10-item symptom screen that was designed for use with survivors of all types of traumatic stress. The TSQ is based on items from the PTSD Symptom Scale—Self Report and has 5 reexperiencing items and 5 arousal items. Respondents are asked to endorse those items that they have experienced at least twice in the past week. The screen is considered "positive" when at least 6 items were endorsed, but is recommended to be conducted 3–4 weeks posttrauma to allow for normal recovery processes to take place. Those screening positive should then be assessed with a structured interview for PTSD. This screening tool is available at Brewin et al. (2002).

Short Screening Scale for PTSD. The Short Screening Scale for PTSD is a 7-item screen designed for all trauma survivors, but was empirically derived in the context of an epidemiological study of PTSD in an urban area of the United States. The screen was designed to be administered after an assessment of trauma exposure and consists of 5 avoidance items and 2 hyperarousal items. The screen is scored by adding the number of "yes" responses, and the suggested cutoff is 4. Those screening positive should then be assessed with a structured interview for PTSD (see Breslau, Peterson, Kessler, & Schultz, 1999).

Interventions for Parents

When working with parents who lose a child to homicide, understand that they, too, are victims with needs. The Office for Victims of Crime (OVC) states that there are three critical needs for all victims:

1. *Victims need to feel safe.* People usually feel helpless, vulnerable, and frightened by victimization. When working with victims, be sure to follow these guidelines:

- Introduce yourself by name and title and briefly explain your role.
- Ensure privacy during your interview. Assure confidentiality when possible (extent of confidentiality depends on your role).
- Reassure victims of their safety. Pay attention to your own words, posture, mannerisms, and tone of voice. Use body language to show concern, such as nodding your head, using natural eye contact,

placing yourself at the victim's level, keeping an open stance, and speaking in a calm, sympathetic voice. Tell victims that they are safe and that you are there for them.

■ Ask victims to tell you in just a sentence or two what happened, and ask if they have any physical injuries. Tend to medical needs first.

■ Offer to contact a family member, friend, victim advocate, or crisis counselor.

■ Ask simple questions to allow victims to make decisions, assert themselves, and regain control over their lives, such as "How would you like me to address you?"

■ Ask victims if they have any special concerns or needs.

■ Develop a safety plan before leaving them. Pull together personal or professional support for the victims. Give victims a pamphlet listing resources available for help or information, including contact information for local crisis intervention centers and support groups; the prosecutor's office and the victimwitness assistance office; the state victim compensation/assistance office; and other nationwide services, including toll-free hotlines and Web addresses.

■ Give them your name and information on how to reach you in writing. Encourage them to contact you if they have any questions or if you can be of further help.

2. *Victims need to express their emotions.* Victims need to express their emotions and tell their story after the trauma. They need to have their feelings accepted and have their story heard by a nonjudgmental listener. They may feel fear, self-blame, anger, shame, sadness, or denial, and most will say, "I don't believe this happened to me." Some may have a reaction formation and act opposite to how they feel, such as laughter instead of crying. Some feel rage at the sudden, unpredictable, and uncontrollable threat to their safety or lives, and this rage can even be directed at the professionals who are trying to help them. When working with victims, be sure to follow these guidelines:

■ Listen. Show that you are actively listening to victims through your facial expressions, body language, and comments such as "Take your time; I'm listening" and "We can take a break if you like. I'm in no hurry."

■ Notice victims' body language, to help you understand and respond to what they are feeling as well as to what they are saying.

- Assure victims that their emotional reactions are not uncommon. Sympathize with the victims by saying things such as: "You've been through something very frightening. I'm sorry."
- Counter self-blame by victims by saying things such as, "You didn't do anything wrong. This was not your fault."
- Ask open-ended questions.
- Avoid interrupting victims while they are telling their story.
- Repeat or rephrase what you think you heard the victims say for validation.

3. *Victims need to know "what comes next" after their victimization.* Victims usually have concerns about their role in the criminal investigation and legal proceedings. They may also be concerned about payment for health care or property damage. You can help relieve some of their anxiety by telling victims what to expect in the aftermath of the crime and by preparing them for upcoming stressful events and changes in their lives. When working with victims, be sure to follow these guidelines:

- Refer the victim to a victim's advocate who will assist the victim through the investigative and legal proceedings.
- Tell victims about subsequent law enforcement interviews or other kinds of interviews they can expect.
- Discuss the general nature of medical forensic examinations the victim will be asked to undergo and the importance of these examinations for the legal proceedings.
- Counsel victims that lapses of concentration, memory losses, depression, and physical ailments are normal reactions for crime victims. Encourage them to reestablish their normal routines as quickly as possible to help speed their recovery.
- Give victims a listing of resources that are available for help and information, as noted above.
- Ask victims whether they have any questions. Encourage victims to contact you if you can be of further assistance.

When working with parents who lost their child to homicide, health care providers should assess and address the following:

The impact of culture on clients' bereavement processes and the need for culturally appropriate interventions

How family members are grieving

The extent to which family systems and processes are functioning

Presence of PTSD reactions in family members

Coping strategies and whether they are working

Degree of social support and the family's use of it

Adequacy of family communication patterns

Changes in family roles

How the family is coping with external agencies, such as the criminal justice system and the media

The need for spiritual support

The need for referrals

Intervention may be needed at any point in the grief continuum. The traumatic nature of losing a child to homicide warrants at least the suggestion that the parents consult a mental health care professional and/or group that can help them through the grieving process.

Treatment of Acute and Posttraumatic Stress Disorders

The American Psychiatric Association (APA) revised its *Practice Guideline for the Treatment of Patients with Acute Stress Disorder and Posttraumatic Stress Disorder* in March 2009. It noted that increasing research attention has been focused on the assessment and treatment of PTSD since the publication of the 2004 guideline and that much work remains to be done. The treatment of these disorders is beyond the scope of this book; however, health care providers can refer to the APA guidelines at www.psychiatryonline.com/content.aspx?aID=156502.

Victim's Compensation

Families may qualify for victim's compensation. Crime victims often incur a significant number of expenses when victimized, yet most health care professionals are unaware of compensation mechanisms. Conviction of the offender is not required, and victims of crime under state, federal, military, and tribal jurisdiction are eligible to apply for compensation. Eligible crime victims include those who have been physically injured and/or who suffer emotional injury as a result of violence or attempted violence, even though no physical injury resulted. Some states also include family members of deceased victims and other individuals who pay for expenses resulting from a victim's injury or death.

According to the National Association of Crime Victim Compensation Boards, each state's eligibility requirements vary slightly, but victims are generally required to report the crime promptly to law enforcement, usually within 72 hours; file a timely application with the compensation program in the state where the crime occurred, and provide any information requested; cooperate in the investigation and prosecution of the crime; and be innocent of any criminal activity or misconduct leading to the victim's injury or death. Many states require that the application be filed within 1 year from the date of the crime, but some states have shorter or longer periods. Applications can be obtained from the state compensation program, police, prosecutors, or victim service agencies. Most state programs have brochures describing their benefits, requirements, and procedures. Health care providers can refer victims to victim service programs for assistance in completing the application. The application should be submitted to the compensation program as soon as possible, where it will be reviewed to determine eligibility and to decide what costs can be paid. The program will notify the applicant of its decision.

Depending on the state, expenses may be covered if they are not paid for by insurance or by another public benefit program, and if they result directly from the crime. These include medical and hospital care, and dental work to repair injury to teeth; mental health counseling; lost earnings due to crime-related injuries; loss of support for dependents of a deceased victim; and funeral and burial expenses. Expenses that are not covered usually include property loss, theft and damage (unless damage is to eyeglasses, hearing aids, or other medically necessary devices), and expenses paid by other sources, such as any type of public or private health insurance, automobile insurance, disability insurance, or workers compensation. A few states may pay limited amounts for the loss of essential personal property during a violent crime and for cleaning up the crime scene.

CHILDREN WHO LOSE A PARENT TO HOMICIDE

Children are at significant risk to develop posttraumatic stress disorder. Accompanying symptoms may be both disturbing and disruptive to their daily routines and can impact the trajectory of their growth and development. Disruption may occur relative to established developmental tasks surrounding issues of understanding moral reasoning, the consequences of one's actions, and the need for family permanence.

A child's ability to cope is related to a number of factors, including cognitive development.

Thus, younger children have a more restricted range of coping skills than older ones and may possess less flexibility and adaptability to traumatic events. Exposure to homicide is uniquely difficult for children because they have yet to navigate the many developmental tasks necessary to function autonomously. Children are at greater risk for traumatic effects because they do not have an established repertoire of coping behaviors. Other factors include children's appraisal of the threat; the intrapsychic meaning they attribute to the event; their emotional means of coping; their capacity to tolerate strong affects; and their ability to adjust to other changes in their lives, including loss and grieving.

Children may feel angry with themselves for not preventing the death or for things left unsaid to loved ones when they were still alive. This "survivors' guilt" is not uncommon and is problematic. There can be confusion and attempts to comprehend that one human could purposefully take the life of another human, especially when that loved one was a family member. Children may express their feelings through their behaviors, including depression, withdrawal or depression, aggression, somatic complaints, and other physical symptoms.

Children experience reactions to trauma and loss for any type of death. However, when death occurs from sudden and unexpected circumstances, especially interpersonal violence and homicide, the reactions are more severe, exaggerated, and complicated. Grief and trauma can become intertwined and can result in posttraumatic stress disorder. (See Chapter 14, "Psychological Effects of Victimization.")

Interventions

Child survivors may have unique circumstances in their grieving processes that need to be addressed in the healing process. They may benefit from support groups, which can provide an outlet for their grief, but the groups should be specific for this type of trauma. They may benefit from an open and safe forum where they can ask questions and express their feelings as they resolve their grief. Education and grief work, including journal writing, drawing, poetry, music, and art, can provide various ways for youths to express the effects of the unexpected changes on their lives. Adolescents view being different from their peers as a threat to their identity; thus, providing a place in which adolescents can socialize with other homicide survivors can minimize the feeling of being "different."

Given the impact of losing a parent to homicide and the possible long-term complications, health care providers should refer children for mental health evaluation and treatment. Since the child is a secondary victim of the event, health care providers can contact their children's advocacy center for referral sources.

RESOURCES

Compassionate Friends: www.compassionatefriends.org
National Center for Victims of Crime: Homicide Survivors: www.ncvc.org/ncvc/main.as
px?dbName=DocumentViewer&DocumentID=32358#1
Parents of Murdered Children: http://www.pomc.com

REFERENCES

American Psychiatric Association. (2000). *Diagnostic and statistical manual of mental disorders* (4th ed., text rev.). Washington, DC: Author.

Breslau, N., Peterson, E. L., Kessler, R. C., & Schultz, L. R. (1999). Short Screening Scale for *DSM–IV* Post-Traumatic Stress Disorder. *American Journal of Psychiatry, 156,* 908–911. Retrieved from http://ajp.psychiatryonline.org/cgi/content/full/156/6/908

Brewin, C. R., Rose, S., Andrews, B., Green, J., Tata, P., McEvedy, C., et al. (2002). Brief Screening Instrument for Post-Traumatic Stress Disorder. *British Journal of Psychiatry, 181,* 158–162. Retrieved from http://bjp.rcpsych.org/cgi/content/full/181/2/158

Clements, P., Faulkner, M., & Manno, M. (2003). Family-member homicide: A grave situation for children. *Topics in Advanced Practice Nursing eJournal.* Retrieved from www.medscape.com/viewarticle/458064

Prins, A., Ouimette, P., Kimerling, R., Cameron, R. P., Hugelshofer, D. S., Shaw-Hegwer, J., et al. (2003). The Primary Care PTSD Screen (PC-PTSD): Development and operating characteristics. *Primary Care Psychiatry, 9,* 9–14. Retrieved from www.ptsd. va.gov/professional/articles/article-pdf/id26676.pdf

Redmond, L. (1989). *Surviving: When someone you love was murdered.* Clearwater, FL: Psychological Consultation and Education Services.

Vigil, G., & Clements, P. (2003). Child and adolescent homicide survivors: Complicated grief and altered worldviews. *Journal of Psychosocial Nursing and Mental Health Services, 41*(1), 30–41.

Worden, J. W. (1991). *Grief counseling and grief therapy.* New York: Springer Publishing.

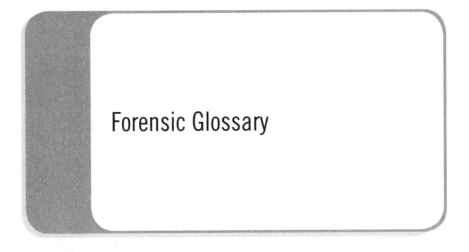

Forensic Glossary

Actuarial Risk Assessment: A risk assessment based upon specific factors that have been researched and demonstrated to be statistically significant in the prediction of risk.

Adjudication: The process for determining a youth's guilt of an offense and the actual finding of involvement.

Adjudicatory Hearing: The phase of a juvenile case in which a judge receives and weighs evidence before deciding whether the youth is responsible for the offense.

Aftercare/Reentry: Activities and tasks that prepare adjudicated youth for reentry into the specific communities to which they will return. Aftercare/Reentry establishes the necessary arrangements with a range of public and private sector organizations and individuals in the community that can address known risk and protective factors,

---

The glossary was compiled from Center for Sex Offender Management Glossary of Terms Used in the Management and Treatment of Sexual Offenders: http://www.csom.org/pubs/glossary.pdf; Garner, B. (2004). *Black's law dictionary* (8th ed.). St. Paul, MN: Thomas West Group; and Merriam-Webster Online: http://www.merriam-webster.com.

and it ensures the delivery of prescribed services and supervision in the community.

Appeal: A formal request to a superior (appellate) court or administrative agency to review the decision of an inferior court (trial or lower appellate) or administrative agency.

Arraignment: An early step in the criminal process in which a defendant is formally charged with an offense and informed of his or her constitutional rights.

Best Interest of the Child: A standard used by child welfare agencies and child welfare courts when determining whether to undertake specific acts regarding a child.

Beyond a Reasonable Doubt: The amount of probability required to find a criminal defendant guilty.

Blunt Force Trauma: Injury caused by force from a blunt object, such as a baseball bat.

Bruise: An injury that causes ruptures of the small underlying vessels with resultant discoloration of tissues but that does not break the skin.

Child Abuse Prevention and Treatment Act (CAPTA): CAPTA was signed into law on January 31, 1974. The Act emphasized multidisciplinary approaches to child abuse and neglect. Codified at 42.

Child Protective Services (CPS): The child welfare department/social service system designed to protect children. Usually the entity that receives and investigates reports of suspected child maltreatment and provides services to children and families to manage past maltreatment and prevent future maltreatment.

Child Welfare and Adoption Assistance Act (Public Law 96–272): A federal law passed in 1980 intended to prevent multiple foster care placements and increase effective permanency planning for children in foster care.

Child Welfare Court: The court that hears child welfare cases, including emergency removal, adjudication, disposition, review and termination of parental rights. Sates have different names for this court, including family court, juvenile court, and dependency court.

Circumstantial Evidence: Evidence of a fact from which another fact can reasonably be inferred.

Clear and Convincing Evidence: An amount of probability less than beyond a reasonable doubt but more than probable cause. It is used in some civil cases, including termination of parental rights cases and sex offender commitment hearings.

Collateral Contacts: Contacts with significant others involved in a case or involved with the offender's life (family, teachers, etc.), to improve the effectiveness and quality of community supervision or for the purpose of completing an evaluation.

Commitment: Placement of a youth under the supervision of the juvenile justice system. Commitment dispositions range from low-risk nonresidential commitment to maximum residential commitment.

Common Law: The system of jurisprudence (the form of law), which developed in England and came to American colonies during colonization. Common law is derived and developed from the decisions of judges instead of statutes or constitutions.

Community Notification: Laws that allow or mandate posting publicly accessible information, or actively informing the public about the identity and other personal information of an adjudicated sex offender.

Community Service: A probation requirement that the youth perform some specific service to the community for a specified period of time.

Competent Intent: The desire to cause an event to happen by someone with the ability to form that intent. Some say a child under age 8 does not have the ability to form competent intent.

Coroner: A jurisdictional official, who is usually elected and whose duty it is to determine the cause and manner of sudden, unexpected, suspicious, or violent deaths. Education requirements vary per jurisdiction.

Coroner's Inquest: An inquiry into the manner and cause of an individual's death, conducted by the Coroner or Deputy Coroner.

Crime Scene: The physical site where a crime may have occurred.

Culpable: Responsible for a wrong or error; accountable and liable.

Custody: Legal right to care and control of a child and the duty to provide that child's food, clothing, shelter, ordinary medical care, education, and discipline. Parents are the natural custodians of their child, but a court may grant temporary custody to someone other than a parent, pending further action or review by the court.

Defendant: In criminal proceedings, the person accused of a crime and synonymous with accused. In civil proceedings, the party responding to the complaint brought by the plaintiff.

Delinquent Act: Any act committed by a juvenile that would be a criminal violation of a federal or state law or local ordinance if committed by an adult. The juvenile age range varies per state.

Delinquent Juvenile: A young person who has been found responsible by a juvenile court judge for having committed a delinquent act and who has been adjudicated delinquent. This is equivalent to an adult being found guilty of a criminal offense.

Dependency Court: Specialized civil court designated to hear matters pertaining to child abuse/neglect.

Detention: Confinement of a juvenile in a secure facility by the state or local authorities. The term is also for home confinement.

Direct Evidence: Evidence that is presented in the testimony of a witness who has direct knowledge of the fact being proved.

Disposition: In Child Protective Services, the finding of the validity of a report of child maltreatment that is made by the caseworker after investigation. Disposition categories vary from state to state.

Disposition Hearing: A court hearing that determines whether a child needs or requires the court's assistance, guidance, treatment, or rehabilitation, and, if so, the nature of that assistance, guidance, treatment, or rehabilitation.

Disposition Review: A hearing in which the court reviews the child's case to ensure that a permanency plan is being implemented in the child's best interest.

Dispositional Hearing: A juvenile case hearing at which the court determines the appropriate sanctions, such as probation, or commitment to the custody of the agency responsible for juvenile justice. It is analogous to a sentencing hearing in criminal court.

Diversion: A less formal or nonjudicial handling of a delinquency case.

Due Process of Law: Peoples' rights under the 5th and 14th Amendments to the U.S. Constitution to procedural and substantive fairness in situations in which the government would deprive the person of life, liberty, or property.

Electronic Monitoring: An automated method of determining compliance with community supervision restrictions through the use of electronic devices.

Evidence: Something that proves or disprove fact.

Examination: The questioning of a witness.

Expungement: Destruction of records. Expungement may be ordered by a court after a specified number of years or when the juvenile, parent, or defendant applies for expungement and shows that his or her conduct has improved. Expungement also means the removal from the Central Registry of certain reports of abuse or neglect.

Family Court: Court designated to hear matters pertaining to family law, such as child custody cases.

Family Reunification: The process of reintroducing a youth back into the home after removal, preferably as part of the youth's treatment program.

Felony: Typically, any criminal offence for which the penalty is imprisonment for more than 1 year. Examples include murder, rape, and armed robbery (usually).

Felony Murder: The unintentional killing of a human being during the commission of a felony, such as an armed robbery.

Forensic Pathologist: A pathologist (physician) with training in criminal pathology.

Foster Care: Placement for children under dependency court jurisdiction.

Graduated Sanctions: A set of integrated intervention strategies designed to enhance accountability, ensure public safety, and reduce recidivism by preventing future delinquent behavior.

Guardian: An adult who is legally responsible for a child.

Guardian ad Litem: A person who has the legal authority (and the corresponding duty) to care for the personal and property interests of another person (or child), called a ward.

Guilty: Responsible for a crime or a civil wrong.

Hearsay: Unverified information from a third party. Hearsay evidence is usually excluded from court proceedings because it is considered unreliable and because the person making the original statement cannot be cross-examined.

Homicide: Death at the hands of another.

Hospital Shopping: The use of different medical facilities so that each individual medical facility's sole contact with the person or family is a single presenting injury.

Incarceration: Confinement in a secure correctional facility.

Incest: Sexual intercourse between persons who are closely related. This also includes other relatives, stepchildren, and children of common-law marriages.

Independent Living: A permanent placement plan for a child in foster care in which the goal is self-sufficiency after discharge from foster care.

Indian Child Welfare Act (ICWA): A federal law that specifies the manner in which child welfare agencies and child welfare courts must handle cases involving Native American and Alaska Native Children.

Infanticide: The killing of one or more infants.

Investigation: The process of actively seeking facts. Investigations are typically conducted by law enforcement and/or child protective services in order to determine whether or not an offense was committed, but can also be conducted by death investigators.

Involuntary Manslaughter: Criminally negligent homicide.

Judgment: A court's final decision.

Jurisdiction: An agency's authority over an incident, investigation, and/or prosecution.

Juvenile: A youth who has not yet attained the age at which he or she should be treated as an adult for purposes of criminal law. Under the federal Juvenile Justice Delinquency Prevention Act, a "juvenile" means an individual who is 17 years of age or younger.

Kinship Care (Relative Placement): Residential caregiving provided to children by nonparental relatives.

Laceration: A torn or jagged wound causing a splitting or tearing in the external skin surface that is caused by blunt trauma.

Late Effects: Conditions or outcomes that may occur at any time after an acute intentional or unintentional injury.

Malice Aforethought: The conscious intent to cause death or great bodily harm to another person before committing the offense.

Mandated Agency: Agency designated by state law to receive and investigate reports of suspected child abuse and neglect.

Mandated Reporters: Persons designated by state law who are legally responsible for reporting suspected child abuse and neglect to the mandated agency within their state. Mandated reporters are usually professionals who have frequent contact with children, such as physicians, nurses, school personnel, and social workers.

Manner of Death: The official vital statistics classification: natural, suicide, homicide, accident, and undetermined.

Manslaughter: Unlawful killing of a person without malice aforethought.

Master: A person appointed by a court in certain cases to hear testimony and make reports that, if approved by the court, become the decision of the court. Masters may hear child welfare court cases. Also called referee or commissioner.

Mechanism of Death: The process that causes one or more vital organs or organ systems to fail when a fatal disease, injury, abnormality, or chemical insult occurs in brain function that caused the heart and/ or lungs to stop functioning. Examples include hemorrhage and hypovolemic shock.

Medical Examiner: An official, usually a physician, whose duty it is to investigate sudden, suspicious, or violent death to determine the cause.

Megan's Law: The first amendment to the Jacob Wetterling Crimes Against Children and Sexually Violent Offenders Act. Megan's Law requires states to allow public access to information about sex offenders in the community. This law was named after Megan Kanka, a 7-year-old girl who was raped and murdered by a twice-convicted child molester in her New Jersey neighborhood. Eleven-year-old Jacob Wetterling was abducted from a group of three boys by a masked gunman; to date, he has never been found and his case remains open.

Minimization: An attempt by the offender to downplay the extent and effect of his or her illegal behavior.

Misdemeanor: Criminal offenses that are less severe than felonies and generally punished by jail terms that do not exceed a year or lesser fines.

Murder: The unlawful killing of a human being with malice aforethought.

National Crime Information Center (NCIC): Criminal justice information systems operated by the Federal Bureau of Investigation in Washington, DC.

Natural Cause: Death resulting from inherent, existing conditions, including congenital anomalies, disease, SIDS, and other medical causes.

Negligence: Doing something that a person of ordinary prudence would not do or the failure to do something that a person of ordinary prudence would do, under given circumstances.

Noncontact Offense: Sexual offenses that do not involve physical contact with the victim such as indecent exposure, making obscene phone calls, and "peeping."

Offense: A violation of federal, state, tribal, or municipal law, statute, or ordinance.

Parens Patriae: "Parent of the country." The role of the state as sovereign and the guardian of persons under legal disability. Parens patriae allows the state to investigate possible child abuse and neglect, and to place a child in foster care.

Perjury: Knowingly and willfully giving false testimony under oath.

Perpetrator: Person who commits an act (usually a crime) against another.

Petition: A formal, written request to the court that it do something.

Physical Evidence: Any tangible piece of proof. Physical evidence usually must be authenticated by a witness who testifies to the connection of the evidence (called an exhibit) with other facts of the case.

Plaintiff: In a civil case, the person who files a lawsuit.

Plea Bargain: The negotiation of charges or dispositions in order to avoid trial on the original charge(s) in return for a guilty plea.

Pleadings: Formal allegations of the claim and defenses raised by the parties to the court case.

Preponderance of Evidence: The proof must be more likely than not. The amount of proof required in most civil cases, including child welfare cases (except for termination of parental rights proceedings).

Prima Facie: Evidence that will suffice as proof of the fact at issue until its effect is overcome by other evidence.

Probable Cause: A requisite element of a valid search and seizure or of an arrest, which consists of the existence of facts and circumstances within one's knowledge that are sufficient to warrant the belief that a crime has been committed (in the context of an arrest).

Probation: A court-ordered disposition through which an adjudicated youth is placed under the control, supervision, and care of a probation field staff member in lieu of confinement, as long as the youth meets certain standards of conduct.

Prosecution: The act of pursuing a lawsuit or criminal trial, and the party initiating a criminal suit.

Recidivism: An officially detected recurrence of illegal behavior after a previous adjudication. Detections may include arrests, charges, convictions, child protection reports, and so forth. There is no widely accepted definition of recidivism.

Reintegration: The gradual reentry from a restricted, highly supervised environment to a less structured environment.

Relapse: Complete or nearly complete return to a former problematic or illegal behavior. Distinguished from reoffense in that it involves both illegal and inappropriate events, and from recidivism in that it involves both detected and undetected events.

Relapse Prevention: A cognitive-behavioral intervention model for risk management that considers internal self-management and external supervision in regard to precipitating and perpetuating factors such as risk situations and risk-related cognitions. This treatment program teaches clients to identify chains of risk factors, thinking patterns, and behavioral and cognitive sequences in order to identify and disrupt offense patterns.

Restitution: Repairing harm caused by a behavior. Restitution may be to the victim (apology, small monetary amount) or community (community service).

Restorative Justice: Focuses on the repair of the harm to the victim and the community, as well as the improvement of prosocial competencies of the offender, as a result of a damaging act. Dispositions are focused on restitution and competency development rather than being exclusively punitive.

Reunification: A well-supervised, gradual procedure in which an adolescent sex offender is reintegrated back into the home where children are present.

Risk Assessment: The process of assigning a probability for a future behavior, such as a sexual offense, to an individual.

Sanctions: Penalty, punishment, loss of reward, or coercive intervention connected to a violation of a law or rule as a means of enforcement.

Search Warrant: An order issued by a judge and directing certain law enforcement officers to conduct a search of specified premises for specified things or persons and to bring them before the court. Search warrants are required by the 4th and 14th Amendment to the U.S. Constitution.

Sex Offender Registration: Laws requiring sex offenders to submit and keep current certain personal identifying information, such as photographs and current address for purposes of maintaining a list of registered sex offenders in the community. Sex offender registration laws may or may not apply to adolescents, and different states have different inclusion criteria and provisions for adolescents. Registration may or may not involve public notification or public access depending upon the jurisdiction.

Standard of Proof: An amount of probability necessary for a court to render a decision regarding the evidence presented to it.

Status Offense: Acts that violate the law but only for individuals with juvenile status, such as underage drinking.

Statute: A law passed by a legislative body.

Subpoena: A command to appear at a certain time and place, on a certain date and give testimony on a certain matter.

Summons: A document used to commence a civil action or special processing. A summons is issued by a court to the sheriff (or other designated official), requiring that official to notify the person named that an action has been commenced against the person and that the person is required to appear on the day named and answer the complaint.

Termination of Parental Rights (TPR): A legal process that severs the legal relationship between parents and the child and vests authority in the child welfare agency.

Testimony: Evidence given by a competent witness under oath or affirmation, as distinguished from evidence derived from written or other sources.

Venue: Locality of the court or courts that possess jurisdiction.

Victims of Crime Fund: Money available to serve crime victims through a federal and/or state program.

Voluntary Manslaughter: An intentional killing committed under circumstances that, although they do not justify the homicide, mitigate it.

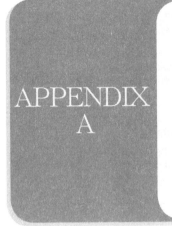

APPENDIX
A

Infant Developmental
Milestones Important for
Sudden Unexplained
Infant Death
Investigations

1 MONTH

Lifts head and chin slightly when lying on stomach on a flat surface.
Keeps hands in fist (closed tightly).
Follows object moved in an arc about 8 inches above face to midline.
Smiles in response to another person.
Responds to noise by startling or crying.
Vocalizes ("eh," "ah").

2 MONTHS

Lifts head (45°) off surface when lying on stomach.
No longer clenches fist all of the time.
Recognizes parents.
Smiles spontaneously.
Makes "cooing" sounds ("ooh," "aah").

3 MONTHS

Lifts head 90° off surface when lying on stomach.
Holds head upright and steady without support when held in sitting position.
Holds hand open at rest.
Grasps (holds onto) rattle placed in hand.
Laughs out loud.

4 TO 5 MONTHS

Raises chest and supports self on out-stretched arms when lying on stomach.
Rolls over from stomach to back and vice versa.
Bears some weight on legs when held upright.
Reaches for objects placed in front of him or her.
Works to get toy by reaching with arm or body.
Turns toward rattling sound.

6 MONTHS

Puts feet in mouth when lying on back.
Sits upright without support (without props) on hard flat surface.
Keeps head level with body when pulled to sitting position when lying on back.
Begins to feeds self.
Turns toward voice.

7 TO 8 MONTHS

Stands holding on to a low table or chair.
Picks up object using raking grasp.
Passes object from one hand to the other.
Imitates sounds and speech.
Says "da," "ma," or vowel-consonant combinations.
Makes razz sound (wet, razzing sound with bubbles coming out mouth).

9 MONTHS

Gets into sitting position from lying, crawling, or standing position.
Pulls self to a standing position from sitting.
Crawls or moves across floor using both legs and arms.
Holds bottle and feeds self using fingers.
Picks up two objects and holds one in each hand.
Says "dada/mama" (not specific).

10 TO 12 MONTHS

Stands without hanging on to anything.
Begins to walk (walks well by 14¾ months).
Bangs two blocks held in hands together.
Uses thumb and finger to pick up small objects.
Plays patty-cake (clap hands).
Indicates what he or she wants.
Combines syllables (e.g., "dadada," "gagaga").
Jabbers or uses unintelligible conversation to self.

Developed from Centers for Disease Control and Prevention Sudden Unexplained Infant Death Investigation Academy Training, and J. Ball and R. Binder, 2005, *Child Health Nursing: Partnering With Children and Families.* Upper Saddle River, NJ: Prentice Hall.

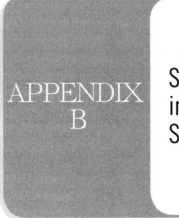

APPENDIX
B

State Age Parameters in the Juvenile Justice System

Table B

STATE	YOUNGEST AGE FOR ORIGINAL JUVENILE COURT JURISDICTION IN DELINQUENCY MATTERS	OLDEST AGE FOR ORIGINAL JUVENILE COURT JURISDICTION IN DELINQUENCY MATTERS	OLDEST AGE OVER WHICH THE JUVENILE COURT MAY RETAIN JURISDICTION FOR DISPOSITION PURPOSES IN DELINQUENCY MATTERS
Alabama	NOT SPECIFIED	17	20
Alaska	NOT SPECIFIED	17	18
Arizona	8	17	20[a]
Arkansas	10	17	20
California	NOT SPECIFIED	17	24
Colorado	10	17	c
Connecticut	NOT SPECIFIED	15	20
District of Columbia	NOT SPECIFIED	17	20
Delaware	NOT SPECIFIED	17	20
Florida	NOT SPECIFIED	17	21
Georgia	NOT SPECIFIED	16	20
Hawaii	NOT SPECIFIED	17	c
Idaho	NOT SPECIFIED	17	20
Illinois	NOT SPECIFIED	16	20
Indiana	NOT SPECIFIED	17	20
Iowa	NOT SPECIFIED	17	18
Kansas	10	17	22
Kentucky	NOT SPECIFIED	17	18
Louisiana	10	16	20
Maine	NOT SPECIFIED	17	20
Maryland	7	17	20
Massachusetts	7	16	20
Michigan	NOT SPECIFIED	16	20
Minnesota	10	17	20
Mississippi	10	17	19
Missouri	NOT SPECIFIED	16	20

Table B

STATE	YOUNGEST AGE FOR ORIGINAL JUVENILE COURT JURISDICTION IN DELINQUENCY MATTERS	OLDEST AGE FOR ORIGINAL JUVENILE COURT JURISDICTION IN DELINQUENCY MATTERS	OLDEST AGE OVER WHICH THE JUVENILE COURT MAY RETAIN JURISDICTION FOR DISPOSITION PURPOSES IN DELINQUENCY MATTERS
Montana	NOT SPECIFIED	17	24
Nebraska	NOT SPECIFIED	17	18
Nevada	NOT SPECIFIED	17	20[b]
New Hampshire	NOT SPECIFIED	16	20
New Jersey	NOT SPECIFIED	17	[c]
New Mexico	NOT SPECIFIED	17	20
New York	7	15	20
North Carolina	6	15	20
North Dakota	NOT SPECIFIED	17	19
Ohio	NOT SPECIFIED	17	20
Oklahoma	NOT SPECIFIED	17	18
Oregon	NOT SPECIFIED	17	24
Pennsylvania	10	17	20
Rhode Island	NOT SPECIFIED	17	20
South Carolina	NOT SPECIFIED	16	20
South Dakota	10	17	20
Tennessee	NOT SPECIFIED	17	18
Texas	10	16	20
Utah	NOT SPECIFIED	17	20
Vermont	10	17	20
Virginia	NOT SPECIFIED	17	20
Washington	NOT SPECIFIED	17	20

(Continued)

Table B

STATE	YOUNGEST AGE FOR ORIGINAL JUVENILE COURT JURISDICTION IN DELINQUENCY MATTERS	OLDEST AGE FOR ORIGINAL JUVENILE COURT JURISDICTION IN DELINQUENCY MATTERS	OLDEST AGE OVER WHICH THE JUVENILE COURT MAY RETAIN JURISDICTION FOR DISPOSITION PURPOSES IN DELINQUENCY MATTERS
West Virginia	NOT SPECIFIED	17	20
Wisconsin	10	16	24
Wyoming	NOT SPECIFIED	17	20

Note. For all states, extended jurisdiction may be restricted to certain offenses or juveniles.
[a]Arizona statute extends jurisdiction through age 20, but a 1979 State Supreme Court decision held that juvenile court jurisdiction terminates at age 18.
[b]Until the full term of the disposition order for sex offenders.
[c]Until the full term of the disposition order.

Developed from *Juvenile Offenders and Victims: 2006 National Report.* Office of Juvenile Justice and Delinquency Prevention. http://ojjdp.ncjrs.org/ojstatbb/nr2006.

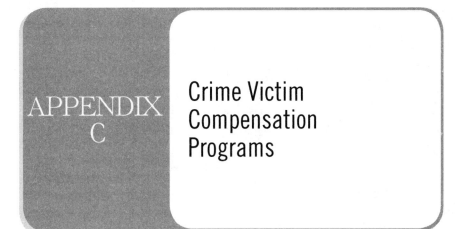

APPENDIX
C

Crime Victim Compensation Programs

National Association of Crime Victim Compensation Boards (NACVCB)
P.O. Box 16003
Alexandria, VA 22302
(703) 313-9500
http://www.nacvcb.org

Alabama
(334) 242-4007

Alaska
(907) 465-3040

Arizona
(602) 364-1155

Arkansas
(501) 682-1020

California
(916) 323-3432

Colorado
(303) 239-4493

Connecticut
(860) 747-4501

Delaware
(302) 995-8383

Florida
(850) 414-3300

Georgia
(404) 559-4949

Guam
(671) 475-3324

Hawaii
(808) 587-1143

Idaho
(208) 334-6080

Developed from the Office for Victims of Crime, Crime Victim Compensation Directory: http://www.ojp.usdoj.gov/ovc/help/progdir.htm.

Illinois
(217) 782-7101/
(312) 814-2581

Indiana
(317) 232-1295

Iowa
(515) 281-5044

Kansas
(785) 296-2359

Kentucky
(502) 573-2290

Louisiana
(225) 925-4437

Maine
(207) 624-7882

Maryland
(410) 585-3010

Massachusetts
(617) 727-2200

Michigan
(517) 373-7373

Minnesota
(651) 282-6256

Mississippi
(601) 359-6766

Missouri
(573) 526-6006

Montana
(406) 444-3653

Nebraska
(402) 471-2828

Nevada
(702) 486-2740/
(775) 688-2900

New Hampshire
(603) 271-1284

New Jersey
(973) 648-2107

New Mexico
(505) 841-9432

New York
(518) 457-8727/
(718) 923-4325

North Carolina
(919) 733-7974

North Dakota
(701) 328-6195

Ohio
(614) 466-5610

Oklahoma
(405) 264-5006

Oregon
(503) 378-5348

Pennsylvania
(717) 783-5153

Puerto Rico
(787) 641-7480

Rhode Island
(401) 222-8590

South Carolina
(803) 734-1900

South Dakota
(605) 773-6317

Tennessee
(615) 741-2734

Texas
(512) 936-1200

Utah
(801) 238-2360

Vermont
(802) 241-1250

Virgin Islands
(340) 774-1166

Virginia
(804) 378-3434

Washington
(360) 902-5355

Washington, DC
(202) 879-4216

West Virginia
(304) 347-4850

Wisconsin
(608) 266-6470

Wyoming
(307) 777-7200

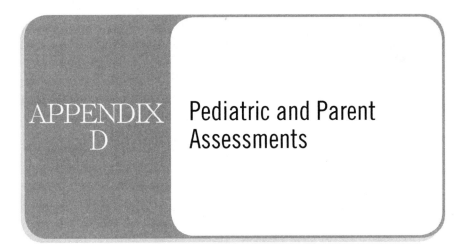

APPENDIX
D

Pediatric and Parent Assessments

The Pediatric and Parent Assessments are used with permission from Melnyk, B.M. & Moldenhauer, Z: The KySS℠ (Keep your children/yourself Safe and Secure) Guide to Child and Adolescent Mental Health Screening, Early Intervention and Health Promotion, © 2006, National Association of Pediatric Nurse Practitioners and the NAPNAP Foundation, Cherry Hill, NJ.

KySS Assessment Questions for Parents of Older Infants and Toddlers

Child's Name_____ DOB_____ Age_____

Parent's/Guardian's Name_____ Relationship to Child_____

Because your child's physical as well as mental/emotional health are very important, please complete each of the following questions. We will have the opportunity to talk about some of these issues during your visit. Please indicate which items are most important to talk about today by placing a check mark in front of those items.

1. What worries or concerns you most about your child's emotions and/or behaviors at this time? _____
   _____

2. Have there been changes in your family in the past year, such as marital separation, remarriage, move, family illness or death? If yes, what?   No   Yes
   _____

3. Are you afraid of anyone in your home?
   If yes, who? _____   No   Yes

4. Do you ever feel so frustrated that you may hit or hurt your child?   No   Yes

5. On a scale of 0 (Not at all) to 10 (a lot), how stressed is your child on a day-to-day basis?   _____

6. Have you been worried about your child being angry, irritable, sad, fearful, or having a change in behavior in the last month? If yes, what is worrying you?   No   Yes
   _____

7. Do you have any worries about your child being sad?   No   Yes

8. Are you concerned about your child's weight? If yes, what concerns you: No   Yes
   _____

9. Who usually watches your child when you are not with him or her? _____

10. What is the easiest part about being your child's parent? _____

11. What is the hardest part about being your child's parent? _____

12. What worries you most about your child? _____

13. On a scale of 0 (Not at all) to 10 (a lot), how stressed are you on a day-to-day basis?   _____

14. On a scale of 0 (Not at all) to 10 (a lot), how depressed are you from day-to-day?   _____

15. How do you discipline your child? _____
_____

16. Do you think that the way that you discipline your child is effective?   No   Yes

17. Do you think that your child has ever been abused? If Yes, when? _____   No   Yes
_____

18. Has your child ever been through a traumatic or very frightening experience (for example, a motor vehicle accident, hospitalization, death of a loved one, watching arguments)? If Yes, when and what was the trauma? _____   No   Yes
_____

19. Has your child ever been diagnosed with an emotional, behavioral, or mental health problem? If yes, what and when? _____   No   Yes

20. Has your child ever been on medication for an emotional, behavioral, or mental health problem? If yes, what medication and when? _____   No   Yes

21. Do you have guns in your home?   No   Yes

22. Are there stressful things that your family has been dealing with recently? If yes, what? _____   No   Yes

23. On a scale of 0 (Not at all) to 10 (very), how emotionally connected do you feel with your child?   _____

24. On a scale of 0 (very easy) to 10 (very difficult), how is
    your child's temperament?   _____

25. Does your child have difficulty sleeping? If yes, what
    specifically (for example, difficulty falling asleep;
    waking up with nightmares)? _____   No   Yes

26. Does anyone in your home smoke?
    If yes, who? _____   No   Yes

27. Does anyone in your home use alcohol or drugs to
    the point that you wish they would stop?   No   Yes

28. On a scale of 0 (None) to 10 (a lot), how much
    arguing goes on in your home?   _____

29. On a scale of 0 (Not at all) to 10 (a lot), do you
    overprotect your child?   _____

30. On a scale of 0 (Not at all) to 10 (very much so), how
    satisfied are you with being a parent to your child?   _____

31. On a scale of 0 (Not at all) to 10 (very much so), how
    consistent are you in setting limits with your child?   _____

32. Have you or any other of your child's blood relatives
    ever been diagnosed with a mental health disorder?
    If yes, who and what? _____   No   Yes

33. What 2 words would you use to best
    describe your child? _____

*This questionnaire may be photocopied (but not altered) and distributed to families. From
Melnyk, B.M. & Moldenhauer, Z: The KySS*^{SM} *Guide to Child and Adolescent Mental Health
Screening, Early Intervention and Health Promotion, © 2006, National Association
of Pediatric Nurse Practitioners and the NAPNAP Foundation, Cherry Hill, NJ.*

KySS Assessment Questions for Parents of Preschool Children

Child's Name_____ DOB_____ Age_____

Parent's/Guardian's Name_____ Relationship to Child_____

Because your child's physical as well as mental/emotional health are very important, please complete each of the following questions. We will have the opportunity to talk about some of these issues during your visit. Please indicate which items are most important to talk about today by placing a check mark in front of those items.

1. What worries or concerns you most about your child's emotions and/or behaviors at this time? _____

2. Have there been changes in your family in the past year, such as marital separation, remarriage, move, family illness or death? If yes, what? _____   No   Yes

3. Are you afraid of anyone in your home?
    If yes, who? _____   No   Yes

4. Do you ever feel so frustrated that you may hit or hurt your child?   No   Yes

5. On a scale of 0 (Not at all) to 10 (a lot), how much does your child worry on a day-to-day basis?   _____

6. What does your child worry most about? _____

7. On a scale of 0 (Not at all) to 10 (a lot), how stressed is your child on a day-today basis? _____

8. Have you been worried about your child being angry, irritable, sad, fearful, or having a change in behavior in the last month? If yes, what is worrying you?   No   Yes

    _____

9. How often does your child complain of headaches or stomachaches?
    a. Never, b. 1x/month, c. 2x/month, d. 1x/week, e. more than 1x/week

10. Do you have any worries about your child being sad or depressed?   No   Yes

11. Are you concerned about your child's weight? If yes, what concerns you?   No   Yes

    _____

12. Who usually watches your child when you are not with him or her? _____

13. Do you talk about safety with your child?   No   Yes

14. What is the easiest part about being your child's parent? _____

15. What is the hardest part about being your child's parent? _____

16. What worries you most about your relationship with your child? _____

17. On a scale of 0 (Not at all) to 10 (a lot), how stressed are you on a day-to-day basis?   _____

18. On a scale of 0 (Not at all) to 10 (a lot), how depressed are you on a day-to-day basis?   _____

19. On a scale of 0 (Not good at all) to 10 (excellent), how does your child cope with stress? _____

20. How do you discipline your child? _____

21. Do you think that the way that you discipline your child is effective?   No   Yes

22. Do you think that your child has ever been abused? If Yes, when?   No   Yes

    _____

23. Has your child ever been through a traumatic or very frightening experience (for example, a motor vehicle accident, hospitalization, death of a loved one, watching arguments)? If Yes, when and what was the trauma?_____   No   Yes

    _____

24. Has your child ever been diagnosed with an emotional, behavioral, or mental health problem? If yes, what and when? _____   No   Yes

25. Has your child ever been on medication for an emotional, behavioral, or mental health problem? If yes, what medication and when? _____   No   Yes

26. Do you have guns in your home?   No   Yes

27. Are there stressful things that your family has been dealing with recently? If yes, what? _____ No Yes

28. On a scale of 0 (poor) to 10 (excellent), how is your child's self-esteem? _____

29. On a scale of 0 (Not at all) to 10 (very), how emotionally connected do you feel with your child? _____

30. On a scale of 0 (very difficult) to 10 (very easy), how is your child's temperament? _____

31. Does your child have difficulty sleeping? If yes, what specifically (for example, difficulty falling asleep; waking up with nightmares)? _____ No Yes

32. Does anyone in your home smoke? If yes, who? _____ No Yes

33. Does anyone in your home use alcohol or drugs to the point that you wish they would stop? No Yes

34. On a scale of 0 (None) to 10 (a lot), how much arguing goes on in your home? _____

35. On a scale of 0 (Not good) to 10 (very good), how well does your child get along with his/her peers or friends? _____

36. On a scale of 0 (Not at all) to 10 (a lot), do you overprotect your child? _____

37. On a scale of 0 (Not at all) to 10 (very much so), how satisfied are you with being a parent to your child? _____

38. On a scale of 0 (Not at all) to 10 (very much so), are you consistent in setting limits with your child? _____

39. Is your child ever cruel to animals? No Yes

This questionnaire may be photocopied (but not altered) and distributed to families. From Melnyk, B.M. & Moldenhauer, Z: The KySS^SM Guide to Child and Adolescent Mental Health Screening, Early Intervention and Health Promotion, © 2006, National Association of Pediatric Nurse Practitioners and the NAPNAP Foundation, Cherry Hill, NJ.

KySS Assessment Questions For
Parents of School-Age Children and Teens

Child's Name_____ DOB_____ Age_____

Parent's/Guardian's Name_____ Relationship to Child_____

Because your child's physical as well as mental/emotional health are very important, please complete each of the following questions. We will have the opportunity to talk about some of these issues during your visit. Please indicate which items are most important to talk about today by placing a check mark before those items.

1. What worries or concerns you most about your child's emotions and/or behaviors at this time? _____

2. Have there been changes in your family in the past year, such as marital separation, remarriage, move, family illness or death? If yes, what? _____   No   Yes

3. Are you afraid of anyone in your home? If yes, who? _____   No   Yes

4. Do you ever feel so frustrated that you may hit or hurt your child?   No   Yes

5. On a scale of 0 (Not at all) to 10 (a lot), how much does your child worry on a day-to-day basis?   _____

6. What does your child worry most about? _____

7. On a scale of 0 (Not at all) to 10 (a lot), how stressed is your child on a day-to-day basis?   _____

8. Have you been worried about your child being angry, irritable, sad, fearful, or having a change in behavior in the last month? If yes, what is worrying you?   No   Yes

_____

9. How often does your child complain of headaches or stomachaches? a. Never, b. 1x/month, c. 2x/month, d. 1x/week, e. more than 1x/week

10. Do you have any worries about your child being depressed?   No   Yes

11. If yes, do you ever think that your child thinks about hurting him- or herself?   No   Yes

12. Are you concerned about your child's weight? If yes, what concerns you?   No   Yes

13. Does your child make negative comments about his or her body or weight?   No   Yes

14. Where does your child spend his/her free time?_____

15. Who usually watches your child when you are not with him or her? _____

16. Do you talk about safety with your child?   No   Yes

17. What is the easiest part about being your child's parent? _____

18. What is the hardest part about being your child's parent? _____

19. What worries you most about your relationship with your child? _____

20. On a scale of 0 (Not at all) to 10 (a lot), how stressed are you on a day-to-day basis?   _____

21. On a scale of 0 (Not at all) to 10 (a lot), how depressed are you on a day-to-day basis?   _____

22. On a scale of 0 (Not good at all) to 10 (excellent), how does your child cope with stress?   _____

23. How do you discipline your child? _____

24. Do you think that the way that you discipline your child is effective?   No   Yes

25. Has your child ever been through a traumatic or very frightening experience (for example, a motor vehicle accident, hospitalization, death of a loved one, rape)? If Yes, when and what was the trauma? _____   No   Yes

26. On a scale of 0 (Not at all) to 10 (a lot), how comfortable do you feel in talking with your child about sexuality?   _____

27. Are you worried about your child becoming sexually active?   No   Yes

28. Are you worried about your child and drug or alcohol use?   No   Yes

29. Are you worried about your child and cigarette smoking?   No   Yes

30. Does your child ever get bullied?   No   Yes

31. Has your child ever been diagnosed with an emotional, behavioral, or mental health problem? If yes, what and when? _____   No   Yes

32. Has your child ever been on medication for an emotional, behavioral, or mental health problem? If yes, what medication and when? _____   No   Yes

33. Do you have guns in your home?   No   Yes

34. Are there stressful things that your family has been dealing with recently? If yes, what? _____   No   Yes

35. On a scale of 0 (poor) to 10 (excellent), how is your child's self-esteem?   _____

36. On a scale of 0 (Not at all) to 10 (very), how emotionally connected do you feel with your child?   _____

37. On a scale of 0 (very difficult) to 10 (very easy), how is your child's temperament?   _____

38. Has your child had a recent decline in his or her school performance/grades? If yes, when and what? _____   No   Yes

39. Does your child have difficulty sleeping? If yes, what specifically (for example, difficulty falling asleep; waking up with nightmares)? _____   No   Yes

40. Does anyone in your home smoke? If yes, who?_____   No   Yes

41. Does anyone in your home use alcohol or drugs to the point that you wish they would stop?   No   Yes

42. On a scale of 0 (None) to 10 (a lot), how much arguing goes on in your home?   _____

43. On a scale of 0 (Not good) to 10 (very good), how well does your child get along with his/her peers or friends?   _____

44. On a scale of 0 (Not at all) to 10 (a lot), do you overprotect your child?   _____

45. On a scale of 0 (Not at all) to 10 (very much so), how satisfied are you with being a parent to your child? _____

46. On a scale of 0 (Not at all) to 10 (very much so), are you consistent in setting limits with your child? _____

47. Is your child ever cruel to animals?   No   Yes

48. Have you or any other of your child's blood relatives ever been diagnosed with a mental health disorder? If yes, who and what?   No   Yes

KySS Worries Questionnaire for Parents (B. Melnyk and Z. Moldenhauer)

Please answer each of the following questions by circling your answers.

Do you wony about any of the following for your child?

	Not at all	Sometimes	Often	Nearly always	Always
1) Depression	1	2	3	4	5
2) Anxiety	1	2	3	4	5
3) Parents separating or divorcing	1	2	3	4	5
4) Violence/being hurt	1	2	3	4	5
5) Physical abuse/neglect	1	2	3	4	5
6) Sexual abuse/rape	1	2	3	4	5
7) Sexual activity	1	2	3	4	5
8) Substance abuse	1	2	3	4	5
9) Eating disorders	1	2	3	4	5
10) Self-esteem	1	2	3	4	5
11) Your relationship with your child	1	2	3	4	5
12) How your child copes with stressful things	1	2	3	4	5
13) Being "bullied" by classmates	1	2	3	4	5
14) Your child's weight	1	2	3	4	5
15) Your child's level of activity/exercise	1	2	3	4	5

16) Do you have any other worries about your child? If yes, please describe them.

17) Do your child's worries interfere with his/her ability to do school work?__Yes __No

18) Do your child's worries interfere with his or her friendships? __Yes __No

KySS Worries Questionnaire
(Ages 10–21 years)
(B. Melnyk and Z. Moldenhauer)

Please answer each of the following questions by circling your answers.

Do you worry about any of the following for yourself?

	Not at all	Sometimes	Often	Nearly always	Always
1) Depression	1	2	3	4	5
2) Anxiety	1	2	3	4	5
3) Parents separating or divorcing	1	2	3	4	5
4) Violence/being hurt	1	2	3	4	5
5) Physical abuse/ neglect	1	2	3	4	5
6) Sexual abuse/rape	1	2	3	4	5
7) Sexual activity	1	2	3	4	5
8) Substance abuse	1	2	3	4	5
9) Eating disorders	1	2	3	4	5
10) Problems with your self-esteem	1	2	3	4	5
11) Your relationship with your parents	1	2	3	4	5
12) Knowing how to copre with things that stress you	1	2	3	4	5
13) Being made fun of by your friends	1	2	3	4	5
14) Your weight	1	2	3	4	5
15) Your level of activity/exercise	1	2	3	4	5

16) Do you have any other worries? If yes, please describe them.

_____

_____

17) Do your worries interfere with your ability
   to do school work?   __Yes __No

18) Do your worries affect your relationship
   with your friends?   __Yes __No

Index